TWO HEMISPHERES–ONE BRAIN
Functions of the Corpus Callosum

Neurology and Neurobiology

TWO HEMISPHERES–ONE BRAIN
Functions of the Corpus Callosum

Proceedings of the Sixth International Symposium of the
Centre de Recherche en Sciences Neurologiques of the
Université de Montréal, Held in Montréal, Canada, May 16–18, 1984

Editors
Franco Leporé

Département de Psychologie
Faculté des Arts et des Sciences and
Centre de Recherche en Sciences Neurologiques
Université de Montréal
Montréal, Québec, Canada

Maurice Ptito

Département de Psychologie
Études Avancées de la Recherche
Université du Québec à Trois-Rivières
Trois-Rivières, Québec, and
Centre de Recherche en Sciences Neurologiques
Université de Montréal
Montréal, Québec, Canada

Herbert H. Jasper

Centre de Recherche en Sciences Neurologiques and
Département de Physiologie
Faculté de Médecine
Université de Montréal and
The Montreal Neurological Institute of McGill University
Montréal, Québec, Canada

ALAN R. LISS, INC. • NEW YORK

Address all Inquiries to the Publisher
Alan R. Liss, Inc., 41 East 11th Street, New York, NY 10003

Copyright © 1986 Alan R. Liss, Inc.

Printed in the United States of America

Library of Congress Cataloging-in-Publication Data
Université de Montréal. Centre de recherche en
   sciences neurologiques. International Symposium
   (6th : 1984 : Montréal, Québec)
   Two hemispheres, one brain.

   Includes bibliographies and index.
      1. Corpus callosum—Congresses. 2. Split brain—
   Congresses. 3. Cerebral hemispheres—Congresses.
   I. Leporé, Franco. II. Ptito, Maurice. III. Jasper,
   Herbert H. (Herbert Henri), 1906–   . IV. Title.
   [DNLM: 1. Cerebral Cortex—physiology—congresses.
   2. Corpus Callosum—physiology—congresses.
   W1 NE3378 v.17 / WL 307 U59 1984t]
   QP382.2.U55 1984   599'.01'88   85-23968
   ISBN 0-8451-2719-5

Contents

SECTION III. ELECTROPHYSIOLOGY

SECTION IV. ANIMAL BEHAVIOR

SECTION V. HUMAN NEUROPSYCHOLOGY I

SECTION VI. HUMAN NEUROPSYCHOLOGY II

Contributors

Hugo O. Adrian, Department of Physiology and Biophysics, University of Chile, Santiago, Chile **[103]**

Antonella Antonini, Istituto di Fisiologia Umana, Università di Verona, Verona, Italy **[171]**

S. Bédard, Département de Psychologie, Université de Montréal, Montréal, Québec H3C 3J7, Canada **[299]**

Giovanni Berlucchi, Istituto di Fisiologia Umana, Università di Verona, Verona, Italy **[171]**

Joseph E. Bogen, Department of Neurological Surgery, University of Southern California and Department of Psychology, University of California, Los Angeles, CA **[21]**

John F. Brugge, Department of Neurophysiology, University of Wisconsin Medical School, Madison, WI 53706 **[103]**

M.P. Bryden, Department of Psychology, University of Waterloo, Waterloo, Ontario N2L 3G1, Canada **[463]**

W.W. Chambers, Department of Anatomy and Institute of Neurological Sciences, University of Pennsylvania, Philadelphia, PA 19104 **[351]**

Alan C. Church, Department of Anatomy and Institute of Neurological Sciences, University of Pennsylvania, Philadelphia, PA 19104; present address: Drug Enforcement Administration, Washington D.C. 20537 **[351]**

M. Colonnier, Department of Anatomy, Faculty of Medicine, Laval University, Quebec, P.Q. G1K 7P4, Canada **[37]**

Catherine G. Cusick, Department of Psychology, Vanderbilt University, Nashville, TN 37240 **[83]**

M. Cynader, Departments of Psychology and Physiology, Dalhousie University, Halifax, Nova Scotia B3H 4J1, Canada **[189]**

Michel Décarie, Division of Neurology and Neurosurgery, Hôpital Sainte-Justine, Université de Montréal, Montréal, Québec H3T IC5, Canada **[361]**

Carole Dion, Groupe de Recherche en Neuropsychologie, Université du Québec, Trois-Rivières, Québec G9A 5H7, Canada **[335]**

M. Di Stefano, Istituto di Fisiologia, Università di Pisa, 56100 Pisa, Italy **[299]**

The number in brackets is the opening page number of the contributor's article.

A. Dobbins, Departments of Psychology and Physiology, Dalhousie University, Halifax, Nova Scotia B3H 4J1, Canada [189]

Robert W. Doty, Center for Brain Research, University of Rochester, Rochester, NY 14642 [269]

Andrea J. Elberger, Department of Neurobiology and Anatomy, The University of Texas Medical School at Houston, Houston, TX 77030; present address: Department of Anatomy, The University of Tennessee Center for the Health Sciences, Memphis TN 38163 [281]

Louis B. Flexner, Department of Anatomy and Institute of Neurological Sciences, University of Pennsylvania, Philadelphia, PA 19104 [351]

Douglas O. Frost, Section of Neuroanatomy, Yale University School of Medicine, New Haven, CT 06510 [255]

J. Gardner, Departments of Psychology and Physiology, Dalhousie University, Halifax, Nova Scotia B3H 4J1, Canada; present address: Research Lab of Electronics, Building 36-873, MIT, Cambridge, MA 02139 [189]

Guy Geoffroy, Division of Neurology and Neurosurgery, Hôpital Sainte-Justine, Université de Montréal, Montréal, Québec H3T IC5, Canada [361]

Jean-Paul Guillemot, Département de Kinanthropologie, Université du Québec à Montréal, Montréal, Québec H3C 3P8, Canada [189, 211]

Charles R. Hamilton, Division of Biology, California Institute of Technology, Pasadena, CA 91125 [315]

D. Hubel, Department of Neurobiology, Harvard Medical School, Boston, MA 02115 [167]

Thomas J. Imig, Department of Physiology, Kansas University Medical Center, Kansas City, KS 66103 [103]

David H. Ingvar, Department of Clinical Neurophysiology, University Hospital, S-221 85 Lund, Sweden [471]

Giorgio M. Innocenti, Institut d'Anatomie, Faculté de Médecine, Université de Lausanne, Lausanne, Switzerland [75, 255]

Herbert H. Jasper, Centre de Recherche en Sciences Neurologiques, Faculté de Médecine, Université de Montreál, C.P. 6128, Succ. A, Montreál, Québec H3C 3J7 and The Montreal Neurological Institute of McGill University, Montreál, Québec, Canada [xiii, 541]

M. Jeannerod, Laboratoire de Neuropsychologie Expérimentale, INSERM-Unité 94, 69500 Bron, France [369]

M.A. Jeeves, Department of Psychology, University of St. Andrews, St. Andrews, Fife, KY16 9JU, Scotland [403]

E.G. Jones, Department of Anatomy, University of California at Irvine, Irvine, CA 92717 [149]

Jon H. Kaas, Department of Psychology, Vanderbilt University, Nashville, TN 37240 [83]

Maryse Lassonde, Groupe de Recherche en Neuropsychologie, Université du Québec, Trois-Rivières, Québec G9A 5H7, and Hôpital Sainte-Justine de Montréal, Québec H3T 1C5, Canada [335, 361, 385]

Franco Leporé, Département de Psychologie, Faculté des Arts et des Sciences, and Centre de Recherche en Sciences Neurologiques, Université de Montréal, Montréal, Québec H3C 3J7, Canada [xiii,139,189,211,299,335]

Jerre Levy, Department of Behavioral Sciences, University of Chicago, Chicago, IL 60637 [511]

Jeffrey D. Lewine, Center for Brain Research, University of Rochester, Rochester, NY 14642 [269]

C.N. Liu, Department of Anatomy and Institute of Neurological Sciences, University of Pennsylvania, Philadelphia, PA 19104 [351]

C.A. Marzi, Dipartimento di Psicologia Generale, Università di Padova, 35139 Padova, Italy [299]

Dom Miceli, Groupe de Recherche en Neuropsychologie Expérimentale, Université du Québec, Trois-Rivières, Québec G9A 5H7, Canada [139,335]

Anne Morel, Department of Physiology, Kansas University Medical Center, Kansas City, KS 66103 [103]

Morris Moscovitch, Department of Psychology and Centre for Studies in Human Development, Erindale College, University of Toronto, Mississauga, Ontario L5L 1C6, Canada [483]

Frank E. Musiek, Sections of Otolaryngology, Audiology and Neurology, Dartmouth-Hitchcock Medical Center, Hanover, NH 03756 [423]

Deepak N. Pandya, Edith Nourse Rogers Memorial Veterans Hospital, Bedford, MA 01730, and Departments of Neurology and Anatomy, Boston University School of Medicine, Boston, MA 02118 [47]

Bertram R. Payne, Department of Anatomy, Medical College of Pennsylvania, Philadelphia, PA 19129; present address: Department of Anatomy, Boston University School of Medicine, Boston, MA 02118 [231]

Karl H. Pribram, Departments of Psychology and of Psychiatry and Behavioral Sciences, Stanford University, Palo Alto, CA 94305 [523]

Maurice Ptito, Centre de Recherche en Sciences Neurologiques, Université de Montréal, Québec H3C 3J7, and Département de Psychologie, Groupe de Recherche en Neuropsychologie, Université du Québec, Trois-Rivières, Québec G9A 5H7, Canada [xiii,139,211,335]

Richard A. Reale, Department of Neurophysiology, University of Wisconsin Medical School, Madison, WI 53706 [103]

Alexander Reeves, Sections of Otolaryngology, Audiology and Neurology, Dartmouth-Hitchcock Medical Center, Hanover, NH 03756 [423]

James L. Ringo, Center for Brain Research, University of Rochester, Rochester, NY 14642 [269]

Hannelore Sauerwein, Groupe de Recherche en Neuropsychologie, Université du Québec, Trois-Rivières, Québec G9A 5H7, Canada [361]

Benjamin Seltzer, Edith Nourse Rogers Memorial Veterans Hospital, Bedford, MA 01730, and Department of Neurology, Boston University School of Medicine, Boston, MA 02118 [47]

Roger Sperry, Division of Biology, California Institute of Technology, Pasadena, CA 91125 [3]

James M. Sprague, Department of Anatomy and Institute of Neurological Sciences, University of Pennsylvania, Philadelphia, PA 19104 **[351]**

Giancarlo Tassinari, Istituto di Fisiologia Umana, Università di Verona, Verona, Italy **[171]**

Betty A. Vermeire, Division of Biology, California Institute of Technology, Pasadena, CA 91125 **[315]**

R. Ward, Département de Psychologie and Groupe de Recherche en Neuropsychologie Expérimentale, Université du Québec, Trois-Rivières, Québec G9A 5H7, Canada **[139]**

Sandra F. Witelson, Departments of Psychiatry, Psychology, and Neurosciences, McMaster University, Hamilton, Ontario L8N 3Z5, Canada **[117]**

Eran Zaidel, Department of Psychology, University of California, Los Angeles, CA 90024 **[435]**

Dedication

ROGER WOLCOTT SPERRY

This monograph entitled "**Two Hemispheres—One Brain: Functions of the Corpus Callosum**" is the report of papers presented at the Sixth International Symposium of Neuroscience of the "Centre de Recherche en Sciences Neurologiques de l'Université de Montréal" May 16–18, 1984. The participants in this symposium have all been inspired by the work of Roger Sperry, who revolutionized our conceptions of the functional importance of the corpus callosum for the integrative activity of the two hemispheres, and the role of each hemisphere in conscious experience and voluntary movement. Although Roger Sperry has made several other important contributions to neuroscience beginning in the 1930s and 40s with his work in developmental neurobiology, it was his work on the corpus callosum and its role in the integration of the separate behavioral and mental functions of the two hemispheres for which he received the Nobel Prize (shared with David Hubel and Torsten Wiesel) in 1981.

Roger Sperry was born in Hartford, Connecticut, August 20, 1913. He received his B.A. in English and his M.A. in Psychology at Oberlin College (1935–1937), and his Ph.D. in Zoology at the University of Chicago with Paul Weiss in 1941. He then became a National Research Council Fellow at Harvard University, 1941–42, and Biology Research Fellow of Harvard at the Yerkes Laboratories of Primate Biology, 1942–46. He returned to the University of Chicago as Assistant Professor in the Department of Anatomy (1946–52) and Associate Professor of Psychology, 1952–53, while serving at the same time as Section Chief, Neurological Diseases and Blindness of the National Institutes of Health in Bethesda, Maryland. It was during this period that he began his classical work with his graduate student Ron Myers on the effects of complete section of the corpus callosum in cats and monkeys. This established the "split-brain" preparation as a revolutionary approach to solving the problems of the function of the corpus callosum. In 1954, Sperry was appointed Hixon Professor of Psychobiology at the California Institute of Technology, where he was able to extend his observations to man in collaboration with neurosurgeons P. Vogel and J. Bogen, together with a number of students, including M. Gazzaniga, J. Levy, C. Trevarthen, and others. We need go no further at this time

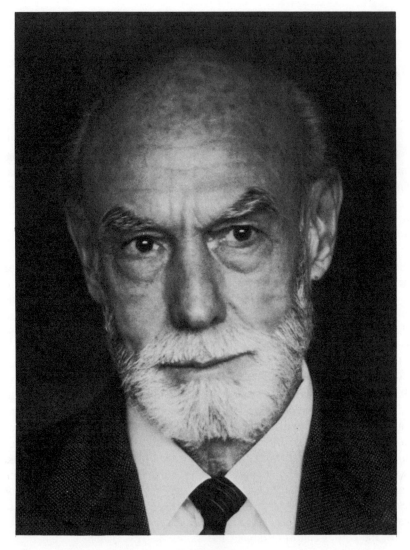

Roger Wolcott Sperry

since we are reprinting the most recent description of this work by Sperry himself, with revisions he has kindly made for this publication.

Rereading this up-to-date version of Sperry's work, with his reflections upon its broader significance places in clear perspective not only the importance of his conceptions of the function of the corpus callosum and hemispheric specialization, but the great impact his work has had upon the whole field of cognitive neuroscience and flowering during recent years as manifest in the contributions to this symposium.

Since the 1970s, Roger Sperry has become more and more interested in the theoretical and philosophical aspects of brain-mind relationships, partly stemming from the challenging problems presented by the "split-mind" aspects of the "split-brain" preparation. His early views were expressed in **Psychological Reviews** in 1969 (Vol. 76), and a recent summary was published as the leading chapter of **The Annual Review of Neuroscience** in 1981 (Vol. 4). In his view, the mind as subjective experience is treated as a scientific reality which may play a leading role in the control of thought and behavior and therefore in the control of the brain mechanisms which underly them. To quote from Sperry's Nobel lecture delivered in Stockholm, December 8, 1981 (**Science,** Vol. 217, 1982) "Cognitive introspective psychology and related cognitive science can no longer be ignored experimentally, or written off as a 'science of epiphenomenon', or as something that must in principle reduce eventually to neurophysiology. The events of inner experience, as emergent properties of brain processes, become themselves explanatory causal constructs in their own right, interacting at their own level with their own laws and dynamics. The whole world of inner experience (the world of the humanities), long rejected by 20th century scientific materialism, thus becomes recognized and included within the domain of science." Sperry goes on to discuss the profound implications of this view for our understanding of human nature and "its societal role as an intellectual, cultural, and moral force . . . . reconciling the traditional scientific and humanistic views of man and the world."

Although Sperry's philosophical views do not play a large role in this publication, we mention them in this dedication to emphasize their far-reaching importance well beyond his contributions to the theme of this symposium "Two Hemispheres—One Brain: Functions of the Corpus Callosum." They represent an additional important reason for our dedication of this work to Roger Sperry.

Franco Leporé
Maurice Ptito
Herbert H. Jasper

SECTION I
GENERAL INTRODUCTION

Two Hemispheres—One Brain:
Functions of the Corpus Callosum, pages 3–20
Published 1986 by Alan R. Liss, Inc.

Consciousness, Personal Identity, and the Divided Brain

ROGER SPERRY

Division of Biology, California Institute of Technology, Pasadena, California 91125

I

It has now become a familiar story in neuroscience that when you divide the brain surgically by midline section of the cerebral commissures the mind also is correspondingly divided. Each of the disconnected hemispheres continues to function at a high level, but most conscious experience generated within one hemisphere becomes inaccessible to the conscious awareness of the other. The parallel mental functions of the separated hemispheres are found to differ further in important ways, the most conspicuous being that the disconnected left hemisphere retains the ability to speak its mind, much as before, whereas the right hemisphere, for most practical purposes, is unable to express itself either in speech or in writing.

In turning to examine more closely these and related phenomena, as they bear on our present topic, I shall be drawing on studies by a long line of associates and myself conducted on a select group of about a dozen so-called commissurotomy or split-brain patients of Drs. Philip Vogel and Joseph Bogen, neurosurgeons at the White Memorial Medical Center in Los Angeles. This commissurotomy operation is performed in rare cases as a last resort measure to help control severe intractable epilepsy.

A few points about the surgery need to be kept in mind: First, it permanently divides in the brain nearly all direct connections mediating crosstalk between the left and right hemispheres (see Fig. 1). This includes those fiber systems that normally interconnect left and right halves of the cortical

Public lecture presented at the Smithsonian Institution, December 1977 in the Frank Nelson Doubleday Lecture Series on "The Human Mind." Published in the Hecaen memorial issue of *Neuropsychologia*, Vol. 22. It is presented here with minor editorial revision and updating.

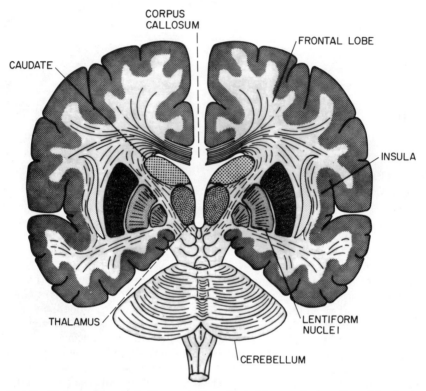

CORPUS
CALLOSUM

FRONTAL LOBE

CAUDATE

INSULA

THALAMUS

LENTIFORM
NUCLEI

CEREBELLUM

Fig. 1. Nature of hemispheric separation effected by surgical section of forebrain commissures. Some indirect cross communication remains possible through intact midbrain and associated brainstem structures.

field for vision. As a result the visual perception of objects in each hemisphere becomes restricted to half the normal field of view, cut off sharply at the vertical midline and center of gaze. The left hemisphere sees things in the right half of the visual field, using either one or both eyes, while things to the left are perceived by the right hemisphere. Interconnections are severed also between the cerebral representations for the right and left hands and feet, including both the primary sensory projections and also the main motor controls for skilled movement. Hence things felt with the right hand are perceived mainly in the left hemisphere, which also governs related motor adjustments of the same hand. Conversely, motor coordination and tactual perception for the left hand are mediated predominantly by the right hemisphere. In addition, the surgery cuts off the functions of the right hemisphere from speech and the main language centers located (in approximately 95% of the population) in the left hemisphere (see Fig. 2).

A leading question with which we shall be concerned can be stated as follows. Are there really in the brain thus divided, two separately conscious minds, in effect two co-conscious selves sharing the one cranium? And, if so, what does this signify regarding the nature and the substrate of mind and the unity of the conscious self in the normal intact brain?

The first point to be emphasized is that these patients following surgery appear in ordinary, everyday behavior to be very typical, single-minded, normally unified individuals. What prompted our studies in the beginning was a series of published reports supporting the conclusion that no definite symptoms are detected after surgery, even with extensive neurological and psychological testing. (For a review of the earlier literature, see [3].) Usually a year or so is required to recover fully from the extensive neural trauma caused by section of the cerebral commissures, which include the largest fiber systems of the brain, estimated to contain well over 200 million nerve fibers. After recovery patients without other brain damage are able to return to school or to household duties, or to an undemanding job assignment. Two years after surgery, a typical commissurotomy patient without complicating disorders could easily go through a complete routine medical examination without revealing to an uninformed practitioner that anything is abnormal. Nor is there any marked change in the verbal scores on the standard IQ test. Complaints about short-term memory are common especially in the early years after surgery. However, the general behavior and conversation during the course of a casual social encounter without special tests typically reveals nothing to suggest that these people are not essentially the same persons that they were before the surgery with the same inner selves and personalities.

Despite the outward seeming normality, however, and the apparent unity and coherence of the behavior and personality of these individuals, controlled lateralized testing for the function of each hemisphere independently (see Fig. 3) indicates that in reality these people live with two largely separate left and right domains of inner conscious awareness. (The basic "split-brain" syndrome in man is reviewed in [28] and [33]; the split-brain animal work is reviewed in [24] and [26].) Each hemisphere can be shown to experience its own private sensations, percepts, thoughts, and memories, which are inaccessible to awareness in the other hemisphere. Introspective verbal accounts from the vocal left hemisphere show a striking lack of awareness in this hemisphere for mental functions that have just been performed immediately before in the right hemisphere. In this respect each surgically disconnected hemisphere appears to have a mind of its own, each capable of controlling the behavior of the body but each cut off from, and oblivious of, conscious events in the partner hemisphere.

Following the surgery these people are unable to recognize by sight something they have just looked at in one visual half-field if it is then

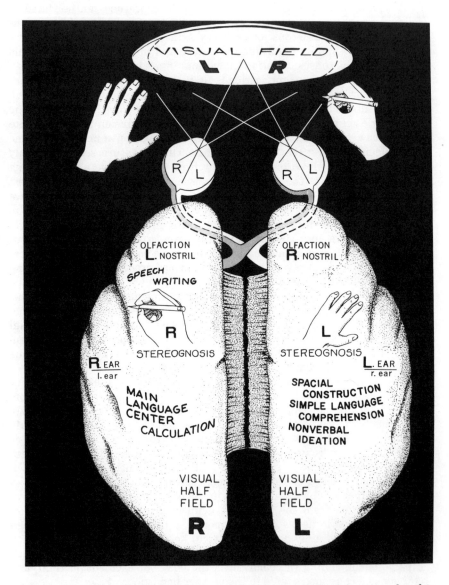

Fig. 2. Schematic representation of some of the main cerebral functions found to be lateralized following hemisphere disconnection.

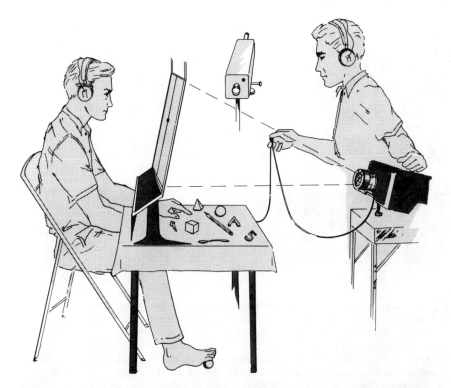

Fig. 3. Testing setup for determining laterality of mental functions in the surgically separated hemispheres.

presented across the vertical meridian in the opposite half-field of view. Objects perceived and identified tactually with one hand out of sight cannot be recognized with the other hand. Such objects also can be recognized in the corresponding half-field of vision but not in the opposite half-field. Similarly, odors identified through one nostril are not recognized through the other. Split-brain subjects fail to identify by verbal report objects felt with the left hand, seen in the left visual field, or smelled through the right nostril—in other words, things experienced within the right hemisphere. In the meantime, good perception and comprehension of these same test stimuli, of which the subject *verbally* disclaims any knowledge, is readily demonstrated *manually,* for example, by selective retrieval with the left hand, or by pointing to the correct picture in a choice array, or by appropriate hand signals or gestures (see Fig. 4).

From the collective results of these and similar kinds of tests, it is inferred that both disconnected hemispheres retain mental function at a

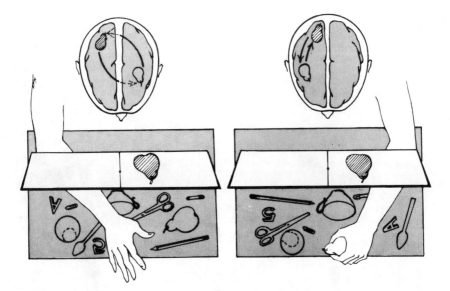

Fig. 4. Visual-tactual associations function correctly within either hemisphere but fail when cross left-right or right-left combinations are involved. Shown an object in left visual field, commissurotomy subjects report verbally that they "did not see" the left field stimulus (projected to right hemisphere). However, the subject then has no difficulty in finding the same stimulus object using the left but not the right hand. In this same setup, objects presented to the left hand for tactual identification cannot then be found with the right hand.

rather high level but are no longer cognizant of most mental functions of the partner hemisphere. The two disconnected hemispheres can further be shown to function concurrently but independently in parallel, by presenting different stimulus items simultaneously to the two hands or to the two visual half-fields. Under these conditions each of the two hemispheres are found to process concurrently their own separate perceptual-cognitive-mnemonic functions, and these may be grossly incompatible or even mutually contradictory [7] without either hemisphere's noticing that anything is wrong—so separate are the inner experiences of the disconnected hemispheres. The basic hemisphere disconnection syndrome is apparent as well in experiments with animals, as shown earlier in extensive studies on cats and sub-human primates during the 1950s [16,24,26,35]. As in man, the surgically separated hemispheres were found to perceive, learn, and remember independently at a high level, apparently with about equal proficiency on left and right sides.

Some authorities, concerned for the essential unity of the conscious self, have been reluctant to accept the conclusion that the mind is divided by commissurotomy, maintaining instead that the mind and self remain unified within the language hemisphere or centered in the intact brain stem or in the person as a whole and that the nonspeaking, subordinate hemisphere operates only as a computer-like, unconscious automaton. (A recent treatment of this controversy may be found in Zangwill [39]; see also [17].) While these alternative interpretations may better conform with common concepts and traditions regarding the usual unity of the inner being, we have not been able to see any real justification in our test findings for denying consciousness to the disconnected mute hemisphere. Everything we have observed in many kinds of task performances over many years of testing reinforces the conclusion that the mute hemisphere has an inner experience of much the same order as that of the speaking hemisphere though differing in quality and cognitive faculties as will be outlined later. Clearly the right hemisphere perceives, thinks, learns, and remembers, all at a very human level. It also reasons nonverbally, makes studied cognitive decisions, and carries out novel volitional actions. Further, it can be shown to generate typical human emotional responses when confronted with affect-laden stimuli and situations.

II

Contrary to prior neurological doctrine based on unilateral lesions, the disconnected mute hemisphere has been found to be neither "word-blind" nor "word-deaf." To our initial surprise the comprehension of spoken instructions proved to be quite good in the right hemisphere, and the reading of printed words was performed moderately well. This comprehension in the minor hemisphere of spoken and written words was demonstrated by selective retrieval or pointing to corresponding objects or pictures. It was possible to go in the reverse direction also, i.e., from objects or pictures to words, written or spoken, and to go from spoken to written words and vice versa [10,28,32,33]. The right hemisphere could also spell simple three- and four-letter words with cut-out letters and read such words presented tactually, in contrast to the strong earlier impressions in neurology that the right hemisphere ordinarily is lacking in this kind of language comprehension and higher cognition.

Our findings are in line with the earlier controversial views of Hughlings Jackson but contradict many other observations that unilateral lesions confined to the left hemisphere alone may cause total global aphasia or leave a person word-deaf and/or word-blind despite the retention of an intact, undamaged right hemisphere. Although this disparity is still not fully resolved, the evidence seems to be settling out in favor of the conclusions drawn from commissurotomy. In particular, the language profile of the right hemisphere after commissure section conforms rather well to that seen after rare surgical removals of the speech hemisphere for malignancy [21]. The vocabulary in the disconnected right hemisphere for comprehension of single spoken words about 10 years after surgery is found to have a mental age rating only slightly below that of the language hemisphere [38].

Earlier interpretations based on the symptoms produced by focal lesions that pictured the minor or subordinte hemisphere as a comparative retardate in brain evolution have had to be revised. The mental performance of this hemisphere after commissurotomy has been found repeatedly to be superior and dominant to that of the speaking hemisphere in a growing series of nonverbal, largely spatial tests. The tasks involved are of the kind where a single spatial image processed as a whole proves to be more effective than a detailed verbal or mathematical description. Examples include the copying of designs, reading faces, fitting forms into molds, discrimination and recall of nondescript tactual and visual forms, spatial transformations and transpositions, judging whole circle size from a small arc, grouping series of different-sized and -shaped blocks into categories, perceiving whole plane forms from a collection of parts, and intuitive apprehension of geometrical properties (this literature is still scattered, but see reviews in [24,26,28,33]; also see [8]).

Commissurotomy makes possible precise left-right comparisons for positive performance within the same brain, where most of the usual confusing background variables cancel out. Also the deceptive interhemispheric interference effects that complicate inferences drawn from focal lesions are eliminated or greatly reduced. Earlier doubts regarding the presence of advanced mental function in the minor hemisphere are now largely dispelled, and the concept of a complementary evolution of both hemispheres has come to replace our older classic view of a single one-sided dominance.

In any case, after watching repeatedly the superior performance of the right hemisphere in tests like the above, one finds it most difficult to think of this half of the brain as being only an automaton lacking in conscious awareness. Especially it is difficult to deny consciousness to the right hemisphere when it proves to be superior in novel tasks that involve logical reasoning and also when it generates typical facial expressions of satisfaction at tasks well done or of annoyance at its own errors or at those made by its uninformed partner hemisphere. Also difficult to reconcile with the concept of an automaton state is the clear ability of the right hemisphere to learn from experience, remembering test items it has seen or felt on prior testing sessions days or even weeks previously.

III

In many kinds of tests it is found that both disconnected hemispheres, regardless of differential speed and proficiency, are able to come up with the correct answers. Further analysis indicates that the answers are arrived at, however, by different processing strategies or modes of thinking on left and right sides. Beyond the more obvious differences like those of speech, writing, and constructive visuospatial manipulation, more subtle organizational differences are indicated that tend to be obscured by individual patient variation in ordinary brain lesion studies, where it is taken for granted that some individuals will be more talkative than others, or more inclined to use verbal logic or visual imagery, etc. Under the conditions of commissurotomy, however, with the same subjects working the same test task with each hemisphere, even slight cognitive differences on left and right sides become meaningful. The same person is observed to employ consistently one or the other of two different kinds of mental strategy much like two different people, depending on whether the right or the left hemisphere is in use. The first evidence for this was obtained by Levy in 1969 [11] and has been repeatedly confirmed many times since. The discovery of complementary cognitive mode asymmetries following commissurotomy has prompted many further studies in normal, in brain-damaged, and in other select populations helping to better pinpoint and delineate the left-right cognitive differences and their variations.

Correlations of cerebral laterality have been extended to handedness, sex, occupational preferences and ability, special innate talents, eye dominance, genetic variations like Turner's syndrome, endocrinology, congenital dyslexia, autism, dreaming, hypnosis, inverted writing—and so on (an introduction and references to this large and rapidly expanding literature can be found in [12]). This has become a rapidly developing and fascinating story in itself of which I mention briefly a few summary points in passing. One important outcome is the increased insight and appreciation, in education and elsewhere, for the importance of nonverbal forms and components of learning, intellect, and communication. By the early seventies it already had become evident, from the standpoint of brain research, that our educational system and modern urban society generally, with its heavy emphasis on linguistic communication and early training in the three Rs, tends increasingly to discriminate against the nonverbal, nonmathematical half of the brain, which has its own perceptual-mechanical-spatial mode of apprehension and reasoning [27,29]. The amount of formal training given to right-hemisphere functions in our public schools traditionally has been almost negligible compared to that devoted to the specialities of the left hemisphere. The need now for better methods by which to detect, measure, and develop the nonverbal components of intellect before their critical development periods have passed is becoming widely recognized.

These and related developments also help bring an increased respect and regard for the inherent individuality in the structure of human intellect. People can no longer be assumed to be qualitatively similar at birth with equal potentiality for becoming a Beethoven or a Shakespeare, an Edison or a Michaelangelo, etc. Different mental disciplines employ qualitatively different forms of cognitive processing that require different patterns of neural circuitry, the basic cerebral requirements for which are largely prewired. Even the potentialities of the two hemispheres of the same brain with respect to verbal and spatial functions are already at birth found to be qualitatively different [4,13,36]. There is strong indication that cognitive spatial ability is partly genetic and correlated with a sex-linked recessive. Evidence is mounting for other genetic and innate developmental variations involved in congenital dyslexia, autism, Turner's syndrome, androgenic females, and the like. Statistically the hemispheres mature earlier and show less lateralization in females, which is thought to account in part for the significant sex differences obtained in large-scale tests for intellectual factors and special abilities, females scoring higher in verbal tests and males in mathematics and tests that demand spatial processing. But many other variables are involved [12].

Actually, the more we learn, the more complex becomes the picture for predictions regarding any one individual, and the more it seems to reinforce the conclusion that the kind of unique individuality we each carry around in our inherent brain wiring makes that of fingerprints or facial features appear gross and simple by comparison. The need for educational tests and policy measures selectively to identify, accommodate, and serve the differentially specialized forms of intellectual potential becomes increasingly evident.

One must caution in this connection that the experimentally observed polarity in right-left cognitive style is an idea in general with which it is very easy to run wild. You can read today that things such as intuition, the seat of the subconscious, creativity, parapsychic sensitivity, the mind of the Orient, ethnocultural disposition, hypnotic susceptibility, the roots of counter-culture, altered states of consciousness—and what not—all reside predominantly in the right hemisphere. The extent to which extrapolations of this kind may eventually prove to be more fact or fancy will require many years to determine. In the meantime it is important to remember that the two hemispheres in the normal intact brain tend regularly to function closely together as a unit and that different states of mind are apt to involve different hierarchical and organizational levels or front-back and other differentiations as well as differences in laterality.

IV

In light of the mounting evidence for higher cognitive faculties and a complementary specialization in the right hemisphere, earlier claims that this hemisphere is not conscious have given way to intermediate positions. One of the latest concedes that the mute hemisphere may be conscious at some levels, but denies that the non-language hemisphere possesses the higher, reflective, and self-conscious type of awareness that characterizes the human mind and is needed, so it is said, to qualify a conscious system as a "person" [5,19]. Self-consciousness is said to be predominantly a human attribute according to present thinking based on evidence drawn mainly from mirror tests for self-recognition [9]. In these terms, self-awareness seems to be largely lacking in animals below the primates and appears only to a limited extent in the great apes. In human childhood, self-consciousness is reported to emerge relatively late, somewhere around 18 months of age. Thus, self-consciousness, by developmental as well as by evolutionary criteria, is rated as a relatively advanced phase of conscious awareness.

We accordingly devised some tasks specifically designed to test for self-consciousness and levels of social awareness in the disconnected minor hemisphere. Procedures were used in which the subject, working with the mute hemisphere, merely has to point manually, on request, to select items in a choice array in order to indicate recognition, identification, personal approval, dislike—or whatever, as requested. The test arrays consist of four to nine pictures, drawings or photographs among which key personal and affect-laden items are inserted irregularly among neutral unknowns. The subject's vision is lateralized throughout to one hemisphere [37] and audio and visual tape recordings are used to analyze the more subtle aspects of responses.

Under these conditions, we found [34] that the right hemisphere can readily recognize and identify, with appropriate emotional reactions and social evaluations, pictures of the subject's self; his or her family, relatives, acquaintances, pets, and other belongings, familiar scenes, and also political, historical, and religious figures and television and screen personalities. The general level of recognition and quality of reaction were quite comparable throughout to those obtained from the same subject using the left hemisphere or free vision. All results to date support the conclusion that the right hemisphere, despite its language deficits, harbors a well-developed, seemingly normal conscious self with a basic personality and social self-awareness that is in close accord with the presurgical character of the patient and also with that of the speaking hemisphere of the same subject. Similar procedures were used to test for a sense of time and concern for the future in the right hemisphere, thus far with no evidence of abnormal deficit. The nonvocal hemisphere appears to be aware of daily and weekly schedules, important dates of the year, holidays, etc., and to make appropriate discriminations with regard to possible future accidents and family losses, life, fire, and theft insurance, and the like.

V

Accepting the dual conscious state of the hemispheres following surgical separation, students of the problem of personal identity and the nature of the conscious self have used the split-brain findings, along with cases of fugue states or multiple personality, to support the argument that it is no longer correct to think of a "person" as being correlated one-to-one with a body, that we need now to sharpen and refine the concept in terms of the critical brain states and neural systems involved. Such refinement becomes important in medicolegal decisions dealing, for example, with prolonged states of coma, stages in fetal development, vital organ transplants and so on.

An extreme position in regard to selfhood and "personal identity" is held by Puccetti [20] and Bogen [2] and others who infer that each hemisphere must have a separate mind of its own, not only after brain bisection but also in the normal intact brain as well. The surgery, they argue, simply reveals what already is there—namely, that we are all of us actually a dual compound of right and left minds, or "persons," as Puccetti puts it— and that this bicameral condition normally goes undetected because the experiences of right and left hemispheres are kept in close synchrony when the commissures are intact. I myself have favored the view that the conscious mind is normally single and unified, mediated by brain activity that spans and involves both hemispheres. This assumes, first, that the fiber systems of the brain mediate conscious awareness as do the switching mechanisms, synaptic interfaces, and other properties of the gray matter; and second, that fiber cross-connections between the hemispheres are not different in this respect from fiber systems within each hemisphere. The bilateral process can be viewed as an integrated mental emergent that, functionally and causally, is qualitatively different from, and more than, the mere sum of the left and right activities and further exerts downward causal control of the neuronal events in both hemispheres. In this view the two hemispheres function together as a closely integrated whole, not as a double, divided, or bicameral system. The two hemispheres, on these terms, normally perceive, think, emote, learn, and remember as a unit. They even speak as a unit in that the right hemisphere during speech is not idling or diverted but is actively focused to aid and sustain the cerebral processing involved in speech, to add tone and expression and to inhibit unrelated activity.

Even in the bisected brain, the question of whether there exists a right/left division of conscious experience is not subject to an unqualified "yes" or "no" answer. While the right/left division of many perceptual, cognitive, and mnemonic processes is clearly evident in lateralized testing, as already described, there are other aspects of consciousness that are not similarly divided. Two principle ways have been recognized in which the conscious mind remains undivided after commissurotomy [28]. The first is attributed to the presence in the brain of bilateral wiring systems that ensure the representation of both left and right components of experience within each hemisphere. The cutaneous sensory system for the face is an example. Sensations from both left and right sides of the face mediated by the trigeminal nerves are each represented in both hemispheres. The kind of separation that applies for right and left halves of the field of vision and for right and left hands does not therefore hold with respect to the face. The same is true for audition and other systems like those mediating crude pain, temperature, pressure, and position sense, especially from the more axial parts of the body. Bilateral motor controls also are extensively present in both hemispheres. For lateralized testing we must necessarily be highly selective and take considerable pains to avoid activity that cannot be reliably confined to a single hemisphere. We thus depend heavily on moderately sophisticated input from the hands and from the half-fields of vision.

Bilateral representation within each hemisphere is further achieved by factors of a more functional kind. Exploratory movements of the eyes, for example, can provide bilateral representation of a perceived scene or object in both disconnected hemispheres. Similarly, exploratory movements of the hands with interchange and overlap can provide for a bilateral unified percept of an object in both hemispheres. These kinds of factors must be routinely guarded against and excluded in our lateralized testing.

Another fundamental way in which the conscious mind is not divided by commissurotomy is illustrated in the tests for self and social awareness mentioned above in which mental-emotional ambience or semantic surround generated in one hemisphere promptly spreads also to the second hemisphere. These "deep structure" components in conscious awareness, which appear to include attitudinal, orientational, emotional, contextual, and even semantic and related cognitive factors, are presumably mediated through undivided deep components of cognition. I have described the structure of the conscious system in the divided brain as being Y-shaped, i.e., divided in its upper, more structured levels but undivided below [31]. Each of the separated hemispheric limbs of the "Y," it should be remembered, contains within itself extensive bilateral representation. Each hemisphere, for example, functions with much the usual sense of awareness of the positions and movements of all body parts on both sides, a sense of being able to initiate and direct motor commands for the whole body, and an awareness also of the environment on all sides. Visceral sensations and central states like those involved in hunger, fatigue, etc., also are bilateralized. Even where the ipsilateral representations are weak or absent, there is good reason to think that there is not direct awareness of the ipsilateral deficits. This accords with a general rule that in many respects brains tend to be oblivious of what they lack.

The brain process responsible for a unified conscious experience need not itself be unified, single, or localized. In addition to the recognized diversity and discontinuity or "graininess" of its neuronal firing patterns, the brain process also is subject to major subdivisions like the left-right and front-back fractionations and the vertical divisions into higher cognitive and deeper emotional components already described. The brain process as such seems to have no counterpart to match the unity, continuity, quality, constancy, and other psychological properties that are experienced subjectively. A hypothesized correlation between mental and neural events based on isomorphic electric fields was suggested by gestalt theory in the 1940s, but was largely abandoned when we found that the insertion of short-circuiting wires or current-distorting dielectric plates all through the visual cortex failed to correspondingly disrupt visual form perception [23,30].

Some years ago we proposed that the answer must lie alternatively in thinking of conscious experience as a functional or operational derivative of the brain process rather than as a spatiotemporal copy or transform [22]. In other words, what counts for subjective unity may lie in the way the brain process functions as a unity or entity regardless of the multilevel and multicomponent make-up of the neural events involved. The overall, holistic functional effect could thus determine the conscious experience. If the functional impact of the neural activity has a unitary effect in the upper-level conscious dynamics, the subjective experience is unified. In these terms the qualities of subjective experience need not correlate with the diverse particulate components of the neuronal infrastructure, only with the function of the active process as a whole. By these operational criteria for generation of subjective meaning the mind may be seen to be largely divided after commissurotomy but unified in the normal intact brain.

VI

Another thing to come out of these concerns for the unity and/or duality of mind, with and without the commissures, is a modified concept of the nature of consciousness. A revised view of the conscious self is involved that includes a formula for mind-brain interaction. For many decades science was traditionally careful to exclude explicitly from its objective explanations any use of conscious or mental forces or phenomena as causal constructs. Mind or subjective experience was accordingly treated in science as an acausal epiphenomenon or as a passive parallel correlate of brain activity, a semantic artifact or most commonly as an inner aspect of the one main physical brain process. In these terms the physiological brain process is assumed to be causally complete in itself with no need or any place for the causal intervention or operation of conscious or mental forces.

The more we learned about the neuronal circuitry and electromechanical mechanisms of brain activity, the more incredible it became to think that the course of these physicochemical events could be influenced in any way by the qualities of conscious experience. As Eccles [6] phrased it in 1964, "We can, in principle, explain all our input-output performance in terms of activity of neuronal circuits; and consequently, consciousness seems to be absolutely unnecessary" and again ". . . as neurophysiologists we simply have no use for consciousness in our attempt to explain how the nervous system works." This was the kind of reasoning that had prevailed widely for more than half a century and had led to the philosophy of scientific materialism with its firm renunciation of consciousness and mentalism in science. Behaviorist psychology, with its rigorous rejection of anything mental or subjective, also relied heavily on this reasoning in neuroscience to overcome the otherwise strong subjectivist pressures in cognitive and humanistic psychology and phenomenological thinking as well as in clinical psychology, the field of perception and other subdisciplines where the contents of introspection were indispensible.

Since the mid-1960s our thinking on these matters has undergone some revolutionary changes. In the course of wrestling with the problem of conscious unity in the presence and absence of the cerebral commissures, I became convinced that consciousness is better conceived as being causal in brain activity rather than noncausal and that science had been wrong in denying this for more than half a century [25]. The classical neuronal reasoning of Eccles was perceived to have a flaw or shortcoming. It correctly emphasized the control exerted by neuronal events in determining subjective experience but had been in error in its predication that the course of these physicochemical events could not be influenced by conscious experience. It had failed to recognize the important "downward control" exerted reciprocally by the resultant mental processes on the course of their component neuronal activities. Thus in direct reversal of earlier thinking, my new logic said that neuronal events in the brain, i.e., when, where, and how neurons fire, are determined not only by physicochemical activity but predominantly by the higher laws and dynamics of mental programming.

In these terms we do not look for conscious awareness in the nerve cells of the brain or in the molecules or atoms of brain processing. Along with the larger as well as lesser building blocks of brain function, these elements are common as well to unconscious, automatic, and reflex activity. For the subjective qualities we look higher in the system at organizational properties that are select and special to operations at top levels of the brain hierarchy and that are seen to supersede in brain causation the powers of their neuronal, molecular, atomic, and subatomic infrastructure. The subsidiary components embodied in the conscious processes, such as the timing of neuronal firing and flow patterns of impulse traffic, as well as the inner molecular and atomic "forces within forces" are all carried along in space and time subject to the overriding higher-level dynamics of the mental programming—just as the flow of electrons in a TV receiver is differentially determined by the program content on different channels.

Without going into further detail, we can see that it follows on this revised scheme that mind does actually move matter within the brain [25], and outside as well, indirectly through physical behavior. Further, it now becomes "mind over matter" in a very real sense. This is all within the brain hierarchy, of course. There is no implication that mind is separate from matter in the dualistic sense. Mentalism is no longer equivalent to dualism in the framework of today's modified paradigm. The revolution of the past decade toward increased scientific acceptance of consciousness does not do anything directly to bolster dualist beliefs in the mystical, the paranormal, or supernatural. At the same time, the new position directly opposes prior materialist doctrine that has been telling us for more than half a century that "Man is nothing but a material object, having none but physical properties" and that "Science can give a complete account of man in purely physiochemical terms." These quotes are from the late 1960s by Armstrong [1], a founding father and leader of the materialist, so-called mind-brain identity theory, which still finds support today, though with major reinterpretations to bring it now into close concordance with the causal emergent views of mind outlined above.

Once science thus modifies its traditional materialist-behaviorist stance and begins to accept in theory, and to encompass in principle, within its causal domain the whole world of inner, conscious, subjective experience (the world of the humanities), then the very nature of science itself is changed. The change is not in the basic methodology or procedures, of course, but in the scope of science and in its limitations, in its relation to the humanities and to values and in its role as a cultural, intellectual, and moral force. The kinds of interpretations that science supports, the world picture and attendant value perspectives and priorities, and the concepts of physical reality that derive from science all undergo substantial revisions on these new terms. We come out with a vastly transformed scientific view of ourselves and the world and of the kinds of forces that are in control. The change is away from the mechanistic, deterministic, and reductionistic doctrines of pre-1965 science to the more humanistic interpretations of the 1970s. Our current views are more mentalistic, holistic, and subjectivist. They give more freedom in that they reduce the restrictions of mechanistic determinism and they are more quality rich and more rich in value and meaning.

The pervasive broad paradigm changes involved are particularly welcomed by all who look to science, not alone for objective knowledge and material advances, but also for worldview perspectives and criteria of ultimate value and meaning; those who see science as the best source of true understanding and the most valid route to an intimate comprehension of "the forces that made and move the universe and created Man." Our new mind-brain paradigm qualifies science to assume a higher and more critical societal role that, hopefully, future science will come increasingly to fulfill.

ACKNOWLEDGMENTS

Work of the author and his laboratory have been supported by the National Institute of Mental Health NIMH grant MH3372 and by the F.P. Hixon Fund of the California Institute of Technology.

REFERENCES

1. Armstrong DM (1968): "A Materialist Theory of the Mind." London: Routledge and Kegan Paul.
2. Bogen JE (1969): The other side of the brain. II. An appositional mind. Bull Los Angeles Neurol Soc 34:135–162.
3. Bremer F, Brihaye J, Andre-Baliseaux G (1956): Physiologie et pathologie du corps calleux. Schweiz Archs Neurol Psychiatry 78:31–87.
4. Dennis M, Kohn B (1975): Comprehension of syntax in infantile hemiplegics after hemidecortication: Left hemisphere superiority. Brain Lang 2:472.
5. Dewitt L (1975): Consciousness, mind and self. Br J Philos Sci 26:41–47.
6. Eccles JC (1966): Conscious experience and memory. In Eccles JC (ed) "Brain and Conscious Experience."
7. Ellenberg L, Sperry RW (1980): Lateralized division of attention in the commissurotomized and intact brain. Neuropsychologia 18:411–418.
8. Franco L, Sperry RW (1977): Hemispheric lateralization for cognitive processing of geometry. Neuropsychologia 15:107–114.
9. Gallup GG (1977): Self-recognition in primates. Am Psychol 32:329–338.
10. Gazzaniga MS, Sperry RW (1967): Language after section of the cerebral commissures. Brain 90:131–148.
11. Levy J (1969): Information processing and higher psychological functions in the disconnected hemispheres of human commissurotomy patients. PhD thesis, California Institute of Technology.
12. Levy J (1974): Psychobiological implications of bilateral asymmetry. In Dimond S, Beaumont JB (eds): "Hemisphere Function in the Human Brain." London: Paul Elek, pp 121–183.
13. Levy J (1976): Cerebral lateralization and spatial ability. Behav Genet 6:171–188.
14. Levy J, Nagalaki T (1972): A model for the genetics of handedness. Genetics 72:117–128.
15. Morgan CL (1923): "Emergent Evolution." New York: Holt.
16. Myers RE (1962): Transmission of visual information within and between the hemispheres. In Mountcastle VB (ed): "Interhemispheric Relations and Cerebral Dominance." Baltimore: John Hopkins Press.
17. Nagel T (1971): Brain bisection and unity of consciousness. Synthese 22:396–413.
18. Neisser U (1966): "Cognitive Psychology." New York: Appleton-Century-Crofts.
19. Popper K, Eccles JC (1977): "The Self and Its Brain." New York: Springer International.
20. Puccetti R (1973): Brain bisection and personal identity. Br J Phil Sci 24:339–355.
21. Smith A (1966): Speech and other functions after left (dominant) hemispherectomy. J Neurol Neurosurg Psychiatry 29:467–471.
22. Sperry RW (1952): Neurology and the mind-brain problem. Am Sci 40:291–312.

23. Sperry RW (1957): Brain mechanisms in behavior. Eng Sci 20:24–29.
24. Sperry RW (1961): Cerebral organization and behavior. Science 133:1749–1757.
25. Sperry RW (1965): Mind, brain and humanist values. In Platt JR (ed): "New Views of the Nature of Man." Chicago: University of Chicago Press, pp 71–92.
26. Sperry RW (1968): Mental unity following surgical disconnection of the cerebral hemispheres. Harvey Lect 62:293–323.
27. Sperry RW (1973): Lateral specialization of cerebral function in the surgically separated hemispheres. In McGuigan FJ, Schoonover RA (eds): "The Psychophysiology of Thinking." New York: Academic Press, pp 209–229.
28. Sperry RW (1974): Lateral specialization in the surgically separated hemispheres. In Schmitt FO, Worden FG (eds): "The Neurosciences: Third Study Program." Cambridge: MIT Press, pp 5–19.
29. Sperry RW (1974): Messages from the laboratory. Eng Sci 37:29–32.
30. Sperry RW (1975): In search of psyche. In Worden FG, Swazey JP, Adelman G (eds): "The Neurosciences: Paths of Discovery." Cambridge: MIT Press, pp 425–434.
31. Sperry RW (1976): Mental phenomena as causal determinants in brain function. In Globus G, Maxwell G, Savodnik I (eds): "Consciousness and the Brain." pp 163–177. (Reprinted in Process Studies 5:247–256, 1976.)
32. Sperry RW, Gazzaniga MS (1967): Language following surgical disconnection of the hemispheres. In Milikan CH and Darley FL (eds): "Brain Mechanisms Underlying Speech and Language." New York: Grune & Stratton, pp 108–116.
33. Sperry RW, Gazzaniga MS, Bogen JE (1969): Interhemispheric relationships: the neocortical commissures. Syndromes of hemisphere disconnection. In Vinken PJ, Bruyn GW (eds): "Handbook of Clinical Neurology." Amsterdam: North Holland, pp 273–290.
34. Sperry RW, Zaidel E, Zaidel D (1979): Self-recognition and social awareness in the deconnected hemisphere. Neuropsychologia 17:153–166.
35. Trevarthen CB (1962): Double visual learning in split brain monkeys. Science 136:258–259.
36. Wada JA, Clarke R, Hamm A (1975): Cerebral hemispheric asymmetry in humans. Cortical speech zones in 100 adult and 100 infant brains. Arch Neurol 32:239–246.
37. Zaidel E (1975): A technique for presenting lateralized visual input with prolonged exposure. Vision Res 15:283–289.
38. Zaidel E (1976): Auditory vocabulary of the right hemisphere following brain bisection or hemidecortication. Cortex 12:191–211.
39. Zangwill OL (1974) Consciousness and the cerebral hemispheres. In Dimond S, Beaumont J (eds): "Hemisphere Function in the Human Brain." London: Paul Elek, pp 264–278.

Two Hemispheres—One Brain:
Functions of the Corpus Callosum, pages 21–34
© 1986 Alan R. Liss, Inc.

One Brain, Two Brains, or Both?

JOSEPH E. BOGEN

Department of Neurological Surgery, University of Southern California and Department of Psychology, University of California, Los Angeles, California 90032

> ...We used, when in trouble, often to comfort ourselves with jokes, among them the old saying of the two kinds of truth. To the one kind belong the statements so simple and clear that the opposite assertion obviously could not be defended. The other kind, the so-called "deep truths," are statements in which the opposite also contains deep truth.
>
> —N. Bohr, 1958

The organizers of this symposium, as indicated by its title, evidently believe that there is a question to be considered. And to judge from the distinguished list of invited scientists, our hosts evidently expect that this particular question can be, if not settled, at least clarified by an experimental approach, a point to which we shall return.

In this chapter I shall present some of the evidence that the one-brain view is inadequate to describe not only the split-brain but also the intact brain. I shall then consider in some detail the possibility of retaining *both* views, as an example of complementarity.

We might rephrase the symposium title as follows: Does an individual having two cerebral hemispheres have, in some important sense, one brain rather than two brains? The "important sense" in which the conference title is intended deserves to be made explicit at the outset. It includes, I believe, the following: that *whatever* may be for physiologists the meaning of the psychological term "mind," the *number* of brains in an individual is the same as the number of minds.[1] If this equivalence of numerosity were

---

[1]And the number of minds is *integral.* Assuming, as considered elsewhere [Bogen, 1981] that "mind" can be fractional (e.g. 1.3 minds?) would provide a quite unorthodox approach to the problem of mental numerosity, probably making any consideration of macroscopic complementarity superfluous.

not agreed upon, we could easily spend all of our time here arguing *that* question as well as its cognates such as, What do we mean by the word "mind"? Such perennial questions are surely not the questions for which our hosts have called us together. We take it for granted, at least for these few days, that what we can learn about mind also tells us about brain and vice versa: or in other words, the mentalistic and physiologic are two different descriptions of the same underlying reality.

It is important to note that in discussing the duality versus singularity of brain, or in shifting back and forth between mentalistic and physiologic vocabularies, we are *not* concerned with a quite different issue, one which is often couched in misleadingly similar terms. That is, we are not here concerned with the ontologic issue of dualism vs. monism, whether the monism be materialistic or idealistic. Whether one professes (as have so many Eastern philosophers and some contemporary quantum physicists: [Wigner, 1967; Mehra, 1973; Bohm, 1981]) that mind begets brain, or whether one supposes [along with Sir Charles Sherrington, 1947] that mind coexists with and interacts with brain, or whether (as I believe) mind is generated by brain, need not concern us here. Our metaphysical views neither entail nor are they entailed by our views on the question at hand. This is because one could easily be on either side of the dualism-monism issue irrespective of one's position on the question of duality or singularity of mind.

HISTORICAL BACKGROUND

How is it that the question at hand (duality versus singularity of brain) has come so forcefully to our attention.

The view that the brain should be considered *not* as a single organ but rather as a pair of organs, in much the same sense that each of us has a pair of kidneys or a pair of lungs, that view is at least as old as the writings of Hippocrates. In his words:

> . . . the human brain, as in the case of all other animals, is double [Chadwick and Mann, 1950, p 183].

This view was urged with utmost conviction by Arthur Ladbroke Wigan, an English physician who published his book, *The Duality of the Mind*, in 1844. Among the many other similar sentiments in this book, he claimed that, "the mind is essentially dual, like the organs by which it is exercised" (p 4). He believed himself able to prove, "that a separate and distinct process of thinking or ratiocination may be carried on in each cerebrum simultaneously" (p 26). Nowadays we call this "the principle of cerebral duality"; it is *not* dependent upon the existence of hemispheric specialization; it is true of cats, monkeys, etc., as well as humans.

The view of the brain as a double was also advanced by others, notably including Brown-Séquard, David Ferrier, and Sir Victor Horsley [Bogen, 1969]. John Hughlings Jackson, in his essay entitled "On the Nature of the Duality of the Brain," wrote as follows:

> That the nervous system is double physically is evident enough. This is a very striking fact, but one so well known that we are in danger of ceasing to think of its significance—of ceasing to wonder at it.
>
> The nervous system, I repeat, is physically double. I wish to show that it is double in function also, and further, in what way it is double in function [Jackson, 1958; p 129].

Such eminent advocates notwithstanding, the view that the brain is double remained in eclipse for nearly a century. It has only recently been disinterred in the light of the split-brain results whose initiation, development, and exposition are largely due to our honoree, Nobel Laureate Roger W. Sperry [Sperry, 1982]. That this view remained in eclipse for so long was probably of multiple causation, but I would suggest that perhaps the strongest of these causes has its origin not in objective science but in subjective intuition—the inner conviction of wholeness, or unity, of singleness felt by each of us here. According to Rene Descartes:

> ". . . there is a great difference between the mind and the body, in that the body is, by its nature, always divisible, and the mind wholly indivisible. For, in fact, when I contemplate it—that is, when I contemplate my own self—and consider myself as a thing that thinks, I cannot discover in myself any parts, but I clearly know that I am a thing absolutely one and complete" [Young, 1970, p 72].

This conviction was elegantly expressed by Sir Charles Sherrington when he wrote:

> "This self is a unity . . . it regards itself as one, others treat it as one. It is addressed as one, by a name to which it answers. The Law and the State schedule it as one. It and they identify it with a body which is considered by it and them to belong to it integrally. In short, unchallenged and unargued conviction assumes it to be one. The logic of grammar endorses this by a pronoun in the singular. All its diversity is merged in oneness" [Sherrington, 1947, p xvii].

However correct or erroneous it may be, *it is this conviction* that offers the greatest resistance to the two-brain view, even now that the split-brain results are so widely appreciated [Bogen, 1984]. One still sees in current print, for example, such sentiments as "the brain is a unity" or "all parts of the brain participate in all of its actions" or [and this may be the canonical form] "the brain works as a whole." This is not a description of an observable fact; it is the slogan, or motto if you will, of a particular philosophic point of view. What *is* the evidence?

The subjective evidence, that is to say, introspection, recurrently reminds each of us that "mind is single." But the objective, experimental evidence increasingly tells us that the intact brain is double. I have summarized much of the evidence in a forthcoming chapter [Bogen, 1985]. I will mention here only a few illustrative examples, having mainly to do with a lack of interhemispheric transfer, beginning with the Sperry and Clark results of 1949.

EXPERIMENTAL EVIDENCE FOR SIGNIFICANT HEMISPHERIC INDEPENDENCE WITH RESPECT TO LEARNING

In 1949, Sperry and Clark reported a clear case of lack of interocular transfer in their training of gobies. (It is worth recalling that the split-brain story started with the question of interocular transfer, i.e., whether learning acquired with one eye was demonstrated with the other.) In this paper Sperry and Clark wrote:

> ... the results seem to support the conclusion that the brain organization of this teleost fish permits interocular transfer, but at the same time the neural mechanisms involved are not so well developed that good transfer is automatically assured in all instances.

In fact, clear-cut savings were observed in only 5 of 16 cases. Lesser degrees of transfer were found in 4, whereas transfer was essentially nil in the rest. The 11 without good transfer had not simply "forgotten" the task, because retesting of the originally trained hemisphere showed approximately the previous (trained) level of correct responses. Then the untrained eye was again tested in 2 cases, and excellent transfer was found in one of them.

In considering the above experiments with fish, we recall that the chiasmal crossing in these animals is essentially complete, so that training with one eye results in training one hemisphere directly and the other only indirectly (if at all). Where chiasmal crossing is complete, lack of interocular transfer is tantamount to lack of interhemispheric transfer; i.e., it is evidence of hemispheric independence. A similar chiasmal crossing is present in the rat and rabbit, which we consider next because some famous mammals of our acquaintance refuse to acknowledge the applicability to them of any experiments on teleost fish.

Russell and Morgan [1979] directed the input in the rat to one hemisphere by restricting the input to one eye. (The white rat's chiasm is almost totally crossed—the wild rat has a little bit less crossing, whereas in the human or monkey it is approximately 50%). Then they tested the other eye. What they concluded was that a failure of interocular transfer in the rat need not represent some sort of anatomical disconnection. On the contrary, as they said:

> . . . these results suggest that under certain conditions an absence of interhemispheric communication is a characteristic of the intact brain.

Using rabbits, Van Hof [1979] repeatedly found "lateralization of the memory trace"; but he cautiously concluded that "it would be premature to regard the rabbit as a 'natural split-brain preparation.' " The rabbit has a corpus callosum, of course; but the engram may not transfer if one sets up the learning situation in a certain way. The same has been found to be true of pigeons, who show interocular transfer for some problems but not for others [Goodale and Graves, 1980].

Some persons have shrugged off these results in "lower animals" and asked: What about primates? Well, in them, too, there is experimental evidence for significant hemispheric independence with respect to learning. In the intact monkey, like monkeys with split-brains, there is often (especially in the unsophisticated animal) a lack of transfer. If one trains a monkey to do something with one hand, he often doesn't straight away do it with the other hand. After a while the monkey transfers better; that is, the lack of transfer typically goes away—unlike the anatomically split condition where the lack of transfer persists.

In a previous review [Bogen and Bogen, 1969], we cited some evidence for lack of interhemispheric transfer of information in the intact brain including a lack of transfer of spatial form discrimination from one hand to the other during early testing of a difficult task in monkeys [Semmes and Mishkin, 1965]. Butler and Francis [1973] reinvestigated this often evanescent phenomenon. They trained baboons to reach through a tube to manipulate stimuli at the other end: this restricted movements at the proximal joints. The animals learned to rotate the stimuli (to get food) in either a clockwise or counterclockwise direction, depending on the stimulus shape. After they learned the task with one hand, the other hand was tested. Two different problems (A and B) were used (three animals learned A first and three learned B first). On the first problem, whether it was A or B, the authors found:

> . . . no animal was able to perform without further training the
> discrimination learned with the other hand; in all cases the
> animals required extensive training with the second hand before
> regaining the proficiency reached with the first one (p 80).

On the second problem (whether B or A), rather than performing at chance as on the first problem, there were often systematic errors because of performance in a mirror-image mode. These results could be interpreted as showing the development of a learning set, that is, the animals may actually *learn* to transfer information, with repeated testing [cf. Berlucchi et al., 1978].

The experiments just described used mainly tactile clues. For visual problems, in the experience of most investigators, monkeys usually show transfer so long as the splenium is intact [Butler, 1979; Hamilton, 1977, 1982; Doty, 1983; Doty et al., 1984]. But even with all commissures intact, lack of transfer has occasionally been evident as a learning deficit on testing of the second hemisphere.

What is important for the purpose of this chapter is that there are certain learning situations giving rise to *certain kinds of information that do not readily transfer in the intact brain.*

Those who dismissed non-primate evidence in their discussions with us have, when presented with evidence such as the foregoing, backed off one more notch and objected, "But what about humans?"

Yes, a lack of interhemispheric transfer in the intact human has been demonstrated in various ways. It seems reasonable to suppose, as did Butler and Francis [1973], that manual manipulations will show less transfer to the other side, the more distal (in the extremity) are the crucial aspects. This could be expected in humans as well as monkeys, and so it is no surprise that it is for fine digital manipulations or detections that savings seem least. A good example is the learning of Braille-like patterns by sighted adults naive to the task. Although there are usually some savings, it requires further training with the second hand to reach the same level of proficiency as with the first hand. Indeed, when going from left to right in right handers, *just as much* training may be needed for the second hand [Harris, 1980].

The amount of transfer probably depends upon what the second hand is doing while the first is being trained, as shown by Hicks et al. [1982]. They had subjects learn a sequence of key presses on a typewriter with one hand while the second hand was either resting or grasping a table leg; partial transfer occurred to the resting hands, but not to the hands occupied with grasping during the original training.

An ingenious study using dichotic listening to digits and tones was reported by Goodglass and Calderon [1977], and their conclusions were supported in another dichotic study by Sidtis and Bryden [1978]. This is not even a situation in which the material is clearly directed to one hemisphere or the other. These experiments were summarized by Bradshaw and Nettleton [1983] in their excellent review, *Human Cerebral Asymmetry*. On page 125 they say:

> These results show that the two hemispheres could concurrently and independently process that component of a complex stimulus for which each is dominant.

Complementing these dichotic experiments is a series of visual half-field experiments by Landis and colleagues [1979, 1981]. I will not describe here their experiments, being content to emphasize their conclusion. In the authors' words: "The result for the emotional expression matching task resembles results obtained with split-brain patients." An alternative approach leading to the same conclusion has been the observation of a different performance pattern in the two visual half-fields of normal subjects doing tasks of the direct access type [Zaidel, 1983].

OF COURSE TWO BRAINS ARE BETTER THAN ONE!

It is understandable that someone would say, (as some do from time to time) that two hemispheres acting together are better than one, especially if we suppose that they are interacting in a mutually supportive manner [Berlucchi, 1983]. That two should be better than one, and moreover that two should incline to act together rather than separately, seems to be in accord not only with our usual intuition but also with some objective, experimental facts. Indeed, we have previously emphasized the crucial importance of hemispheric interaction [Bogen and Bogen, 1969]. Of course, in the human the two hemispheres are different [Gordon, 1985]; this might well incline to interference rather than simple reinforcement, something to be determined, in all likelihood, for each particular circumstance.

That two brains should incline to work together and that when they do they are better than one does not, however, demonstrate that there was but one brain to begin with. In fact, it seems actually to be a sort of back-handed argument for the two-brain view, an argument of interest even if a bit redundant for those who have already found the fore-handed evidence more persuasive.

BOTH ONE BRAIN *AND* TWO BRAINS: A CASE OF COMPLEMENTARITY?

Descriptions of human behavior in terms of "one brain" or of *"the* mind" (singular) have been with us for a very long time. Indeed, they have been in use for so long, and have been so often helpful that we can rest assured that such usage will continue. This is not merely a matter of custom since there are so many situations, both naturally arising and experimental, in which the "one brain" view has seemed both simpler and more useful than any alternative way of explaining behavior.

On the other hand, the very existence of this conference testifies to the fact that there are circumstances for which the "one brain" interpretation has *not* sufficed. More and more people find it not only convenient, but fruitful, to attribute to each hemisphere the qualities of a mind [Bogen, 1977]. The number of such persons is growing. Moreover, since in science as elsewhere one finds what one looks for, we can expect that observations consonant with or even demanding of such "two brain" usage will continually accrue. Those who find such usage uncongenial could find themselves in a progressively shrinking minority.

It seems to be necessary to change from one usage to another, depending on the circumstances. We might then ask if this is merely a matter of verbal usage. Is it possible (as Professor A. Van Harreveld has suggested) that our describing the brain as sometimes single and other times double is related to our vacillation between mentalistic and physiologic explanations of behavior? Most of us *do* resort to both of these approaches, emphasizing one or the other as it seems to suit our needs.

How can we hold simultaneously two seemingly incompatible (and occasionally conflicting) descriptions? There is, of course, a well-known precedent in particle physics, whose practicioners learned to hold *both* the wave and particle views simultaneously. Einstein expressed it in 1924 as follows:

> We now have two theories of light, both indispensable, but it must be admitted, without any logical connection between them, despite twenty years of colossal effort by theoretical physicists.

A half-century later Holton wrote: "One cannot construct an experiment that simultaneously exhibits the wave and particle aspects of atomic matter. A particular experiment will always show only one view or [the other]" [1973, p 119].

If the mentalism/physicalism pair persists not simply as verbal usage but because no experiment can decide between them, we might consider that they make up what Niels Bohr [1958] called a "complementarity." As pointed out by Holton [1973, p 148 ff.], Bohr felt that the concept of complementarity could be particularly helpful in psychology. The idea that quantum theoretical concepts could help us understand brain states has often been argued by D.O. Walter [1971a,b]. What is complementarity?

By the term "complementarity," we refer to the existence of two conflicting interpretations, such that either interpretation provides a useful but incomplete description. As a result, both interpretations must be utilized (usually by alternating or oscillating between them) in order to have the fullest possible account. We do not say that a complementarity exists whenever we have two conflicting explanations of something. Indeed, the overwhelming majority of such pairs are *not* complementary. It is a prominent aspect of scientific endeavor to devise experiments that will help us decide between one or the other explanation, to choose what we call the "correct" interpretation. In order for a mutually conflicting pair to be considered a "complementarity," at least two conditions must be fulfilled:

I. After numerous attempts to formulate a decisive test, either in actual practice or by thought experiment, it gradually becomes accepted by workers in the field that no such experiment is possible [Feynman, 1963, Vol 1, pp 37–38]. Since this conclusion is necessarily dependent upon the somewhat dubious belief that current workers in a field are as knowledgeable as they will ever be, a certain reserve inevitably accompanies any belief that no such crucial experiment will be forthcoming. Such doubts as continue to exist in spite of the lack of a decisive experiment can to some extent be allayed by adding a compelling, rational argument, such as the following:

II. Someone shows how the two conflicting views possess certain essential properties in common, whatever may be their superficial differences, so that no crucial "distinguishing test" should be expected. Such a criterion for wave-particle complementarity was reached when it was realized that a mathematical formulation of the wave theory (the wave equation of Schrödinger) was of sufficient scope and power to account for both aspects. Not only was Schrödinger's equation shown to be isomorphic with the matrix algebra of Heisenberg, but it could be used to predict discontinuous intervals (i.e., quantum jumps) in spite of being a differential equation involving only continuous functions of continuous variables [Feynman, 1963, vol III, pp. 16–14].

III. There is a third, more narrow criterion to be discussed below, after some further generalities.

It is their apparent incompatibility when the two views are expressed in ordinary language, but not when expressed in mathematical terms, that is crucial. As Holton wrote: "What Bohr had done in 1927, was to develop a point of view which would allow him to accept both members of the $(\theta, \bar{\theta})$ couple as valid pictures of nature, accepting the continuity-discontinuity (or wave-particle) duality as an irreducible fact, instead of attempting to dissolve one member of the pair in the other' . . . Bohr asked that physicists accept both θ and $\bar{\theta}$—though both would not be found in the same plane of focus at any given time' . . . We see at once why all parties concerned, both those identified with θ and those identified with $\bar{\theta}$, would not easily accept a new thema which saw a basic truth in the existence of a paradox that the others were trying to remove."

It is worth reiterating how important is the difference between the mathematical formalism (in this case, quantum mechanics) and descriptions in natural language. As Rohrlich [1983] wrote,

... we find that our common language is utterly inadequate for the description of the quantum world and that the mathematical language is much more suitable. [In quantum mechanics an electron] is "just like a particle" or "just like a wave" only in limiting cases depending on the particular experiment (p 1253).

There is a nice way to picture the wave-particle complementarity and its dependence upon our choice of observational method. This was recently pointed out to me by Professor F. Zachariasen and can be described as follows: consider that the event to be observed has a distribution of definite width (we would ordinarily describe the width as a function of the variance). Then, if the resolving power of the observational method were quite wide compared to the width of the observable, one could consider the latter to be negligible; i.e., we would see the observable as a spike with a definite size (height) and a definite location, but no area (i.e., extension) in the ordinary sense. However, if our observational method had a very narrow field of view, we would appear to be confronted (as we move our aperture around) with a standing wave of essentially infinite extent whose height would be different at various locations and whose area we could determine between any two reasonably close locations, but for which the ordinary concept of location would be inapplicable.

If we could formulate a resolution of what we see now as continual vacillation, between two different views, what might be the quantitative concomitants? Does it make sense that "mind" resonates between the two states: "single" or "double"? Could it make sense to describe hemispheric interaction in terms of a phase angle whose size represented the amount of hemispheric synchrony (or disparity)? Does the method of testing (for example, psychological testing) actually affect in some degree whether we see the mind as double or single? This sounds at first like something we might accept. What most of us may not yet be prepared to accept is that the *same* observable will differ from time to time and that this indeterminacy is not observational deficiency but is, indeed, the *real* nature of mind.

ARGUMENTS AGAINST COMPLEMENTARITY

As was forcibly pointed out by Professor M. Adelson, abrupt transitions from one state to another (as from a "one-brain state" to a "two-brains state") certainly do not require the assumption of an underlying complementarity; abrupt transitions of water to ice or vapor are familiar examples. Complementarity could be relevant if it were the case (which it is not for water) that a gradual increase in temperature (or other variable) could have on different trials different results, each with a certain probability but none fully determined. Accepting complementarity (i.e., accepting simultaneously two mutually incompatible views) is something most scientists will not do unless it is forced upon them in each specific case by experimental evidence. (No matter how convenient, seemingly rational, or esthetically pleasing it might be!) So we come to the third criterion alluded to above.

This third criterion is essential to any actual application of quantum mechanics; and it is thought, by some at least, that this criterion should be satisfied *whenever* one wishes to introduce the idea of complementarity. The criterion is that when there are two or more routes to arrive at some result, the probability distribution of the result must be predictable *on the assumption of superposition* rather than classical additivity. In other words, one must add probability amplitudes (expressed in complex numbers) rather than probabilities. This is the case when the probabilities of the alternative routes are not essentially independent. There is a substantial body of opinion [e.g., Putterman, 1983] that no such interaction should be expected on the macroscopic level. If that is so, not only would the concept of complementarity be inapplicable to the one-brain/two-brain issue, but indeed (Niels Bohr notwithstanding) to almost *any* problem of brain function.

Although the assumption of superposition is necessary, it is not sufficient. Suppose we found that a behavior having a Gaussian distribution when exhibited by persons with hemispherectomy had, when exhibited by intact individuals, an interferencelike distribution (more or less W-shaped); then we could conclude that there was an interference *reminiscent* of quantum mechanics. But this would not justify the conclusion that there was a "deep complementarity" in the physicists' sense. This objection can be expressed more generally as follows: although acceptance of contradictory models, using sometimes one and sometimes another, may be necessary in a wide variety of complex situations (indeed, it is typical of real life), one should not consider this to be "complementarity" in the physicists' sense. For physicists, complementarity asserts a fundamental limitation on our ability to describe the basics of nature in ordinary language, whereas in the complex situations of real life the alternating use of contradictory models, and the airing of a diversity of views, merely reflects our current lack of understanding [Iberall, 1979].

This is an enlightening argument but one wonders if we can ever feel we know it all about anything. As pointed out by Dr. J. Johnstone, if complementarity or superposition (or any other idea) can be used to throw light on a subject, who is to say that it is unappropriate only because in *that* subject (unlike physics) we are not yet "fully knowledgeable"?

Even if a quantum theoretic approach were useful, it might not be needed, since there are now available a number of other methods for dealing in a classical, deterministic way with the problem of more than one stable outcome of shared probabilities. These include, for example, variations on the population equation [Kadanoff, 1983]. Should such approaches be workable, we might still have (without complementarity) the possibility of both singularity and duality of mind at different times. But then, as in the case of a continuum between one mind and two, all of the observable states would be interpretable in terms of just two minds and their combinations, including overlap or intersection in varying degree.

CONCLUDING REMARKS

Among neuroscientists there remain some who still find the two-brain view uncongenial. To them we say: Find an experimental situation that is explained by the one-brain view and *not* by the double brain. There are now available data that are inexplicable in terms of the one-brain view; are there also objective data that are incompatible with the two-brain view? If not, considering complementarity may not be necessary, or even reasonable. And we can then look forward to the eventual demise of the doctrine that our two hemispheres make up but one brain.

REFERENCES

Berlucchi G, Buchtel E, Marzi CA, Mascetti GG and Simoni A (1978): Effects of experience on interocular transfer of pattern discriminations in split-chiasm and split-brain cats. J Comp Physiol Psych 92:532–543.

Berlucchi G (1983): Two hemispheres but one brain. Behav Brain Sci 6:171–172.

Bogen JE (1969): The other side of the brain II: An appositional mind. Bull Los Angeles Neurol Soc 34:135–162.

Bogen JE (1977): Further discussion on split-brains and hemispheric capabilities. Br J Philos Sci 28:281–286.

Bogen JE (1981): Mental numerosity: Is one head better than two? Behav and Brain Sci 4:100–101.

Bogen JE (1984): Split-brain syndromes. In Frederiks JAM (ed): "Handbook of Clinical Neurology," Vol 45. (in press).

Bogen JE (1985): Partial hemispheric independence with the neocommissures intact. In Trevarthen C (ed): "Brain Circuits and Functions of the Mind." Cambridge: Cambridge University Press (In press.)

Bogen JE, Bogen GM (1969): The other side of the brain III: The corpus callosum and creativity. Bull Los Angeles Neurol Soc 34:191–220.

Bohm D (1981): "Wholeness and the Implicate Order." London: Routledge and Kegan Paul.

Bohr N (1958): "Atomic Physics and Human Knowledge." New York: John Wiley & Sons.

Bradshaw JL, Nettleton NC (1983): "Human Cerebral Asymmetry." Englewood, New Jersey: Prentice-Hall.

Butler SR (1979): Interhemispheric transmission of visual information via the corpus callosum and anterior commissure in the monkey. In Russell IS, Van Hof MW, Berlucchi G (eds): "Structure and Function of Cerebral Commissures." Baltimore: University Park Press.

Butler CR, Francis AC (1973): Split-brain behavior without splitting. Tactile discriminations in monkeys. Isr J Med Sci 9 (Suppl):79–84.

Chadwick J, Mann WN (1950): "The Medical Works of Hippocrates." Oxford: Blackwell, p 183.

Doty RW (1983): Some thoughts, and some experiments on memory. In Butters N, Squire L (eds): "The Neuropsychology of Memory." New York: Guilford Press.

Doty RW, Lewine JD, Ringo JL (1984): Mnemonic interaction between and within cerebral hemispheres in macaques. In Allen DL, Woody CD (eds): "Neural Mechanisms of Conditioning." New York: Plenum Publishing Corp. (in press).

Einstein A (1924): Quoted by Holton (1973), p 117.

Feynman RP, Leighton RB, Sands M (1963): "The Feynman Lectures on Physics." Reading, Mass: Addison Wesley.

Goodale MA, Graves JA (1980): Failure of interocular transfer of learning in pigeons (columba livia) trained on a jumping stand. Bird Behav 2:13–22.

Goodglass H, Calderon M (1977): Parallel processing of verbal and musical stimuli in right and left hemispheres. Neuropsychology 15:397–407.

Gordon H (1985): The neurological basis of hemisphericity. In Trevarthen C (ed): "Brain Circuits and Theories of Mind." Cambridge: Cambridge University Press.

Hamilton CR (1977): Investigations of perceptual and mnemonic lateralization in monkeys. In Harnad S, Doty RW, Goldstein L, Jaynes J, Krauthamer G (eds): "Lateralization in the Nervous System." New York: Academic Press.

Hamilton CR (1982): Mechanisms of interocular equivalence. In Ingle, DJ, Goodale, MA, Mansfield RJW (eds): "Analyses of Visual Behavior." Cambridge: MIT Press.

Harris LJ (1980): Which hand is the "eye" of the blind?—A new look at an old question. In Herron J (ed): "The Neuropsychology of Left Handedness." New York: Academic Press.

Hicks RE, Frank JM, Kinsbourne M (1982): The locus of bimanual skill transfer. J Gen Psychol 107:277–281.

Holton G (1973): "Thematic Origins of Scientific Thought." Cambridge: Harvard University Press.

Iberall AS (1979): On complementarity—A rebuttal. J Soc Biol Struct 2:173–174.

Jackson JH (1958): On the nature of the duality of the brain. Med Press Circ 1:19,41,63 (1874). Reprinted in Brain Vol 38, 1915. In Taylor J (ed): "Selected Writings of John Hughlings Jackson." New York: Basic Books.

Kadanoff LP (1983): Roads to chaos. Physics Today: December: 46–53.

Landis T, Assal G, Perret E (1979): Opposite cerebral hemispheric superiorities for visual associative processing of emotional facial expressions and objects. Nature 278:739–740.

Landis T, Graves R, Goodglass H (1981): Dissociated awareness of manual performance on two different visual associative tasks: A "split-brain" phenomenon in normal subjects? Cortex 17:435–440.

Mehra J (1973): Quantum mechanics and the explanation of life. Am Sci 61:722–728.

Putterman S (1983): Impossibility of observing coherent macroscopic quantum superposition: A new law of thermodynamics? Physics Letters 98A:324–328.

Rohrlich F (1983): Facing quantum mechanical reality. Science 221:1251–1255.

Russell IS, Morgan SC (1979): Interocular transfer of visual learning in the rat. In Russell IS, Van Hof MW, Berlucchi G (eds): "Structure and Function of Cerebral Commissures." Baltimore: University Park Press.

Semmes J, Mishkin M (1965): A search for the cortical substrate of tactual memories. In Ettlinger G (ed): "Functions of the Corpus Callosum." London: Ciba.

Sherrington C (1947): "The Integrative Action of the Nervous System." Cambridge: Cambridge University Press, p xvii.

Sidtis JJ, Bryden MP (1978): Asymmetrical perceptions of language and music: Evidence for independent processing strategies. Neuropsychology 16:627–632.

Sperry R (1982): Some effects of disconnecting the cerebral hemispheres. Science 217:1223–1226.

Sperry RW, Clark E (1949): Interocular transfer of visual discrimination habits in a teleost fish. Physiol Zool 22:372–378.

Van Hof MW (1979): Interocular transfer and interhemispheric communication in the rabbit. In Russell IS, Van Hof MW, Berlucchi G (eds): "Structure and Function of Cerebral Commissures." Baltimore: University Park Press.

Walter DO (1971a): Alternatives to continuity, observability, and passivity in biological modeling: A tribute to McCulloch. Math Biosci 11:85–94.

Walter DO (1971b): Objectivity revised: Models from 20th-century physical science for use in the human sciences. Int J Neurosci 1:243–249.

Wigan AL (1844): "The Duality of the Mind: A New View of Insanity." London: Longman, Brown, Green and Longmans.

Wigner EP (1967): "Symmetries and Reflections." Cambridge: MIT Press, p 176.

Young RM (1970): "Mind, Brain and Adaptation in the Nineteenth Century." Oxford: Clarendon Press.

Zaidel E (1983): Disconnection syndrome as a model for laterality effects in the normal brain. In: Hellige J (ed): "Cerebral Hemisphere Asymmetry: Method, Theory and Application." New York: Praeger.

SECTION II
ANATOMY

Two Hemispheres—One Brain:
Functions of the Corpus Callosum, pages 37–45
© 1986 Alan R. Liss, Inc.

Notes on the Early History of the Corpus Callosum With an Introduction to the Morphological Papers Published in This Festschrift

M. COLONNIER

Department of Anatomy, Faculty of Medicine, Laval University, Quebec, P.Q., Canada G1K 7P4

Before the pioneering studies of Myers [1955, 1956] and Sperry [1961], in the late 1950s, on the interhemispheric transfer of information through the corpus callosum, there existed widely diverging opinions about the function of that structure. In the 18th century some authors believed that this "callous body" or "hard part" of the brain was the "seat of the soul," i.e., that it was the "center" for rationality or, as we would say today, for higher mental functions. In contrast, in the first half of this century it seemed to have no function at all.

An interesting account of the 18th-century view is given by Thomas Southwell in a book published in 1764, which can be found in Montreal at McGill's Osler Library. It consists of personal transcriptions of papers presented at the "Académie royale des sciences de Paris" in the first half of the 18th century. In a chapter entitled "On the Seat of the Soul," Southwell recounts a report read by Monsieur de la Peyronie in 1741.

At the time, neither Monsieur de la Peyronie, nor Mr. Southwell knew of the existence of neurons and of their axons. They had never, of course, heard of Sperry's experimental work, nor did they have the benefit of his views [Sperry, 1980] on the emergence of mind and of consciousness. And indeed neuroanatomists at the time all seem to have been inveterate dualists, for Southwell says that, "All anatomists are now agreed that the soul is seated in the brain, but are not agreed as the particular part, there being no one part but some writer or other has made it the seat of the soul. The best method to guide us thro' this intricate inquiry seems to be to consider whether, when most parts of the brain happen to be sphacelated or otherwise destroyed, there yet remained one part sound, and that while this part remained sound and untouched, reason subsisted; it is evident that the soul can be seated in this part only that remained sound, and by no means in those parts that had rotted, or were otherwise consumed. . . ." The essay continues by describing a number of clinical cases in which selected parts of the brain having been destroyed, from the cerebral cortex to the midbrain tectum, the patient "retained his senses." It concludes that the soul cannot be seated in any of them. Descartes is especially taken to task for his suggestion of the pineal gland as a likely candidate, for as everyone knows "it is often found petrified," with no effect on rationality. Monsieur de la Peyronie is then reported to have "related several cases ... of his own knowledge, whereby it appears that the corpus callosum cannot be either compressed, sphacelated or otherwise injured, but for both reason and all sensations are abolished, from all of which he concludes that the corpus callosum must necessarily be the immediate seat of the soul." In contrast to this view, by the middle of the present century, McCulloch and Garol [1941] summarized the then current literature by stating that lesions of the corpus callosum or even surgical section of that structure "have failed to produce any characteristic disorders except, possibly, impairment of coordination of the hemispheres in complicated symbolic activity."

Obviously in both cases a useful paradigm and an appropriate methodology is lacking. Until Sperry, useful methods were also lacking for studies on the anatomy of the corpus callosum, for the days before Sperry are also the days before Nauta, whose silver technique for degenerating axons will also be published in the 1950s [Nauta and Gygax, 1954]. Before that time anatomists had to rely largely on gross dissection, on the observation of histological sections stained for Nissl bodies or normal myelin, on the Golgi method, or on the Marchi stain for the selective staining of degenerating myelin.

By the 19th century, neurons and their processes had, of course, been described, and once this concept was established even gross dissection could demonstrate that the fibers of the corpus callosum linked the cortex of the two hemispheres. At the beginning of this century, van Valkenburg [1913] clearly formulated several of the anatomical questions posed by such a cortical commissural system. Does a commissure, he asks (1) ensure connections only between homotopical parts of the cortex or between both homotopical and heterotopical areas? (2) are all homotopical areas interconnected? and (3) from what cortical cells do these callosal fibers arise and to what cortical cells do they project? Several authors (Pandya, Imig, Kass and Cusik, Innocenti) in this book have extensively applied themselves to these questions.

Even before Valkenburg, and before Marchi had published his method for degenerating myelin, some authors had already begun to give tentative answers. Sherrington [1889], after lesions of what he called the "cord area" of the cortex of macaque and dog, described a zone of degenerating axons in the corpus callosum. This zone, he said, "tends to scatter and does not pass chiefly between 'identical' areas of the two hemispheres." Beevor [1891], on normal material stained for myelin, did a study of the posterior part of the corpus callosum in the marmoset monkey. Following the orientation of the small segments of myelinated fibers, meticulously, from section to section, he concludes that though the fibers of the splenium cannot be traced into the gray matter, their direction within the occipital lobe is such that "it apparently does not supply the calcarine cortex." These first studies thus suggest on the one hand that heterotopic connections do exist, and on the other that not all regions are interconnected by the corpus callosum. It is interesting to note that van Valkenburg agrees with Beevor about the lack of callosal fibers between right and left striate areas and he is very impatient with those who would believe otherwise. "I fail to see any ground for assuming a connection by which one half of the visual field, after arrival in the cortex must immediately be placed in connection with the center for the other half . . ."

Ramón y Cajal [1911] speaks very little of the corpus callosum in his many studies on the cerebral cortex. In "Histologie du système nerveux" he states that because of the length of the pathway he is unable to follow the axons from their origin to their termination in large gyrencephalic mammals. On small young lissencephalic hemispheres he did describe connections between corresponding areas, adding that during their trajectory, collaterals were sometimes found going to other areas. He also speaks of two types of callosal axons: those coming "directly" from cortical cells of the other side, and those which are collaterals of association or projection neurons.

Cajal raised another interesting question in regard to the corpus callosum when he considers its possible functional role. Perceptual cortical centers, he says, are present on both sides of the brain, each representing their half of the perceptual field, while memory centers for language are found only on one side of the brain. The memory centers must obviously receive their input from both right and left perceptual centers: consequently those from the opposite side must cross the commissure to reach the memory center. Cajal concludes that the corpus callosum must therefore necessarily exist: "La disposition bilatérale des centres percepteurs et unilatérale des centres de mémoire justifie, à notre avis, l'existence du corps calleux. Elle entraîne, en effet, la *nécessité* [italics added] de deux sortes de fibres d'associations ou, pour le moins, de deux sortes de collatérales: les unes *directes* [Cajal's italics], conduisant la moitié homolatérale de l'image au centre de mémoire, les autres *commissurales* ou *calleuses* [Cajal's italics], qui apportent à ce même centre la partie de l'image projetée sur le centre percepteur de l'autre hémisphère."* Note that he is also implying that there may be a

---

*The existence of the corpus callosum is justified in my view by the fact that the centers for perception are organized bilaterally while that of the centers for memory are organized unilaterally. Indeed this arrangement requires (literally: entails the necessity of) two types of association fibers or at least two types of collaterals: some *direct* for the transmission of the homolateral half of the image to the memory center, the others *commissural* or *callosal* transmitting to this same center the portion of the image projected on the perception center of the other hemisphere.

relationship between brain asymmetry and the size of the corpus callosum. Dr. Sandra Witelson addresses this long-standing question, in her chapter on the size of the corpus callosum [this volume].

It was with the Marchi technique that the first convincing experimental studies were done on the projection of specific cortical areas to the other side of the brain. Polyak [1927], after small selective cortical lesions, concludes that most degenerating commissural fibers go to homotopical areas, while fewer reach heterotopical regions. In 1932 and 1935, using the same technique, Mettler published a number of remarkable papers on the connections of the auditory cortex of cat and of the frontal, parietal, temporal, and occipital regions of *Macaca mulatta* [Mettler, 1932, 1935a–d]. In these papers he formulated his principle of heterolateral cortical association which states that the heterotopical fields correspond to the site of short association fibers ipsilaterally. He concludes that activation of a limited cortical field will result in the activation of outlying areas by the short association fibers, and that "no more steps are necessary in the exciting of a corresponding crossed field, since the initial field of one side sends callosal fibers . . . to an extensive zone corresponding with the ipsilateral short association area."

On the question of whether all areas project equally through the corpus callosum, Sunderland [1939], in a study on the exact localization of fibers from different areas in the corpus callosum, concluded that some regions seemed to give rise to more fibers than others.

In the same year, the question of the cells of origin was also considered by Pines and Maiman [1939]. By means of retrograde degeneration of neuronal cell bodies after destruction of the opposite hemispheres, they reached the surprisingly accurate conclusion that callosal fibers take their origin from cells in layers III and VI.

A series of electrophysiological experiments in the early 1940s confirmed most of these anatomical findings. The authors also concluded that commissural fibers are mainly homotopical [Curtis, 1940], adding that some areas give rise only to homotopical fibers, while others did not project in the callosum at all [McCulloch and Garol, 1941], and emphasizing that the striate area of cat, and that the arm and leg portion of motor area 4 do not give rise to such fibers [Garol, 1942].

And that is how things were at the beginning of the 1940s; and for about 20 years, until the work of Myers and Sperry rekindled interest in the corpus callosum, anatomists seemed to have almost completely lost interest in the structure.

Interestingly, during that hiatus one of the first papers written by Nauta [Nauta and Bucher, 1954] using the technique that was to bear his name [Nauta and Gygax, 1954] was on the efferent connections of area 17 in the rat. He noted that commissural fibers could only be seen leaving a lateral strip of visual cortex, adjoining area 18a, and that the medial portion of 17 did not send fibers through the corpus callosum. He also stated that the commissural fibers extended up into the cortex as high as the second layer.

The renaissance of anatomical papers begins with Myers [1962] and Ebner and Myers [1965]. In the first paper, removal of an occipital lobe in monkey was said to give rise to degenerating commissural fibers in area 18 and in a strip of area 17 immediately adjoining 18, but not in other parts of 17. In 1965, a clean cut through the corpus callosum and the anterior commissure of cat and racoon permitted a complete account of the distribution of these commissural fibers. The authors describe important differences in the density of fibers in different cytoarchitectonic areas, emphasizing again the absence of fibers in 17, plus their absence from the forelimb and distal hindlimb regions of the sensory and motor area, as well as their small number in parts of the auditory area. The strip of area 17 receiving callosal fibers corresponds to the vertical meridian, and this gave rise to the view that the function of the callosum was here to ensure the continuity of large receptive fields across the midline. This seminal work was to be followed by a large number of papers in the late 1960s and early 1970s in which many authors would use the Nauta technique to describe in great detail the commissural connections of specific cortical areas. Two authors of this book were important contributors to the literature of the time. Jones co-authored several papers on the interhemispheric connections of the auditory cortex of cats [Diamond et al., 1968], and on the somatic sensory cortex of cat [Jones and Powell, 1968] and monkey [Jones and Powell, 1969]. It was at this time that Pandya [Pandya and Kuypers, 1969; Pandya and Vignolo, 1968, 1969; Pandya et al., 1969a,b 1971a,b] began his magnum opus on cortico-cortical connections in the macaque monkey, exploring literally the whole cortical surface, describing in great detail ipsilateral intrahemispheric associations as well as interhemispheric commissural connections [see Pandya, 1984].

The early 1970s saw the appearance of many new precise and reliable techniques for the tracing of neuronal pathways by anterograde and retrograde axonal transport. Because of the new techniques, anatomists could ask more refined questions about the connections of the corpus callosum, and the first results using these techniques suggested still more questions that have proven to be increasingly stimulating and meaningful in terms of cortical functions. It was at this time that neurobiologists discovered that many afferent systems terminated in the form of discontinuous patches, columns, or slabs. The first such a description was that of the periodic terminations of geniculocortical afferents to the striate cortex by Hubel and Wiesel [1972]. These were immediately correctly identified as the basis of the previously described functional ocular dominance columns. In 1979 Jones et al. showed that the callosal projections also terminate in the form of columns or slabs. The significance of this patchy distribution, the exact form of the patches, their relation to other afferent inputs and to other anatomical patches, columns, and slabs, and especially their relation to the various functional columns described in different areas have become the questions of the day.

This has been superbly explored by Imig [Imig and Brugge, 1978; Imig et al., 1982, this volume] in the auditory system. While studying the commissural connections in this way, he came to realize that the maps of the patches of callosal terminations were highly individual, as indeed, were, the maps of the functional columns. He concluded that correlations of the anatomical and functional maps would only be really meaningful if the correlation was done in the same individual. This he has done, and the results yield very significant insights into the contribution of the corpus callosum to information processing in the neocortex.

Kaas also has recently combined anatomical and electrophysiological mapping of the somatosensory areas with fascinating results [Gould and Kaas, 1981; Killackey et al., 1983]. He reviews these in his chapter [this volume] and adds new data on the visual system in which the whole question of the callosal input to area 17 is reopened, forcing us to take a new look at the significance of this projection.

Innocenti, at the Institute of Anatomy in Lausanne, has also been applying modern anatomical techniques to the study of the postnatal development of callosal connections in the visual and somatosensory cortices. He has found that the final selective interconnections of the corpus callosum are largely determined postnatally [Innocenti, 1978, 1981; Innocenti and Clarke, 1983; Koppel and Innocenti, 1983] and, with Frost, that the connections are plastic and can be set differently by different environmental factors [Innocenti and Frost, 1979]. The interindividual differences between callosal maps might thus in part be related to early environmental experiences. In this book he adds new, exciting data on exuberant cortical connections in the cat [Innocenti, 1984].

Witelson has also been interested in interindividual differences and especially in the correlation of individual lateralization of function to brain asymmetries in humans. She has been able to test a large number of terminally ill men and women for lateralization of function and to obtain their brains at autopsy. As a first report on the correlation between behavioral lateralization and brain morphology, her chapter [this volume] gives new data on variations of the size of the corpus callosum in a number of subjects.

The following anatomical papers thus represent important recent contributions to the continuing story of the corpus callosum. They open new ways of thinking about the function of that structure and about the manner by which it acquires its final adult configuration.

REFERENCES

Beevor CE (1891): On the course of the fibres of the cingulum and the posterior parts of the corpus callosum and fornix in marmoset monkey. Philos Trans Roy Soc Lond 182:135–199.

Curtis HJ (1940): Intercortical connections of corpus callosum as indicated by evoked potentials. J Neurophysiol 3:407–413.

Diamond IT, Jones EG, Powell TPS (1968): Interhemispheric fiber connections of the auditory cortex of the cat. Brain Res 11:177–193.

Ebner FF, Myers RE (1965): Distribution of corpus callosum and anterior commissure in cat and racoon. J Comp Neurol 124:353–366.

Garol HW (1942): Cortical origin and distribution of corpus callosum and anterior commissure in cat. J Neuropathol Exp Neurol 1:422–429.

Gould HJ, Kaas JH (1981): The distribution of commissural terminations in somatosensory areas I and II of the grey squirrel. J Comp Neurol 196:489–504.

Hubel DH, Wiesel TN (1972): Laminar and columnar distribution of geniculocortical fibers in the macaque monkey. J Comp Neurol 146:421–450.

Imig TJ, Brugge JF (1978): Source and terminations of callosal axons related to binaural and frequency maps in primary auditory cortex of the cat. J Comp Neurol 182:637–660.

Imig TJ, Morel A, Kauer CD (1982): Covariation of distribution of callosal cell bodies and callosal axon terminals in layer III of cat primary auditory cortex. Brain Res 251:157–159.

Innocenti GM (1978): Postnatal development of interhemispheric connections of the cat visual cortex. Arch Ital Biol 116:463–470.

Innocenti GM (1981): Growth and reshaping of axons in the establishment of visual callosal connections. Science 212:824–827.

Innocenti GM, Frost DO (1979): Effects of visual experience on the maturation of the efferent system to the corpus callosum. Nature 200:231–234.

Innocenti GM, Clarke S (1983): Multiple sets of visual cortical neurons projecting transitorily through the corpus callosum. Neurosci Lett 41:27–32.

Jones EG, Powell TPS (1968): The commissural connections of the somatic sensory cortex in the cat. J Anat 103:433–455.

Jones EG, Powell TPS (1969): Connections of the somatic sensory cortex of the rhesus monkey. II: Contralateral connections. Brain 92:717–730.

Jones EG, Burton H, Porter R (1979): Commissural and corticocortical "columns" on the sensory-motor cortex of monkeys. J Comp Neurol 188:133–136.

Killackey HP, Gould HJ III, Cusik CG, Pons TP, Kaas JH (1983): The relation of corpus callosum connections to architectonic fields and body surface maps in sensorimotor cortex of new and old world monkeys. J Comp Neurol 219:384–419.

Koppel H, Innocenti GM (1983): Is there a genuine exuberancy of callosal projections in development? A quantitative electron microscopic study in the cat. Neurosci Lett 41:33–40.

McCulloch WS, Garol HW (1941): Cortical origin and distribution of corpus callosum and anterior commissure in the monkey (Macaca mulatta). J. Neurophysiol 4:555–563.

Mettler FA (1932): Connections of auditory cortex of the cat. J Comp Neurol 55:139–183.

Mettler FA (1935a): Cortifugal fiber connections of the cortex of the *Macaca mulatta*. The occipital region. J Comp Neurol 61:221–256.

Mettler FA (1935b): Cortifugal fiber connections of the cortex of the *Macaca mulatta*. The frontal region. J Comp Neurol 61:509–542.

Mettler FA (1935c): Cortifugal fiber connections of the cortex of the *Macaca mulatta*. The parietal region. J Comp Neurol 62:263–291.

Mettler FA (1935d): Cortifugal fiber connections of the cortex of the Macaca mulatta. The temporal region. J Comp Neurol 63:25–47.

Myers RE (1955): Interocular transfer of pattern discrimination in cats following section of crossed optic fibers. J Comp, Physiol Psychol 48:470–473.

Myers RE (1956): Function of corpus callosum in interocular transfer. Brain 79:358–363.

Myers RE (1962): Commissural connections between occipital lobes of the monkeys. J Comp Neurol 118:1–16.

Nauta WJH, Gygax PA (1954): Silver impregnation of degenerating axons in the central nervous system: A modified technique. Stain Technol 29:91–93.

Nauta WJH, Bucher VM (1954): Efferent connections of the striate cortex in the albino rat. J Comp Neurol 100:257–286.

Pandya DN, Vignolo LA (1968): Interhemispheric neocortical projections of somatosensory area I and II in the rhesus monkey. Brain Res 7:300–303.

Pandya DN, Vignolo LA (1969): Interhemispheric projections of the parietal lobe in the rhesus monkey. Brain Res 15:49–65.

Pandya DN, Kuypers HGJM (1969): Cortico-cortical connections in the rhesus monkey. Brain Res 13:13–36.

Pandya DN, Gold D, Berger T (1969): Interhemispheric connections of the precentral motor cortex in the rhesus monkey. Brain Res 15:594–596.

Pandya DN, Hallett M, Mukherjee SK (1969): Intra- and interhemispheric connections of the neocortical auditory system in the rhesus monkey. Brain Res 14:49–65.

Pandya DN, Dye P, Butters N (1971): Efferent cortico-cortical projections of the prefrontal cortex in the rhesus monkey. Brain Res 31:35–46.

Pandya DN, Karol EA, Heilbronn D (1971): The topographical distribution of interhemispheric projections in the corpus callosum of the rhesus monkey. Brain Res 32:31–43.

Pines LJ, Maiman RM (1939): Cells of origin of the corpus callosum. Arch Neurol Psychiatr (Chic) 42:1076–1081.

Polyak S (1927): An experimental study of the associational, callosal, and projection fibers of the cerebral cortex of the cat. J Comp Neurol 44:197–258.

Ramón y Cajal S (1911): Histologie du système nerveux de l'homme et des vertébrés. Vol 2. "Consejo Superior de Investigaciones Cientificas." (Madrid 1954: Instituto Ramón y Cajal).

Sherrington MA (1889): On nerve-tracts degenerating secondarily to lesions of the cortex cerebri. J Physiol 10:429–432.

Southwell T (1764): On the seat of the soul. In: "Medical Essays and Observations, Abridged from the Memoirs of the Royal Academy. Vol 3." London: J. Knox, pp 86–99.

Sperry RW (1961): Cerebral organization and behavior. Science 133:1749–1757.

Sperry RW (1980): Mind-brain interaction: Mentalism, yes; dualism, no. Neuroscience 5:195–206.

Sunderland S (1939): The distribution of commissural fibres in the corpus callosum in the macaque monkey. J Neurol Psychiatr 3:9–18.

van Valkenburg CT (1913): Experimental and pathologicoanatomical researches on the corpus striatum. Brain 36:119–165.

Two Hemispheres—One Brain:
Functions of the Corpus Callosum, pages 47–73
© 1986 Alan R. Liss, Inc.

The Topography of Commissural Fibers

DEEPAK N. PANDYA AND BENJAMIN SELTZER

*Edith Nourse Rogers Memorial Veterans Hospital, Bedford, Massachusetts
01730 and Departments of Neurology (D.N.P., B.S.) and Anatomy (D.N.P.),
Boston University School of Medicine, Boston, Massachusetts 02118*

INTRODUCTION

The forebrain commissures represent the axons of cortical neurons that cross from one hemisphere to the other. Commissural fibers constitute one of the major sets of extrinsic connections of the cerebral cortex. As stressed by Roger Sperry, whom we honor today, interhemispheric connections are crucial to many forms of complex behavior [Sperry, 1961; Myers, 1965; Geschwind, 1965, 1967; Gazzaniga, 1970; Russell et al., 1979].

The cerebral cortex is heterogeneous with respect to the density of commissural connections. That is to say, some regions of the hemisphere have numerous contralateral connections, while others have virtually none [Ebner and Myers, 1962; Myers, 1965; Jones and Powell, 1969; Karol and Pandya, 1971; Van Essen et al., 1982]. There are also interspecies differences, as well as differences between neonates and adults, in density of interhemispheric fibers [Innocenti, 1980]. As a general rule, the higher the species on the phylogenetic scale, or the more mature the organism, the more restricted are the commissural connections. In the adult rhesus monkey, for example, some cortical areas, such as certain sectors of the pre- and postcentral gyri, the inferior parietal lobule, and the caudal superior temporal gyrus, have extensive interhemispheric connections, while other areas have few, if any. These latter areas include portions of the pre- and postcentral gyri, certain regions of the prelunate gyrus, and the primary visual cortex (Fig. 1). Those areas of sensorimotor cortex that contain the somatic sensory or motor representation of axial, or midline, parts of the body tend to have the most numerous commissural connections, while those that deal with sensory and motor functions of extreme distal parts of the extremities appear to have relatively few [Jones and Powell, 1969; Karol and Pandya, 1971; Killackey et al., 1983]. Higher-order association areas, in the frontal lobe and at the parieto-temporo-occipital junction, have variable densities of contralateral connections.

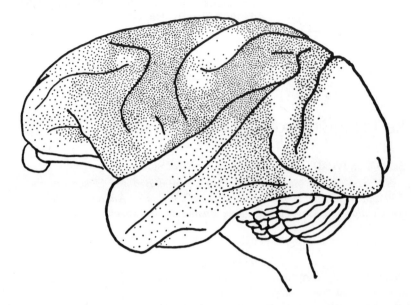

Fig. 1.   Diagram of the lateral surface of the cerebral hemisphere of *Macaca mulatta* to show the distribution (dots) of commissural projections [Myers, 1965].

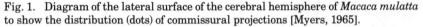

Contralateral projections are directed to both homotopic and heterotopic sites in the opposite hemisphere. All cortical areas that have contralateral connections send fibers to homotopic zones. Projections to heterotopic zones are more variable. For example, the contralateral projections of primary auditory cortex in the rhesus monkey are mainly with the opposite primary auditory cortex. The primary somatic sensory (SI) cortex, on the other hand, projects not only to the contralateral SI but to the nearby second (SII) and supplementary (SSA) sensory areas as well (Fig. 2A) [Pandya and Vignolo, 1969]. Similarly, the inferior parietal lobule projects not only to the contralateral inferior parietal lobule, but also to the opposite superior temporal sulcus, cingulate gyrus, and parahippocampal area (Figs. 2B,3) [Hedreen and Yin, 1981]. Since these latter areas also receive ipsilateral projections from the inferior parietal lobule [Pandya and Kuypers, 1969; Jones and Powell, 1970; Seltzer and Pandya, 1976, 1978, 1984], it is apparent that contralateral connections parallel ipsilateral cortical connections [Hedreen and Yin, 1981]. The contralateral connections, however, are less dense than ipsilateral ones. Furthermore, certain ipsilateral projections, e.g., from the inferior parietal lobule to the frontal lobe, do not have contralateral counterparts (Fig. 3). As a rule, termination zones in the opposite hemisphere are more restricted than those in the ipsilateral hemisphere.

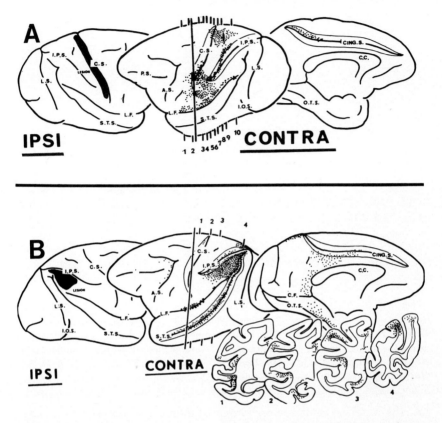

Fig. 2. Diagrams of the lateral and medial surfaces of the cerebral hemisphere to show the homotopic and nonhomotopic callosal projections of the postcentral gyrus (A) and the inferior parietal lobule (B) [Pandya and Vignolo, 1969].

Commissural fibers originating in isocortex have their cells of origin principally in layer III and terminate, in columnar fashion, in and around layer IV of the contralateral target zone [Jacobson and Trojanowski, 1974; Jones et al., 1975, 1979; Jouandet and Gazzaniga, 1979; Hedreen and Yin, 1981]. Fibers coming from the "proisocortex" and "periallocortex," which are cytologically simpler than the isocortex, originate in cells scattered through both supra- and infragranular cortical layers. These latter fibers terminate in the first layer of the opposite hemisphere [Amaral et al., 1984; Demeter et al., 1985]. Whatever their source, or eventual destination, commissural fibers are clearly identified with the autoradiographic technique as a distinct bundle, separate from ipsilateral cortico-cortical and subcortical fibers (Fig. 4), and cross the midline in one of the forebrain commissures,

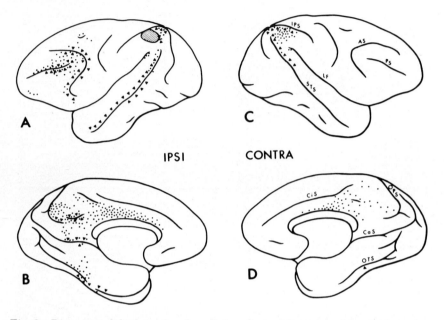

Fig. 3. Diagrams of the lateral and medial surfaces of the cerebral hemispheres to show the sites of commissural neurons (triangles) projecting to the opposite inferior parietal lobule (C) as well as the sites of callosal projections (dots) of the inferior parietal lobule (D) [Hedreen and Yin, 1981]. Ipsilateral connections of the inferior parietal lobule are shown in panels A and B.

viz., the anterior commissure, corpus callosum, and dorsal and ventral hippocampal commissures.

One important morphological issue regards the topography of commissural fibers. What route is taken by the interhemispheric fibers coming from different anatomical and functional regions of the hemisphere? By way of which commissure do they cross the midline? What are the relationships among commissural fibers originating in different cortical areas? Is there a strict topography of fibers with respect to their site of origin or do fibers from different regions travel together as they cross from one hemisphere to the other?

These questions have practical significance. Lesions of the forebrain commissures in humans are seldom complete. One must know which particular interhemispheric connections have been interrupted in order to understand the nature of the deficits they produce. Furthermore, if the precise topography of these fibers were known, it might be possible to perform selective transections to control epilepsy in cases where the epileptogenic focus is located to a particular cortical region. It would also be possible to

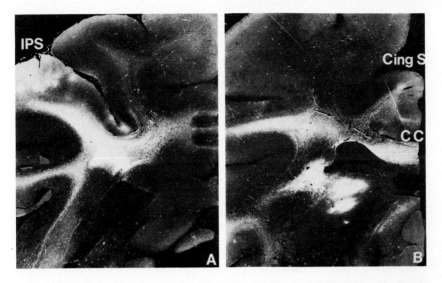

Fig. 4. Photomicrographs to show the course of different fiber bundles following an isotope injection of the inferior parietal lobule. The course of callosal fibers is shown by arrows.

produce discrete, dissociable, behavioral syndromes in experimental species by selective sections of the commissures.

Previous studies of the topography of commissural fibers were based either on an analysis of the distribution of terminal degeneration in the cerebral cortex following partial sections of the commissures or by analyzing the distribution of degenerated fibers in the commissures following selective cortical ablations [Sunderland, 1940; Luttenberg and Marsala, 1963; Zeki, 1970; Pandya et al., 1971, 1973]. Although these studies provided preliminary information on the topography of commissural fibers, the development of the autoradiographic method [Cowan et al., 1972] in recent years now allows for a more precise delineation of the course of these fibers. Using this technique, a number of studies have traced the topography of commissural fibers.

The basic strategy of these studies has been to inject radiolabeled amino acids into various discrete sectors of the cerebral cortex. Next, following an appropriate survival time, the animal is sacrificed, and autoradiograms of coronal sections of the hemisphere are prepared. Under darkfield light microscopy, the course of labeled fiber bundles is traced from the injection site, through the subcortical white matter, into one or more of the forebrain commissures. The position of labeled fibers in the mid-sagittal plane is then reconstructed onto a tracing of a photograph of the medial surface of the hemisphere (Fig. 6 illustrates the location of the forebrain commissures and the divisions of the corpus callosum in the mid-sagittal plane). In this review, we will present a summary of the observations derived from a large number of different experiments. For details of individual studies, the reader is referred to the literature: [Pandya et al., 1971; Seltzer and Pandya, 1983; Amaral et al., 1984; Barbas and Pandya, 1984; Cipolloni and Pandya, 1985; Demeter et al., 1985; Rockland and Pandya, in preparation].

It should be noted at the outset that the information to be presented bears directly only on the *efferent* contralateral connections of a given region. Nevertheless, for reasons described in the discussion, we assume that the *afferent* contralateral connections of the cortical region traverse essentially the same route as the efferent connections. Finally, the nature of this material does not allow any conclusions as to whether there is any significant asymmetry of commissural connections. That is to say, whether there is any topographical or numerical difference between right-to-left and left-to-right commissural fiber systems.

FRONTAL LOBE

For the purpose of this presentation, we will consider separately the commissural connections of the prefrontal, premotor, and precentral cortex. The prefrontal region will be further subdivided into medial, ventral (orbital), and lateral sectors. The lateral sector includes area 46 and the region within the concavity of the arcuate sulcus, area 8. "Premotor cortex" will be defined as that portion of the frontal lobe that lies caudal to the arcuate sulcus, but rostral to the precentral gyrus, and extends onto the medial surface of the hemisphere. The dorsomedial portion of the premotor cortex contains the supplementary motor area (MII).

As shown in Figure 5, the medial prefrontal cortex, below the rostral tip of the cingulate sulcus (areas 25 and 32), sends interhemispheric fibers through the ventral part of the genu of the corpus callosum [Barbas and Pandya, 1984]. The caudal orbitofrontal cortex (areas 13 and 14) also sends fibers through the ventral part of the genu, as well as through the rostrum, of the corpus callosum. The orbitofrontal cortex, however, gives rise to some additional fibers that cross to the other hemisphere by way of the anterior commissure. Turning to the lateral surface of the prefrontal region, the dorsal portion of area 46 also projects to the contralateral hemisphere by way of the genu of the corpus callosum. At the mid-sagittal level, however, these fibers are situated slightly dorsal to those originating in medial and ventral prefrontal sectors. Fibers from the cortex *ventral* to the principal sulcus (ventral area 46 and area 12) occupy the same region of the corpus callosum. The cortex of the arcuate concavity (dorsal and ventral area 8), by contrast, projects through the corpus callosum in a slightly more caudal location, at the border of the genu and the body. In summary, prefrontal commissural fibers traverse the genu and rostrum of the corpus callosum (Fig. 6).

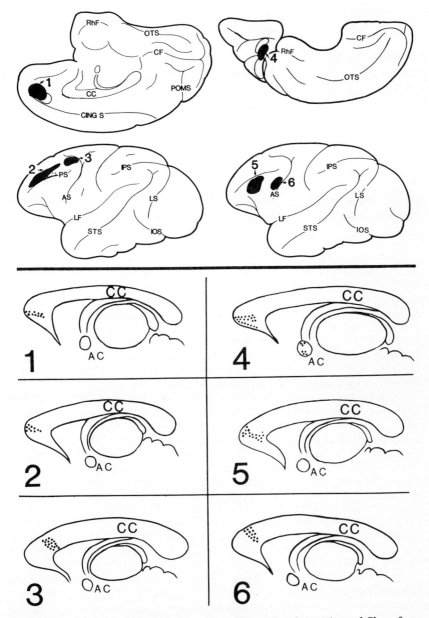

Fig. 5. Diagrammatic representation of the topography of commissural fibers from different parts of the prefrontal cortex. The lower part of the figure depicts midline views of the corpus callosum with the distribution of commissural fibers shown by dots.

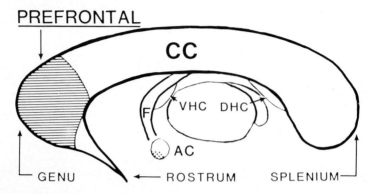

Fig. 6. Mid-sagittal diagram of the corpus callosum, as well as other cerebral commissures, to show the subdivisions of the corpus callosum and the location of prefrontal commissural fibers.

With regard to the premotor region, the dorsolateral surface caudal to the arcuate sulcus (area 6) sends fibers through the rostralmost sector of the body of the corpus callosum, immediately caudal to fibers from prefrontal cortex (Fig. 7). These premotor fibers portray a dorsal/ventral topography according to whether they originate in dorsal or ventral sectors of the lateral premotor region. Axons from the *medial* surface of the premotor region, including the supplementary motor area (MII), cross the midline in the same general location. The lower part of Figure 7 shows the relative positions of prefrontal, premotor, and supplementary motor callosal fibers. The location of precentral fibers is discussed below.

Thus there is a definite rostral-to-caudal topography in the distribution of frontal callosal fibers. Prefrontal fibers are situated rostral to premotor fibers. Furthermore, within the category of prefrontal fibers, those emanating from the medial and ventral surfaces are most rostral; those originating in the region of the arcuate concavity most caudal. Interhemispheric fibers from the region around the principal sulcus occupy an intermediate position. Fibers are also segregated in the dorsal/ventral dimension. For example, those coming from the dorsal portion of area 46 are dorsal to those originating in the ventral portion. Note, however, that there is also overlap of callosal fibers, particularly between those coming from the ventral and medial surfaces of the prefrontal region, between the dorsal and ventral sectors of the principal sulcus region, and between the dorsolateral and medial premotor regions. Finally, although the majority of frontal fibers cross the midline in the corpus callosum, some orbitofrontal axons also traverse the anterior commissure.

POSTERIOR PARIETAL LOBE

Commissural fibers of the posterior parietal lobe are restricted to the corpus callosum. As in the frontal lobe, there is a general segregation of

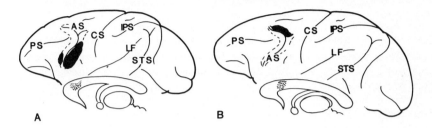

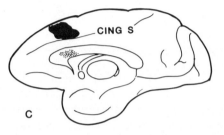

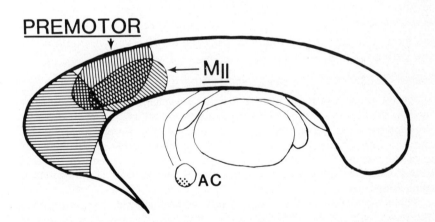

Fig. 7. The upper diagram illustrates the topography of callosal fibers from premotor (A,B) and supplementary motor (MII) (C) regions. The lower diagram shows the relative positions of prefrontal, premotor, and supplementary motor (MII) callosal fibers in the mid-sagittal plane.

fibers with respect to their place of origin in the cerebral cortex, although overlap of fibers from different posterior parietal regions does occur [Seltzer and Pandya, 1983]. As shown in Figure 8, both the superior and inferior parietal lobules send interhemispheric fibers through the caudal part of the body of the corpus callosum. Superior parietal lobule fibers, however, are concentrated dorsally, while those from the inferior parietal lobule are located ventrally. Furthermore, fibers derived from rostral sectors of both the superior and inferior parietal lobules cross the midline slightly rostral to those originating in caudal sectors. The callosal fibers of the medial surface of the parietal lobe, however, spread from the dorsal border of the corpus callosum ventrally into the central presplenial area, where they overlap, to some extent, the callosal trajectory of fibers from the caudal inferior parietal lobule (Fig. 8, mid-sagittal sections 3 and 6). The possible significance of this phenomenon is described below.

SENSORIMOTOR CORTEX

Since we do not have autoradiographic material prepared specifically for somatic sensory and motor areas, we must rely on previous ablation/degeneration studies [Pandya et al., 1971] in order to outline the topography of their commissural fibers. Those studies showed that fibers from both primary motor (MI) and primary (SI) and second (SII) somatic sensory areas cross the midline in the central sector of the body of the corpus callosum. Motor fibers are rostral; somatic sensory fibers are caudal. Figure 9 shows the location of sensorimotor callosal fibers in relation to frontal and posterior parietal commissural axons.

TEMPORAL LOBE

For the present purpose we will divide the temporal lobe into two major sectors: the superior temporal region (comprising the supratemporal plane, superior temporal gyrus, and upper bank of the superior temporal sulcus); and the inferotemporal area (including the lower bank of the superior temporal sulcus). As will be seen, a further distinction between rostral and caudal temporal areas also has relevance to the pattern of commissural connections.

The dorsal portion of the temporal pole, rostral superior temporal gyrus, and upper bank of the adjacent superior temporal sulcus, as far caudal as the rostral tip of the central sulcus, send fibers to the opposite hemisphere by way of the anterior commissure (Fig. 10). They do not project through the corpus callosum [Whitlock and Nauta, 1956; Jouandet and Gazzaniga, 1979; Cipolloni and Pandya, 1985]. By contrast, interhemispheric fibers from primary and second auditory (AI and AII) cortexes, which, in the rhesus monkey, are located in the supratemporal plane, form a compact bundle situated, at the mid-sagittal level, in the caudal portion of the body of the corpus callosum (Fig. 10, mid-sagittal section 8). Commissural fibers

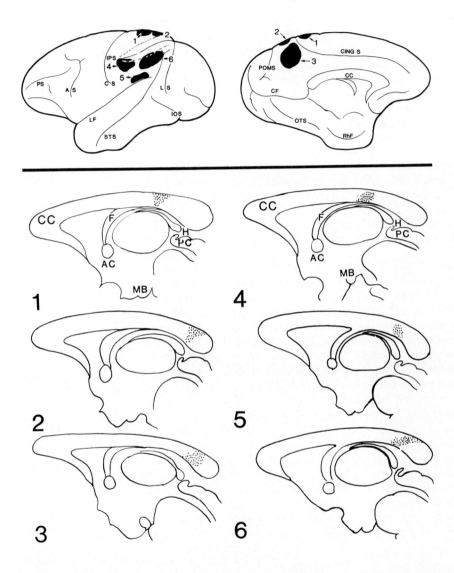

Fig. 8. Diagrammatic representation of the topography of callosal fibers from different parts of posterior parietal cortex.

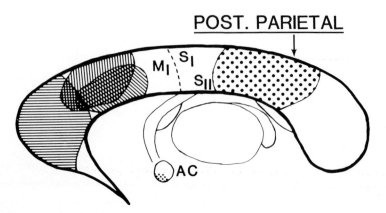

Fig. 9. Summary diagram to show the locations of commissural fibers of posterior parietal cortex, the precentral (MI), and postcentral (SI and SII) gyri, as well as prefrontal and premotor regions.

from the *caudal* superior temporal gyrus and adjacent upper bank of the superior temporal sulcus are also restricted to the caudal part of the body. The mid-portion of the superior temporal gyrus and adjoining superior temporal sulcus, however, has a dual pattern of interhemispheric connections, viz., both the anterior commissure and the caudal part of the body of the corpus callosum (Fig. 10, mid-sagittal section 5). The general location of superior temporal and auditory fibers in relation to those commissural fibers previously discussed is shown in Figure 11.

The commissural connections of the inferotemporal area parallel those of the superior temporal region. The ventral temporal pole, rostral inferotemporal area, and rostral segment of the lower bank of the superior temporal sulcus transmit fibers by way of the anterior commissure alone [Pandya et al., 1973; Zeki, 1973; Demeter et al., 1985]. More caudal areas send interhemispheric fibers that traverse the caudal corpus callosum, specifically, the area immediately rostral to the splenium (Fig. 12). The lower portion of Figure 12 illustrates the overall location of inferotemporal commissural fibers.

OCCIPITAL LOBE

Interoccipital fibers connecting both the juxta- and peristriate cortexes (areas 18 and 19) of the two hemispheres traverse the splenium of the corpus callosum. In the rhesus monkey, the primary visual cortex (area 17) does not have commissural connections.

Area 18 sends interhemispheric fibers through the ventral sector of the caudalmost portion of the splenium, as shown in Figure 13 [Rockland and Pandya, in preparation]. Within this sector there is some evidence for

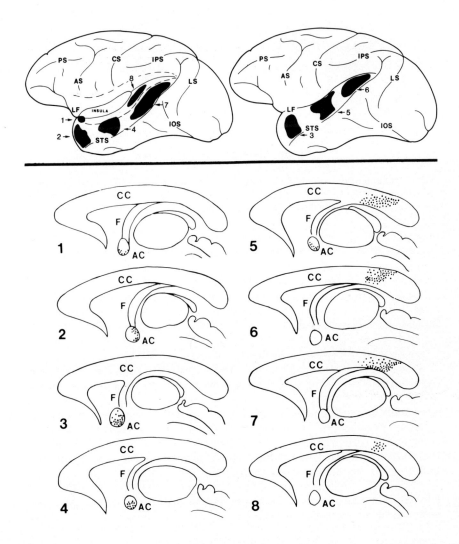

Fig. 10. Diagrammatic representation of the topography of commissural fibers from different parts of the superior temporal region.

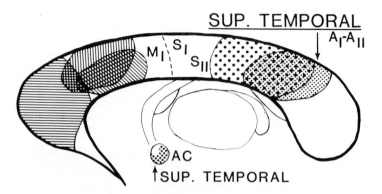

Fig. 11. Summary diagram to show the locations of commissural fibers from different subdivisions of the superior temporal region in addition to those from prefrontal, premotor, MI, SI, SII, and posterior parietal regions.

topographical segregation of fibers coming from different sectors, e.g., dorsal vs. ventral, of area 18, but there is also overlap of these fibers as well. Commissural fibers emanating from area 19 are situated dorsal and rostral to those coming from area 18, but also in the splenium of the corpus callosum. As in area 18, callosal fibers originating in different subsectors of area 19 also intermingle at the mid-sagittal level. The relative positions of interoccipital fibers are shown in Figure 14.

CINGULATE GYRUS AND INSULA

These cortical areas both send commissural fibers through the corpus callosum alone. The rostral cingulate gyrus (area 24) projects through the anterior half of the body of the corpus callosum; the caudal cingulate gyrus (area 23) through the posterior half, as far caudal as the junction with the splenium (Fig. 15). In both instances fibers are concentrated in the dorsal sector of the corpus callosum. A similar rostral/caudal dichotomy exists for the contralateral pathways of the rostral and caudal insular cortex (Mufson and Pandya, unpublished observations). These fibers, however, are restricted to the ventral sector of the corpus callosum (Fig. 16). The lower portion of Figure 16 shows the trajectories of rostral and caudal cingulate and insular commissural fibers.

VENTRAL TEMPORAL LOBE

The ventral temporal lobe consists of the parahippocampal gyrus, entorhinal cortex, presubiculum, and hippocampus. Data on the commissural connections of these regions come from the studies of Demeter et al. [1985] and Amaral et al. [1984]. As shown by these investigators, the routes taken by interhemispheric fibers of the parahippocampal gyrus are complex. The

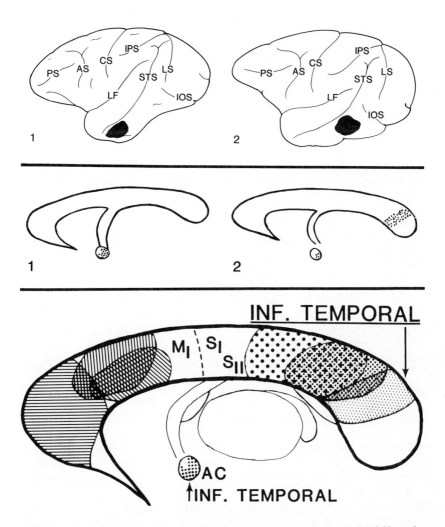

Fig. 12.   Diagrammatic representation of the topography of commissural fibers from different subregions of inferotemporal cortex. The lower part of the figure is a summary diagram to show the locations of the commissural fibers from the inferotemporal cortex in addition to those from prefrontal, premotor, MI, SI, SII, posterior parietal, and superior temporal regions.

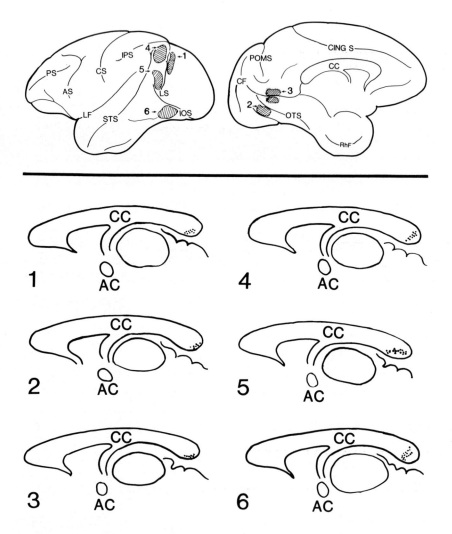

Fig. 13. Diagrammatic representation of the topography of commissural fibers from different parts of the occipital lobe.

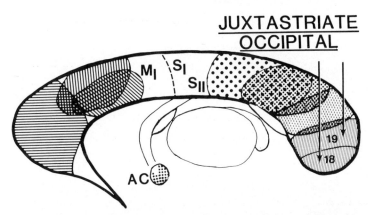

Fig. 14. Summary diagram to show the locations of commissural fibers from different subdivisions of the occipital lobe in addition to those from prefrontal, premotor, MI, SI, SII, posterior parietal, superior temporal, and inferotemporal areas.

caudal part of the parahippocampal gyrus sends fibers through the splenium of the corpus callosum (Fig. 17, mid-sagittal section 3). The *lateral* parahippocampal gyrus (area TF) projects predominantly through the anterior commissure (mid-sagittal sections 1 and 2). The *medial* portion of the parahippocampal gyrus (area TH), by contrast, sends most of its interhemispheric fibers via the dorsal hippocampal commissure (DHC), with a small additional contingent through the anterior commissure (mid-sagittal section 4). The commissural fiber trajectories of the parahippocampal gyrus are presented schematically in the lower portion of Figure 17.

Unlike parahippocampal fibers, interhemispheric axons of the entorhinal cortex and presubiculum pass entirely through the dorsal hippocampal commissure (DHC) as shown in Figure 18. Although the amygdala and most of the hippocampus proper do not have commissural connections, the rostral uncal portion of the hippocampus does send fibers across the midline in the ventral hippocampal commissure (Fig. 18). These results are summarized in the lower part of Figure 18.

DISCUSSION

Interhemispheric fibers originating in different regions of the cerebral cortex consistently cross the midline in specific locations. Most of these fibers are found in the *corpus callosum.* Medial and ventral prefrontal fibers traverse the rostrum and the ventral genu of the corpus callosum; lateral prefrontal fibers, the dorsal portion of the genu. Premotor fibers, including those of the supplementary motor region, traverse the rostralmost portion of the body of the corpus callosum. The midportion of the body is occupied by fibers interconnecting sensorimotor areas of the two hemispheres. Cau-

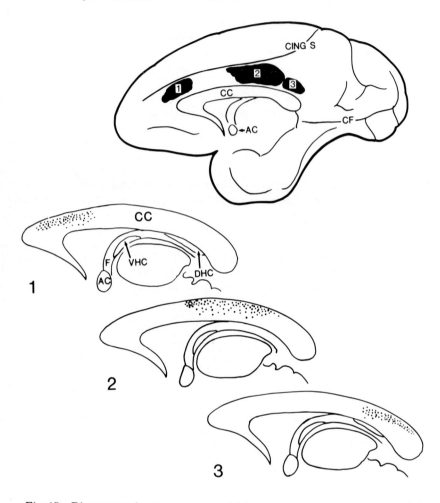

Fig. 15. Diagrammatic representation of the topography of commissural fibers from different sectors of the cingulate gyrus.

dal to sensorimotor fibers, in the posterior part of the body of the corpus callosum, are fibers originating in posterior parietal cortex and the mid- and caudal superior temporal region. Fibers from the caudal inferotemporal area, as well as from the caudal parahippocampal gyrus, are located at the junction of the body and the splenium, while those interconnecting the occipital lobes (areas 18 and 19) are restricted to the splenium. Fibers from the cingulate gyrus and the insula traverse the body of the corpus callosum; cingulate fibers are located dorsally, insular fibers ventrally. The *anterior*

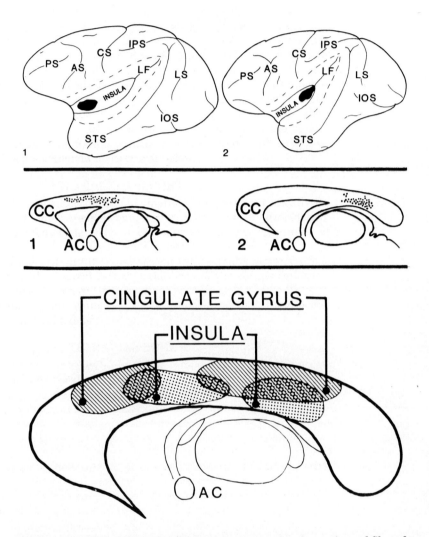

Fig. 16.   Diagrammatic representation of the topography of commissural fibers from subdivisions of insular cortex. The lower diagram is a summary illustration to show the location of commissural fibers from the cingulate gyrus and insula.

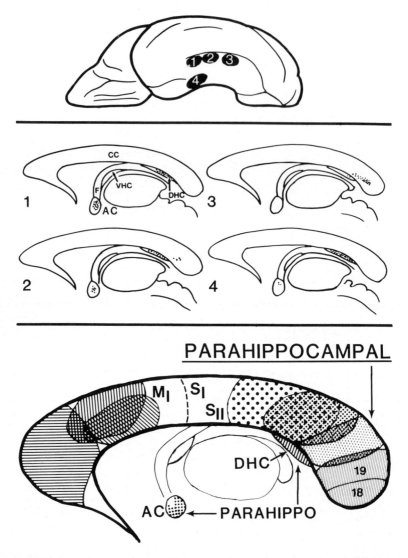

Fig. 17. Diagrammatic representation of the topography of commissural fibers from different sectors of the parahippocampal gyrus. The lower diagram summarizes the location of parahippocampal commissural fibers in addition to those from prefrontal, premotor, MI, SI, SII, posterior parietal, superior temporal, inferotemporal, and occipital cortexes.

commissure transmits fibers from the orbital surface of the frontal lobe, the rostralmost superior and inferior temporal gyri, and lateral and rostral sectors of the parahippocampal gyrus. The *dorsal hippocampal commissure* contains interhemispheric fibers of entorhinal cortex, the presubiculum, and the medial sector of the parahippocampal gyrus, while the *ventral hippocampal commissure* conveys fibers from the rostral portion of one hippocampus to the other (Figs. 16,18).

In the rhesus monkey, a relationship appears to exist between the cytoarchitectonic features of a given cortical area and the commissure by which it sends its interhemispheric axons. The allocortex of the hippocampus transmits fibers through the ventral hippocampal commissure. Fibers from periallocortical structures, viz., the entorhinal cortex and presubiculum, traverse the dorsal hippocampal commissure. The anterior commissure contains fibers from periallocortical and proisocortical, e.g., temporal pole and caudal orbitofrontal cortex, as well as some isocortical areas while the corpus callosum transmits fibers exclusively from isocortex.

In general, commissural fibers from a given cortical region tend to occupy a distinct location in one of the forebrain commissures. This is particularly true for the interhemispheric fibers of primary motor and somatic sensory cortexes as well as the occipital lobe. They do not overlap the trajectories of other fiber systems. On the other hand, fibers from certain cortical areas tend to intermingle with fibers coming from other regions.

Several factors may contribute to this overlap. One relates to the architectonic features of the regions of origin. Based on a comparative study of cerebral architectonics, Sanides [1969] has divided the cerebral cortex into several different subtypes, each representing a different stage in evolutionary development. An analysis of the present data reveals that, in many instances, overlap of callosal trajectories occurs between areas that have similar architectonic features and are at the same stage of development even though they may not be geographically contiguous. Thus, fibers from medial prefrontal cortex and the orbitofrontal region, which are architectonically similar, have overlapping trajectories in the genu of the corpus callosum [Barbas and Pandya, 1982, 1984]. Similarly, the caudal inferior parietal lobule and the cortex on the medial surface of the parietal lobe, although geographically separate from each other, are architectonically at a similar stage, and their fibers overlap each other in the caudal portion of the body of the corpus callosum [Pandya and Seltzer, 1982; Seltzer and Pandya, 1983].

Another factor to explain overlap is the connectional pattern of the cerebral cortex. Overlap of callosal trajectories tends to occur between those cortical areas that have contralateral interconnections. Thus, not only are the caudal inferior parietal lobule and the medial parietal lobe architectonically similar, as mentioned above, but they are also reciprocally interconnected contralaterally [Pandya and Vignolo, 1969; Hedreen and Yin, 1981].

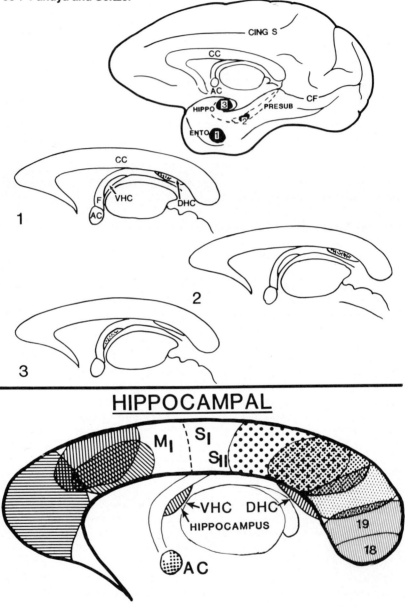

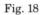

Fig. 18

The overlap of their callosal trajectories may therefore reflect their inter-hemispheric connections. Moreover, inferior parietal lobule and medial pa-rietal fibers not only overlap each other, but also overlap fibers from the caudal superior temporal gyrus. This latter region has contralateral connec-tions with the posterior parietal lobe [Pandya and Vignolo, 1969; Hedreen and Yin, 1981]. Posterior parietal fibers do not, however, overlap frontal fibers in the corpus callosum. This may be because the posterior parietal lobe and frontal cortex, although ipsilaterally connected [Chavis and Pan-dya, 1976; Petrides and Pandya, 1984], do not have contralateral connec-tions [Pandya and Vignolo, 1969; Hedreen and Yin, 1981].

Cingulate gyrus and insular fibers overlap a number of different frontal, temporal, and parietal fiber systems. Both of these regions have extensive ipsilateral connections with frontal, temporal, and parietal areas [Mesulam et al., 1977; Baleydier and Mauguiere, 1980; Pandya et al., 1981; Mesulam and Mufson, 1982], although their contralateral connections have not, to the best of our knowledge, been studied. The overlapping trajectories of their commissural projections suggests, however, that they might have extensive contralateral connections as well. Since there is overlap then between the callosal trajectories of heterotopically connected zones in the two hemispheres, and since fibers from homotopic zones in the two hemi-spheres presumably traverse the same location in the forebrain commis-sures, we assume that efferent and afferent, homotopical and heterotopical, commissural connections of a given region occupy the same general location in the corpus callosum in the mid-sagittal plane.

A corollary of these anatomical observations is that different topograph-ical regions of the forebrain commissures contain fibers relating to different functional specializations. Somatic sensory and motor functions are local-ized to the central portion of the body of the corpus callosum; the splenium deals mainly with visual-related functions. A similar localization may also be true for certain "higher cortical functions." Reference has been made above to the overlap between posterior parietal and superior temporal fibers in the caudal part of the body of the corpus callosum. These two cortical regions are part of a more widespread system of ipsilateral and contralateral connections that ties together various higher-order association areas and may be involved in attentional and other complex functions [Mesulam, 1981; Hyvarinen, 1982]. The posterior part of the body of the corpus cal-losum appears, then, to be a nodal point in this system of connections. Disruption of an analogous site in the human corpus callosum might there-

Fig. 18. Diagrammatic representation of the topography of commissural fibers from entorhinal cortex, the presubiculum, and hippocampus. The lower diagram summa-rizes the locations of commissural fibers from entorhinal cortex, the presubiculum, and hippocampus in addition to those from prefrontal, premotor, MI, SI, SII, poste-rior parietal, superior temporal, inferotemporal, occipital, and parahippocampal cortexes.

fore cause specific attentional and/or language deficits [Geschwind, 1965; 1967].

Clinical and experimental evidence indicates that discrete lesions of the forebrain commissures differentially disrupt cortical functions. These observations are in keeping with the topographical organization of the commissures. For example, in humans, tumors of the anterior corpus callosum cause behavioral syndromes resembling schizophrenia, while tumors encroaching upon other parts of the corpus callosum do not [Nasrallah and McChesney, 1981]. Likewise, anterior lesions result in certain forms of apraxia, while posterior callosal lesions may cause selective deficits of reading and writing [Geschwind, 1965]. Selective section of posterior parts of the corpus callosum results in impairment of auditory function in humans [Musiek, this volume]. In the primate, lesions of the splenium of the corpus callosum and of the anterior commissure both selectively disrupt visual functions, but the visual deficits from the two types of ablations are qualitatively different, reflecting the different sets of commissural fibers disconnected [Doty and Negrao, 1973; Butler, 1977; Gross et al., 1977]. Thus, an understanding of the precise topography of commissural fibers allows one to assess the nature of functional deficits following selective commissural lesions and to predict the localization of functions within cerebral commissural systems.

ACKNOWLEDGMENTS

We thank Mr. Brian O. Butler and Ms. Valerie Knowlton for technical assistance. This work was supported by the Edith Nourse Rogers Memorial Veterans Hospital, Bedford, Massachusetts, and NIH grant NS14018.

REFERENCES

Amaral DG, Insausti R, Cowan WM (1984): The commissural connections of the monkey hippocampal formation. J Comp Neurol 224:307–336.

Baleydier C, Mauguiere F (1980): The duality of the cingulate gyrus in monkey: Neuroanatomical study and functional hypothesis. Brain 103:525–554.

Barbas H, Pandya DN (1982): Cytoarchitecture and intrinsic connections of the prefrontal cortex of the rhesus monkey. Soc Neurosci Abstr 8:933.

Barbas H, Pandya DN (1984): Topography of commissural fibers of the prefrontal cortex in the rhesus monkey. Exp Brain Res 55:187–191.

Butler SR (1977): Interhemispheric transfer of visual information via the corpus callosum and anterior commissure in the monkey. In Russell IS, Van Hof MW, Berlucchi G (eds): "Structure and Function of Cerebral Commissures." Baltimore: University Park Press, pp 343–357.

Chavis DA, Pandya DN (1976): Further observations on corticofrontal connections in the rhesus monkey. Brain Res 117:369–386.

Cipolloni PB, Pandya DN (1985): Topography and trajectories of commissural fibers of the superior temporal region in the rhesus monkey. Exp Brain Res. 57:381–389.

Cowan WM, Gottlieb DI, Hendrickson AE, Price JL, Woolsey TA (1972): Autoradiographic demonstration of axonal connections in the central nervous system. Brain Res 37:21–51.

Demeter S, Rosene DL, Van Hoesen GW (1985): Interhemispheric pathways of the hippocampal formation, presubiculum, and entorhinal and posterior parahippocampal cortices in the rhesus monkey: The structure and organization of the hippocampal commissures. J Comp Neurol 233:30–47.

Doty RW, Negrao N (1973): Forebrain commissures and vision. In Jung DR (ed): "Handbook of Sensory Physiology. Vol. VII.3b. Central Processing of Visual Information." Berlin: Springer, pp 543–559.

Ebner FE, Myers RE (1962): Commissural connections in the neocortex of the monkey. Anat Rec 142:229.

Gazzaniga MS (1970): "The Bisected Brain." New York: Appleton-Century-Crofts, pp 1–168.

Geschwind N (1965): Disconnexion syndromes in animals and man. Brain 88:237–294, 585–644.

Geschwind N (1967): Brain mechanisms suggested by the study of interhemispheric connections. In Millikan CH, Darley FI (eds): "Brain Mechanisms Underlying Speech and Language." New York: Grune and Stratton, pp 103–108.

Gross CG, Bender DB, Mishkin M (1977): Contributions of the corpus callosum and the anterior commissure to visual activation of inferior temporal neurons. Brain Res 131:227–240.

Hedreen JC, Yin TCT (1981): Homotopic and heterotopic callosal afferents of caudal inferior parietal lobule in Macaca mulatta. J Comp Neurol 197:605–621.

Hyvarinen J (1982):"The Parietal Cortex of Monkey and Man." New York: Springer.

Innocenti GM (1980): The primary visual pathway through the corpus callosum: Morphological and functional aspects in the cat. Arch Ital Biol 118:124–188.

Jacobson S, Trojanowski JQ (1974): The cells of origin of the corpus callosum in rat, cat, and rhesus monkey. Brain Res 132:235–246.

Jones EG, Burton H, Porter R (1975): Commissural and cortico-cortical "columns" in the somatic sensory cortex of primates. Science 190:572–574.

Jones EG, Coulter JD, Wise SP (1979): Commissural columns in the sensory-motor cortex of monkeys. J Comp Neurol 188:113–136.

Jones EG, Powell TPS (1969): Connexions of the somatic sensory cortex of the rhesus monkey. II. Contralateral connexions. Brain 92:717–730.

Jones EG, Powell TPS (1970): An anatomical study of converging sensory pathways within the cerebral cortex of the monkey. Brain 93:793–820.

Jouandet ML, Gazzaniga MS (1979): Cortical field of origin of the anterior commissure of the rhesus monkey. Exp Neurol 66:381–397.

Karol EA, Pandya DN (1971): The distribution of the corpus callosum in the rhesus monkey. Brain 94:471–486.

Killackey HP, Gould JH III, Cusick CG, Pons TP, Kaas JH (1983): The relation of corpus callosum connections to architectonic fields and body surface maps in sensorimotor cortex of new and old world monkeys. J Comp Neurol 219:384–419.

Luttenberg J, Marsala J (1963): Lokalisace komisuralnich vlaken v corpus callosum kocky. Ceskoslovenska Morfologie 11:166–175.

Mesulam MM (1981): A cortical network for directed attention and unilateral neglect. Ann Neurol 10:309–325.

Mesulam MM, Mufson EJ (1982): Insula of the old world monkey. III. Efferent cortical output and comments on function. J Comp Neurol 212:38–52.

Mesulam MM, Van Hoesen GW, Pandya DN, Geschwind N (1977): Limbic and sensory connections of the inferior parietal lobule (area PG) in the rhesus monkey: A study with a new method for horseradish peroxidase histochemistry. Brain Res 136:393–414.

Musiek FE (In Press): The effects of partial and complete commissurotomy on central auditory function. This volume.

Myers RE (1965): The neocortical commissures and interhemispheric transmission of information. In Ettlinger EG (ed): "Functions of the Corpus Callosum." Boston: Little Brown, pp 1–17, 133–143.

Nasrallah HA, McChesney CM (1981): Psychopathology of corpus callosum tumors. Biol Psychiatry 16:663–669.

Pandya DN, Karol EA, Heilbronn D (1971): The topographical distribution of interhemispheric projections in the corpus callosum of the rhesus monkey. Brain Res 32:31–43.

Pandya DN, Karol EA, Lele PP (1973): The distribution of the anterior commissure in the squirrel monkey. Brain Res 49:177–180.

Pandya DN, Kuypers HGJM (1969): Cortico-cortical connections in the rhesus monkey. Brain Res 13:13–36.

Pandya DN, Seltzer B (1982): Intrinsic connections and architectonics of posterior parietal cortex in the rhesus monkey. J Comp Neurol 204:196–210.

Pandya DN, Van Hoesen GW, Mesulam MM (1981): Efferent connections of the cingulate gyrus in the rhesus monkey. Exp Brain Res 42:319–330.

Pandya DN, Vignolo LA (1969): Interhemispheric projections of the parietal lobe in the rhesus monkey. Brain Res 15:49–65.

Petrides M, Pandya DN (1984): Projections to the frontal cortex from the posterior parietal region in the rhesus monkey. J Comp Neurol 228:105–116.

Rockland KS, Pandya DN (in preparation): The trajectory and topography of occipital lobe commissural connections in the rhesus monkey.

Russell IS, van Hof MW, Berlucchi G (1979): "Structure and Functions of Cerebral Commissures." Baltimore: University Park Press.

Sanides F (1969): Comparative architectonics of the neocortex of mammals and their evolutionary development. Ann NY Acad Sci 167:404–423.

Seltzer B, Pandya DN (1976): Some cortical projections to the parahippocampal area in the rhesus monkey. Exp Neurol 50:146–160.

Seltzer B, Pandya DN (1978): Afferent cortical connections and architectonics of the superior temporal sulcus and surrounding cortex in the rhesus monkey. Brain Res 149:1–24.

Seltzer B, Pandya DN (1983): The distribution of posterior parietal fibers in the corpus callosum of the rhesus monkey. Exp Brain Res 49:147–150.

Seltzer B, Pandya DN (1984): Further observations on parieto-temporal connections in the rhesus monkey. Exp Brain Res 55:301–312.

Sperry RW (1961): Cerebral organization and behavior. Science 133:1749–1757.

Sunderland S (1940): The distribution of commissural fibers in the corpus callosum in the macaque monkey. J Neurol Psychiatry 3:9–18.

Van Essen DC, Newsome WT, Bixby JL (1982): The pattern of interhemispheric connections and its relationship to extrastriate visual areas in the macaque monkey. J Neurosci 2:265–283.

Whitlock DG, Nauta WJH (1956): Subcortical projections from the temporal neocortex in Macaca mulatta. J Comp Neurol 106:183–212.

Zeki SM (1970): Interhemispheric connections of prestriate cortex in monkey. Brain Res 19:63–75.

Zeki SM (1973): Comparison of the cortical degeneration in the visual regions of the temporal lobe following section of the anterior commissure and the splenium. J Comp Neurol 148:167–176.

ABBREVIATIONS

AC	Anterior commissure
AS	Arcuate sulcus
CaS	Calcarine sulcus
CC	Corpus callosum
CF	Calcarine fissure
CING S(CiS)	Cingulate sulcus
CS	Central sulcus
DHC	Dorsal hippocampal commissure
ENTO	Entorhinal cortex
F	Fornix
H	Habenula
HIPPO	Hippocampus
IOS	Inferior occipital sulcus
IPS	Intraparietal sulcus
LF	Lateral fissure
LS	Lunate sulcus
MB	Mammillary body
OPS	Occipito-parietal sulcus
OTS	Occipitotemporal sulcus
PC	Posterior commissure
POMS	Parieto-occipital medial sulcus
PRESUB	Presubiculum
PS	Principal sulcus
RhF	Rhinal fissure
STS	Superior temporal sulcus
VHC	Ventral hippocampal commissure

Two Hemispheres—One Brain:
Functions of the Corpus Callosum, pages 75–81
© 1986 Alan R. Liss, Inc.

What Is so Special About Callosal Connections?

GIORGIO M. INNOCENTI

Institut d'Anatomie, Université de Lausanne, 1005 Lausanne, Switzerland

INTRODUCTION

In the last few years, the widespread interest in the organization of callosal connections as the substrate for interhemispheric integration, owing largely to the neuropsychological studies of Sperry and collaborators, has been paralleled by a growth of interest in the development of these connections. In this recent work, some of the events and mechanisms underlying the formation of specific connections in the central nervous system have come into focus. It is a curious coincidence that the leading theory on the mechanisms responsible for the specificity of connections, the so-called "chemoaffinity hypothesis," should be due to Sperry's other major, and earlier, line of research.

Callosal connections are "specific" in four different ways (for references see Innocenti [1986]):

i. Each area projects to and receives from a characteristic, restricted set of areas in the other hemisphere.

ii. Different sets of neurons project from one area to each of the contralateral target areas, although a few neurons send bifurcating axons to more than one of those areas. Furthermore, still different sets of neurons project ipsilaterally.

iii. The various sets of callosal neurons and those of ipsilaterally projecting neurons occupy restricted, and often different, radial positions in the cortex.

iv. Connections between two areas are point-to-point. In general, tangentially defined subunits ("columns") of two areas are interconnected in a characteristic, orderly manner. A special case of such specificity is that of areas only partially connected through the corpus callosum as, for example, the visual and the somatosensory areas (see below).

Information is beginning to emerge on how these "specificities" appear in development [see also Frost and Innocenti, this volume]. It must be noticed that similar "specificities" characterize other cortico-cortical and cortico-subcortical connections. And there is evidence that both sets of connections may develop in a manner similar to that of callosal connections.

ELIMINATION OF CALLOSAL CONNECTIONS IN NORMAL DEVELOPMENT

Using horseradish peroxidase (HRP) as a retrograde tracer [Innocenti et al., 1977], it was observed that while in adult cats callosal connections originate and terminate only near the boundary between the areas 17 and 18, in newborn kittens they originate from throughout each of these areas. At the end of the first postnatal week, acallosal gaps appear in medial 17 and in lateral 18 and progressively enlarge, leading to the normal adult distribution of callosal efferents during the second and third postnatal month [Innocenti and Caminiti, 1980]. With a few exceptions [see Innocenti and Clarke, 1984b] the radial distribution of callosal neurons is similar at birth and in the adult.

These observations were soon generalized to other areas and species [for references see Innocenti, 1985], in particular, in the cat, to the somatosensory [Innocenti and Caminiti, 1980] and auditory [Feng and Brugge, 1983] areas.

Nevertheless, the use of retrograde tracers for this kind of developmental study suffers of the following drawbacks: (i) Loss of callosal connections can be readily detected only in regions that become acallosal or partially acallosal in the adult. (ii) Even in these areas, the apparent loss cannot always be trusted and even less quantified. Most probably, a tracer normally reveals only a proportion of the afferents to the area where it has been injected, and not necessarily the same proportion at different ages. Moreover, the number of labeled neurons depends on the location and size of the injections, and it is difficult to obtain identical or even comparable injections in animals of different ages. In fact, probably the only brain region where the loss of callosal connections can certainly not be ascribed to their incomplete visualization in the adult may be the visual cortex of the cat. Here, unequivocal electrophysiological evidence supports the repeatedly confirmed anatomical finding of a restricted origin of callosal connections in the adult [Choudhury et al., 1965; Berlucchi et al., 1967; Hubel and Wiesel, 1967; Shatz, 1977].

To circumvent these difficulties, we counted the axons in the corpus callosum during development, using electron microscopy [Koppel and Innocenti, 1983]. This approach offers a number of potential pitfalls, such as the sampling difficulties, possible differential shrinkage of the electron microscopic material where axon density is obtained and of the light microscopic material used to determine the total callosal surface, etc. [see Koppel and Innocenti, 1983]. However, a much more precise estimate of the number of callosal axons than that derived from light microscopy can be obtained. In fact, the electron microscopic estimate of callosal axons in adult cats (23 million) turned out to be more than four times larger than the previously accepted light-microscopic figure.

The loss of callosal axons assessed with this method in the cat is enormous. About 70% of the 79 million axons present at birth are eliminated by adulthood. A similar proportion of callosal axons are also eliminated in the monkey in development [LaMantia and Rakic, 1984]. In the cat, this loss greatly exceeds the proportion of cortical surface lacking callosal connections in the adult (see, for example, Fig. 1 in Ebner and Myers [1965]).

Therefore, one must assume that certain regions of cortex lose callosal connections but without becoming fully acallosal (see below).

AXONAL ELIMINATION VERSUS NEURONAL DEATH

The question of whether the elimination of transitory callosal connections is due to the death of a specific set of cortical neurons or to elimination of a set of transitory axons was resolved in favor of the second possibility in the visual cortex of the cat [Innocenti, 1981] and subsequently in the somatosensory cortex of the rat [O'Leary et al., 1981; Ivy and Killackey, 1982]. The fluorescent tracer fast blue was injected into the visual cortex of newborn kittens, and the animals were sacrificed during the second postnatal month, when callosal neurons have already become focussed near the 17-18 border. Labeled neurons turned out to be as widely distributed as at the time of injection. A few days before sacrifice, many of the neurons near the 17-18 border, but none away from the border, could be relabeled by a second injection of a different tracer in the hemisphere that had received the first injection.

At the time when callosal neurons are widely distributed, callosal axons have entered specific parts of the gray matter, those that will also receive callosal afferents in the adult. A more widely distributed population of axons exists in the white matter, but most of them appear not to enter the gray matter, at least not postnatally [Innocenti, 1981].

The fact that the restricted distribution of callosal terminals precedes that of the callosal neurons may mean that the former determines the latter. In other words, crucial events for the fate of juvenile callosal projections may occur at their terminal site. With this perspective, it became necessary to find out which part of the visual areas give rise to the axons that enter the cortex and to those that do not.

THE ORGANIZATION OF JUVENILE CALLOSAL CONNECTIONS

In a new series of experiments, the injection of retrograde tracers was restricted to parts of the gray matter, of the white matter, or of both [Innocenti and Clarke, 1984b]. Although we had tried a similar experiment with HRP, only the retrograde fluorescent tracers, probably because of their low solubility in water, gave sufficiently localized injections.

In these kittens, injections (on postnatal days 0–10) restricted to the gray matter labeled callosal neurons only when regions were involved, such as the 17-18 border, where the anterograde transport studies had revealed terminating callosal axons. Such regions also receive from the medial part of the dorsal lateral geniculate nucleus (dLGN), and therefore from the retinal midline. The pattern of retro-grade labeling obtained in the contralateral hemisphere by such injections was very similar to that of the adult. Labeled neurons were concentrated at the 17-18 border and in the retinotopically corresponding parts of other visual areas, i.e., at the vertical meridian representations. In addition, a few neurons were often labeled in parts of cortex, e.g., medial area 17, destined to become acallosal. At the moment it is uncertain whether these neurons do indeed send an axon into the cortex or whether limited spread of dyes to the white matter has occurred.

Injections extending into the white matter, or restricted to it, labeled callosal neurons with a different tangential distribution. Labeled neurons were in an irregular crescent-shaped territory (Fig. 1), including visual areas that will become partly acallosal and even areas that will completely lose their callosal projection to areas 17 and 18 (see below). The shape of the labeled territory is constant in different animals and varies only little for different injection sites along the lateral gyrus. However, its rostrocaudal position shifts systematically with that of the injection along the lateral gyrus (Fig. 1). Simultaneous injections of different fluorescent tracers at different and nonoverlapping positions along the lateral gyrus label extensively overlapping territories in the contralateral hemisphere. In the region of overlap, neurons are labeled by one or the other dye but very seldom by both. Thus, there is a major divergence-convergence in the juvenile callosal projections, but this is not due to an abundance of single neurons with widely bifurcating axons.

Similarly, simultaneous injections of different fluorescent tracers in the 17-18 region and in more lateral visual areas labeled mediolaterally overlapping territories. In particular, injections in 19-21a or in posteromedial lateral suprasylvian area (PMLS) labeled neurons throughout contralateral area 17, including its transitorily callosal part, but there were few double-labeled neurons. Thus, the mediolateral divergence-convergence seems also not to be due to the collateralization of single axons. Particularly surprising is the presence of several distinct populations of transitory callosal neurons in medial area 17, each projecting specifically, but transiently to a different target [Innocenti and Clarke, 1983, 1984b].

Perhaps the most striking new finding emerging from this series of experiments was that the territory labeled by injections reaching the white matter under areas 17 and 18 extended beyond the visual areas, i.e., it included areas that do not project to areas 17 and 18 in the adult. The widest and most conspicuous of those projections originates from the auditory cortex, including fields A1, A2, and EP and possibly some other auditory

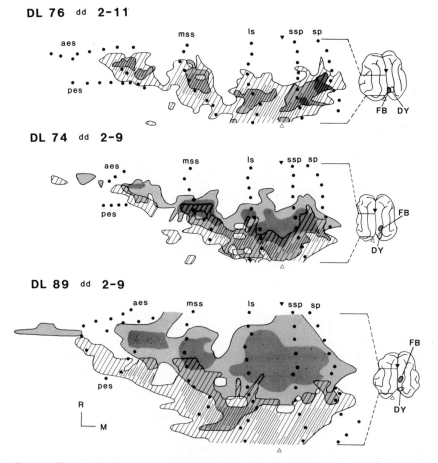

Fig. 1. Flat reconstructions of the occipital portion of the brains of three kittens (identified by code number, age at injection, and age at death), showing regions containing layer II–VI callosal neurons retrogradely labeled by diamidino yellow (DY; hatching) or by fast blue (FB; shading). The region reconstructed is that between bars on brain insets. The reconstructions are based on hand-drawn sketches of cell distributions. Only two arbitrary levels in density of labeled neurons are indicated, i.e., high density (dark shading or hatching) and low density (light shading or hatching). Location of injection sites is marked on brain insets. In DL 76, the FB injection was restricted to the white matter under area 17; the DY injection was in the gray and white matter near the 17-18 border. In DL's 74 and 89 all injections were in the gray and white matter near the 17-18 border. Filled and empty triangles point to corresponding positions on the brain surface and on the reconstructions; they denote the axis along which coronal sections were aligned. Dotted lines correspond to sulci, the most important of which are also marked by abbreviations. aes, anterior ectosylvian sulcus; pes, posterior ectosylvian sulcus; mss, middle suprasylvian sulcus; ls, lateral sulcus; ssp, suprasplenial sulcus; sp, splenial sulcus. R is rostral, M is medial. Bars = 2 mm (reproduced from Innocenti and Clarke [1984]).

subdivisions of the middle and anterior ectosylvian gyrus [Innocenti and Clark, 1984a,b].

Labeled neurons were found in the auditory region not only contralaterally, but also ipsilaterally to the injected visual cortex. Transitory ipsilateral projections to the visual cortex originate also from somatosensory areas [Clarke and Innocenti, 1984, and in preparation]. Thus, not only callosal, but also ipsilateral association connections develop through a phase of exuberancy.

Simultaneous injections of different tracers showed that the transitory callosal and ipsilateral auditory-to-visual projections originate from different sets of neurons at different levels in the cortex [Innocenti and Clarke, 1984a]. The ipsilateral projection comes predominantly from layer II and the upper part of layer III, the callosal projection mostly from layer III. The auditory-to-auditory callosal projection originates still deeper, in layer III and in upper layer IV. At least part of this projection will be preserved into adulthood [Feng and Brugge, 1983].

Both transitory auditory-to-visual projections disappear around the end of the first postnatal month, apparently by axonal elimination [Innocenti and Clarke, 1984a]. A reciprocal visual-to-auditory projection is not present at birth.

CONCLUSIONS

Although callosal connections are already present at birth, they lack many of their adult, specific features. Nevertheless, what is found at birth is not a diffuse or "random" connectivity. It is as if the adult organization was preceded by a different organization reflecting the needs and the constraints of juvenile functions, especially of morphogenesis. Later, the organization of callosal connections will conform to the adult function.

Some of the developmental concepts that are emerging from the study of callosal connections can be extended to corticocortical connections in general. And, indeed, they may be valid for other corticosubcortical connections as well, where similar phenomena are beginning to be described [Stanfield et al., 1982; Adams et al., 1983; Tolbert and Panneton, 1983; Mihailoff et al., 1984].

ACKNOWLEDGMENTS

I am grateful to Dr. Peter Clarke for his help with this text. This work was supported by the Swiss National Science Foundation grant 3.422.0.83.

REFERENCES

Adams CE, Mihailoff GA, Woodward DJ (1983): A transient component of the developing corticospinal tract arises in visual cortex. Neurosci Lett 36:243–248.

Berlucchi G, Gazzaniga MS, Rizzolatti G (1967): Microelectrode analysis of transfer of visual information by the corpus callosum. Arch Ital Biol 105:583–596.

Choudhury BP, Whitteridge D, Wilson ME (1965): The function of the callosal connections of the visual cortex. J Exp Physiol L:214–219.

Clarke S, Innocenti GM (1984): Exuberant intrahemispheric projections to the visual cortex in young kittens. Neurosci Lett [Suppl] 18:S291.

Ebner FF, Myers RE (1965): Distribution of corpus callosum and anterior commissure in cat and raccoon. J Comp Neurol 124:353–366.

Feng JZ, Brugge JF (1983): Postnatal development of auditory callosal connections in the kitten. J Comp Neurol 214:416–426.

Hubel DH, Wiesel TN (1967): Cortical and callosal connections concerned with the vertical meridian of visual fields in the cat. J Neurophysiol 30:1561–1573.

Innocenti GM (1981): Growth and reshaping of axons in the establishment of visual callosal connections. Science 212:824–827.

Innocenti GM (1986): The general organization of callosal connections. In Jones EG, Peters AA (eds): "Cerebral Cortex." New York: Plenum Press (in press).

Innocenti GM, Caminiti R (1980): Postnatal shaping of callosal connections from sensory areas. Exp Brain Res 38:381–394.

Innocenti GM, Clarke S (1983): Multiple sets of visual cortical neurons projecting transitorily through the corpus callosum. Neurosci Lett 41:27–32.

Innocenti GM, Clarke S (1984a): Bilateral transitory projection to visual areas from auditory cortex in kittens. Dev Brain Res 14:143–148.

Innocenti GM, Clarke S (1984b): The organization of immature callosal connections. J Comp Neurol 230:287–309.

Innocenti GM, Fiore L, Caminiti R (1977): Exuberant projection into the corpus callosum from the visual cortex of newborn cats. Neurosci Lett 4:237–242.

Ivy GO, Killackey HP (1982): Ontogenetic changes in the projections of neocortical neurons. J Neurosci 2:735–743.

Koppel H, Innocenti GM (1983): Is there a genuine exuberancy of callosal projections in development? A quantitative electron microscopic study in the cat. Neurosci Lett 41:33–40.

LaMantia AS, Rakic P (1984): The number, size, myelination, and regional variation of axons in the corpus callosum and anterior commissure of the developing rhesus monkey. Neurosci Abs 10:1081.

Mihailoff GA, Adams CE, Woodward DJ (1984): An autoradiographic study of the postnatal development of sensorimotor and visual components of the corticopontine system. J Comp Neurol 222:116–127.

O'Leary DDM, Stanfield BB, Cowan WM (1981): Evidence that the early postnatal restriction of the cells of origin of the callosal projection is due to the elimination of axonal collaterals rather than to the death of neurons. Dev Brain Res 1:607–617.

Shatz C (1977): Abnormal interhemispheric connections in the visual system of Boston siamese cats: A physiological study. J Comp Neurol 171:229–246.

Stanfield BB, O'Leary DDM, Fricks C (1982): Selective collateral elimination in early postnatal development restricts cortical distribution of rat pyramidal tract neurones. Nature 298:371–373.

Tolbert DL, Panneton WM (1983): Transient cerebrocerebellar projections in kittens: Postnatal development and topography. J Comp Neurol 221:216–228.

Two Hemispheres—One Brain:
Functions of the Corpus Callosum, pages 83–102
© 1986 Alan R. Liss, Inc.

Interhemispheric Connections of Cortical Sensory and Motor Representations in Primates

CATHERINE G. CUSICK AND JON H. KAAS

Department of Psychology, Vanderbilt University, Nashville, Tennessee 37240

INTRODUCTION

Corpus callosum connections were among the first cortical pathways to be studied intensively with the advent of sensitive degeneration methods for revealing axons and axon terminations [Myers, 1962; Ebner and Myers, 1965; Ebner, 1969]. These early studies led to the general conclusions that corpus callosum pathways united separate representations of the right and left visual hemifields and the separate representations of the right and left body midline surfaces in the two cerebral hemispheres. Thus, callosal connections were described as along the representation of the zero vertical meridian between the primary and secondary visual representations (V-I and V-II) and along the representations of the body midline in the primary and secondary somatosensory areas (S-I and S-II), and in the motor cortex (M-I). Other parts of visual, somatic, and motor representations, especially those dealing with peripheral vision or distal limbs, were thought to be devoid or nearly devoid of callosal connections. Callosal connections for sensory and motor areas, then, were thought to provide what would normally be local connections between representations of adjoining sensory surfaces that happen to be widely separated in the two cerebral hemispheres. We now have considerable anatomical and electrophysiological evidence that this view of function of the corpus callosum is too limited, and that callosal connections have much broader significance in sensory and motor areas. This evidence is consistent with the extensive behavioral findings stemming from the now classical studies of Myers and Sperry [1953] that the corpus callosum transfers sensory and perceptual information from one hemisphere to the other.

Current conclusions regarding callosal connections depend on several recent advances. First, it is now apparent from electrophysiological mapping studies that advanced mammals, such as monkeys, have a number of sensory representations in the cortex. Thus, conclusions about the functions of the callosal pathway need not be based only on primary and secondary fields, but can be deduced from the connections of other sensory representations as well. Second, the use of horseradish peroxidase (HRP) as an anatomical tracer, in conjunction with sensitive methods for revealing HRP, has allowed a much more complete picture of the total distribution of callosal connections, including both the locations of projecting cells and the terminal arbors of these cells in the opposite hemisphere. Third, there are clear advantages to studying brain sections cut in nonstandard planes. In particular, surface-view patterns of label are most obvious in brain sections cut parallel to the surface of artificially flattened brains.

In the following review, we describe the surface-view distributions of interhemispheric connections for subdivisions of somatic, motor, and visual cortices for several species of primates, and relate these patterns to those found in more generalized mammals. Connections are characterized for tree shrews and Virginia opossums as examples of generalized mammals, and for prosimian primates (galagos), New World monkeys (owl monkeys), and Old World monkeys (macaques) to provide a range of primate species. The observations support at least seven major conclusions: (1) In higher primates with many sensory representations, parts of the primary representations are largely devoid of interhemispheric connections, while more generalized mammals with fewer sensory representations have more widely distributed connections in the primary representations. (2) Within primates there are significant species differences in the details of connection patterns in both primary and "higher-order" cortical representations. (3) In general, later stages in cortical processing sequences have more widely distributed callosal connections than earlier stages. (4) However, some "higher-order" areas have few callosal connections. (5) Each cortical field has a unique pattern of callosal connections, suggesting that callosal connections perform different roles in different cortical fields. Often the typically uneven distribution of connections forms a semiregular pattern that may reflect the presence of repeating processing modules within a field. (6) Callosal connections from a given representation characteristically include the same representation and one or more adjacent representations in the processing sequence in the opposite hemisphere. (7) Callosal connections often relate mismatched parts of sensory maps, especially in "higher-order" areas. In this manner, callosal connections contribute not only to extending contralateral excitatory receptive fields past the midline and to the creation of large bilateral receptive fields, but also to large antagonistic surrounds of receptive fields. Some of the evidence to support these conclusions is presented below.

INTERHEMISPHERIC CONNECTIONS IN GENERALIZED MAMMALS

Comparative studies indicate that early mammals had proportionately little neocortex and relatively few cortical subdivisions [Kaas, 1982]. The brain of the Virginia opossum represents a primitive stage of cortical development [Ebner, 1969], comparable to that of many insectivores, and the brain of the tree shrew, a somewhat distant relative of primates, represents a slight advance, with some overall expansion of the neocortex and probably an increase in the number of cortical areas [Sesma et al., 1984a; Cusick et al., 1985].

The distribution of interhemispherically projecting cells, as revealed by multiple HRP injections in the opposite cerebral hemisphere, are shown on sections from a flattened cortex for a tree shrew and an opossum in Figure 1. The distributions of labeled cells can be related to known sensory areas as determined by comparisons with alternate myelin-stained sections and previous electrophysiological mapping studies. The primary and secondary visual areas and primary somatosensory cortex are shown for both mammals. S-II is indicated for the tree shrew, and the motor cortex is just rostral to S-I. The occipital-temporal cortex has several visual areas, including the temporal dorsal area (TD) [see Sesma et al., 1984a,b], but the organization of this cortex is not completely known. The opossum does not have a separate motor area, and S-II adjoins S-I caudolaterally [Pubols et al., 1976].

The results shown in Figure 1 indicate that interhemispheric connections originate from much or most of the primary and secondary sensory fields in opossums and tree shrews, and from most of the motor cortex in tree shrews. Distributions of interhemispheric terminations follow a similar pattern. Clearly, the distributions of interhemispheric connections are not restricted to the representations of the vertical midline of the visual field (zero vertical meridian) or the midline of the body. Comparisons of these connection patterns with those for the same fields in primates (Figs. 2–5) indicate that interhemispheric connections are more broadly distributed in primary fields in these generalized mammals than in higher primates.

THE PRIMARY SENSORY AND MOTOR AREAS OF PRIMATES

In primates, the callosal connections of primary somatic and motor areas are sparse in the representations of the distal limbs, and dense in the representations of the trunk and parts of the face. The primary visual cortex has dense callosal connections along the V-II border. Prosimian primates have more broadly distributed connections, and Old World monkeys have more restricted connections than New World monkeys.

Somatosensory Cortex (S-I)

In monkeys, S-I has traditionally been regarded as including four architectonic fields, areas 3a, 3b, 1, and 2. However, it is now apparent that each of these fields contains a separate representation of the body, and several lines of evidence argue that only area 3b is the homologue of S-I in nonprimates [see Kaas, 1983 for review]. The details of the representations of the body surface in area 3b have been described for New World and Old World monkeys and for S-I of prosimian galagos [see Kaas, 1983]. More recently,

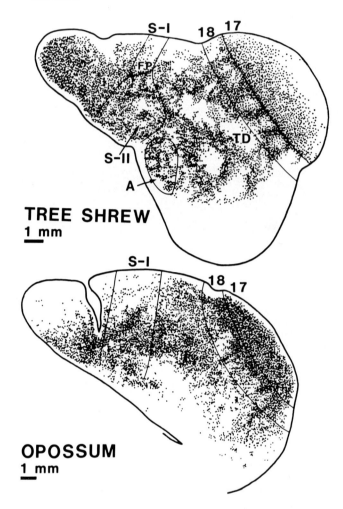

Fig. 1.   Distributions of neurons projecting to multiple horseradish peroxidase injection sites in the opposite cerebral hemisphere of a tree shrew and opossum. Each drawing shows a section cut parallel to the surface of cortex that had been separated from rest of the brain and flattened. Labeled cells are compiled from three or more sections through superficial cortical layers. The locations of primary and secondary visual (17 and 18) and somatosensory (S-I and S-II) fields, as well as the auditory cortex (A) are based on architectonic criteria. FP indicates the representation of the forepaw in S-I of tree shrews. Rostral, left; medial, up. The opossum is from unpublished studies of Krubitzer, Cusick and Kaas. The tree shrew is a composite of two cases from Cusick et al. [1985]. For further explanation, see text.

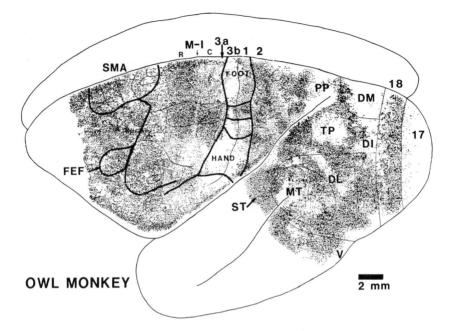

Fig. 2. Callosally projecting neurons in owl monkeys. Visual areas include 17 (V-I), 18 (V-II), middle temporal (MT), dorsolateral (DL), dorsointermediate (DI), dorsomedial (DM), posterior parietal (PP), temporal parietal (TP), superior temporal (ST), and ventral (V) fields [see Cusick et al., 1984]. The medial area, M, is hidden from view. Areas 3a and 2 form mediolateral bands along areas 3b and 1 of approximately 1 and 2 mm in width, respectively. Rostral and caudal portions of motor cortex, the supplementary motor area (SMA), and the frontal eye fields (FEF) are indicated. Fine lines mark represented body parts with face, hand, shoulder-trunk, and hind-limb in a lateromedial progression in M-I, and eye movements, face, hand, body, and hindlimb in a rostrocaudal sequence in SMA. The lateromedial parallel se-quences of representation in 3b and in 1 are face, hand, forelimb, trunk, and hindlimb (foot). The callosal connections of the unlabeled regions in the frontal lobe and temporal cortex were not determined (based on Cusick et al. [1984], Gould et al. [1983], and Killackey et al. [1983]).

patterns of callosal connections have been studied in owl and macaque monkeys where the organization of S-I (area 3b) was determined by micro-electrode mapping methods in the same cases [Killackey et al, 1983]. In addition, we have determined callosal connection patterns for S-I in galagos (Cusick and Kaas, unpublished) and related results to the previously pub-lished maps.

In owl monkeys, callosal connections are sparse but present in the repre-sentations of the glabrous hand and foot (Figs. 2,3). Connections are denser

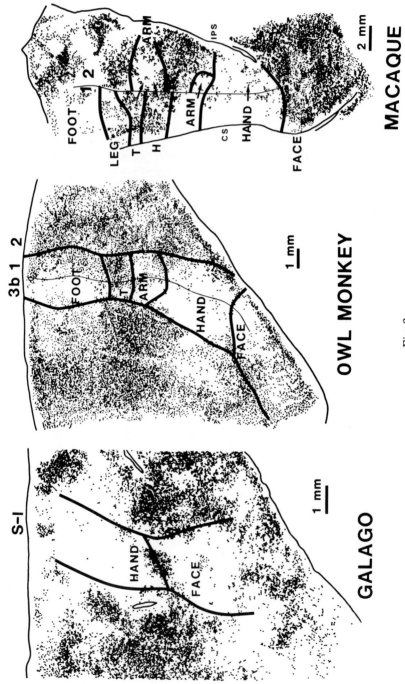

GALAGO   OWL MONKEY   MACAQUE

Fig. 3

in the representation of the face, trunk, and part of the arm. Concentrations of label rostrally and caudally in the trunk representation are consistent with the notion that representations of the body midline have callosal connections, but these are not the only parts of the S-I with connections. The distribution of callosal connections in area 3b of macaque monkeys is roughly similar to that in owl monkeys, but the connections are more restricted. In macaque monkeys, the hand representation is almost devoid of both projecting cells and terminations, and connections are mainly associated with the representations of the face and trunk.

Callosal connections in S-I of prosimian galagos resemble the connections found in area 3b of owl monkeys (Fig. 3). At least a few labeled cells are found in all parts of the body representation and more cells and terminations occur in the trunk and face regions. Thus, primates generally appear to have fewer callosal connections for S-I than generalized nonprimates, and macaque monkeys have the fewest connections, suggesting that a loss of callosal connections in area 3b accompanied the development of an enlarged brain in advanced monkeys. Monkeys also appear, however, to have retained features that may be common to more generalized mammals, such as connections associated with the hand-face border in the S-I (Figs. 1–3).

Motor Cortex (M-I)

Patterns of callosal connections have been directly related to the organization of motor cortex in owl monkeys by combining microstimulation motor mapping techniques with the anatomical tracing of callosal connections in the same animals [Gould et al., 1983]. An important observation is that the rostral part of M-I contains more callosal connections than the caudal part (Fig. 2). This arrangement of connections may be correlated with the segregation of deep and cutaneous sensory input to rostral and caudal zones of M-I described for other monkeys [Wise and Tanji, 1981; Strick and Preston, 1982]. In addition, the representations of some body parts have fewer callosal connections than others. In the caudal portion of motor cortex, only sparse callosal connections are found in cortex related to movements of the

Fig. 3. Callosally projecting neurons in somatosensory cortex of three primates. The callosal connections of S-I in galagos and area 3b in owl monkeys and macaque monkeys are mainly restricted to portions of the trunk and face representations. All body parts in galagos and owl monkeys have at least some callosally projecting neurons, while the connections of the area 3b representation of the hand in macaque monkeys (not shown) has virtually no connections. In monkeys, areas 1 and 2 have progressively more connections. For further explanation, see text. All three examples are from flattened hemispheres. The representation of body parts in the galago brain was estimated based on sections stained for myelin. The body representations for the owl and macaque monkeys were determined by detailed electrophysiological recording in these same animals [modified from Killackey et al., 1983]. CS, central sulcus. IPS, intraparietal sulcus. T, trunk. H, head. Orientation as in previous figures.

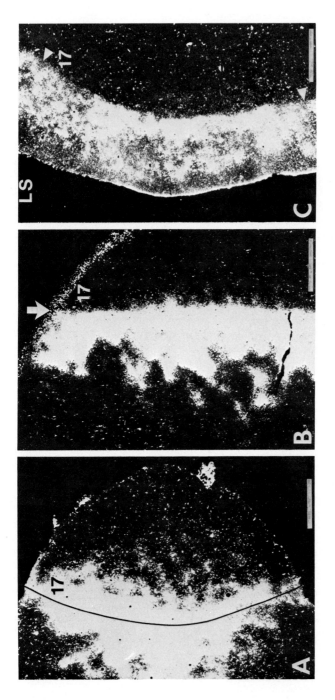

Fig. 4. Callosal connections of areas 17 and 18 in three primates. Darkfield photomicrographs of single flattened sections showing anterograde and retrograde label from a galago (A), owl monkey (B), and newborn macaque monkey (C). The 17–18 border is indicated for each case. Note patches of label in A and B, and progressively more restricted connections in area 17 in A–C. The callosal connections extend somewhat further into area 17 in A and B on deeper sections. For further explanation, see text. Orientation as in previous figures, except for C, where lateral is toward the top. Scale = 1 mm. LS, lunate sulcus. Tetramethyl benzidine (TMB) stain.

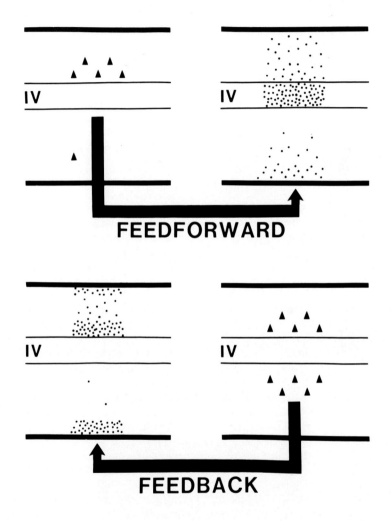

Fig. 5. Feedforward and feedback types of corticocortical connections. Triangles indicate projecting cells and dots indicate terminal fields. For further explanation, see text.

hand. Dense connections occur in parts of M-I where movements of the head and trunk are evoked, and less dense connections are found in the cortex related to hindlimb and proximal forelimb movements. Thus, the caudal part of the motor cortex in owl monkeys is similar to the primary somatosensory cortex, area 3b, in the relative density of connections with respect to representation of different body parts.

A general trend for the loss of callosal connections related to distal body parts with advanced brain organization is apparent when callosal connections of the motor forepaw region are compared in tree shrews (Fig. 1), owl monkeys (Fig. 2), and macaque monkeys [Zant and Strick, 1978]. In the motor representation of the forepaw, just rostral to the somatosensory representation, tree shrews have moderate numbers of projecting cells, while owl monkeys and especially macaque monkeys have reduced numbers of projecting cells.

Visual Cortex (V-I or area 17)

The earliest descriptions of interhemispheric connections of the visual cortex in primates were made for macaque monkeys, and they described an almost complete absence of connections in area 17. Later studies obtained similar results, although some terminations were demonstrated within area 17 up to 1 mm from the area 17–18 border. Experiments using HRP tracing in macaque monkeys revealed virtually no callosally projecting cells within area 17 [see Cusick et al., 1984, for a review]. Recently, however, callosally projecting cells in area 17 of macaques have been described for a region near foveal vision [Spatz and Kunz, 1984]. Thus, callosal connections of area 17 appear to be extremely limited in macaque monkeys. Our observations on two newborn macaques [Cusick and Kaas, unpublished] indicate that this restriction of connections is present near the time of birth (Fig. 4).

Not all primates have such limited callosal connections for area 17. Weyand and Swadlow [1980] first demonstrated that a large extent of area 17 in galagos has callosally projecting cells. More recently, we found callosally projecting cells and terminations up to 5 mm within area 17 of galagos [Cusick et al., 1984]. Furthermore, these connections are not uniformly distributed. Near the area 17–18 border, callosal connections are nearly even in area 17. However, away from the border, the connections in layer III have a clustered arrangement (Fig. 4) corresponding in location to regions with dense concentrations of cytochrome oxidase, a mitochondrial enzyme reflecting high levels of metabolic activity. The widespread and periodic callosal connections of area 17 in galagos appear to relate to the W-cell system [see Stone, 1983], which projects from the koniocellular layers of the lateral geniculate nucleus [Norton and Casagrande, 1982] to the cytochrome oxidase concentrations in layer III of area 17.

The distribution of callosal connections in area 17 of New World owl monkeys is intermediate between the very restricted pattern in macaques and the widespread connections in galagos. Terminations extend into area 17 for about 1 mm, and projecting cells occur up to 2 mm from the border [Cusick et al., 1984]. As in galagos, terminations away from the border in layer III of owl monkeys are concentrated in small pufflike regions (Fig. 4). Thus, callosal connections of area 17 of both galagos and owl monkeys tend to be clustered, and this may reflect aspects of modular organization in area 17. A tendency for clustering of callosal connections within area 17 has also been described for pigmented rats [Cusick and Lund, 1982] and squirrels [Gould, 1984].

THE CALLOSAL CONNECTIONS OF SUBSEQUENT STATIONS IN CORTICAL PROCESSING SEQUENCES

Studies of ipsilateral connections in sensory and motor cortices suggest that cortical subdivisions can be arranged in hierarchical sequences that emphasize the serial processing of information from area to area. Since cortical processing includes parallel components as well, postulated cortical sequences are based on "strengths" of connections, as well as the laminar patterns of connections (Fig. 5) [see Maunsell and Van Essen, 1983]. Briefly, "feedforward" connections terminate mainly in layer IV of the higher area and originate mainly in layer III. "Feedback" terminations avoid layer IV and arise from both layer III and infragranular layers. Observations on different fields in sensory and motor cortices support the conclusion that higher stages in cortical processing sequences have more interhemispheric connections. Thus, information from "non-midline" parts of sensory surfaces may be relayed through a processing sequence in the ipsilateral hemisphere before being transferred across the corpus callosum.

Somatosensory Sequences

In the somatosensory cortex of monkeys, patterns of ipsilateral cortical connections suggest that information is largely processed in an area 3b, 1, 2, 5 sequence, although parallel thalamic inputs and other sequences of cortical connections also exist as complications [see Mountcastle, 1984 for review]. In owl monkeys (Fig. 2), callosal connections are the least dense in area 3b, more dense in area 1, and quite dense in area 2. In addition, they are unevenly distributed in area 3b, so that some parts of the representation are almost devoid of connections. Callosally projecting cells are less uneven in area 1, and almost uniform in area 2. Area 5, between area 2 and PP, resembles area 2 in its pattern of callosal connections. The pattern across areas in macaque monkeys is similar, except that macaque monkeys have fewer callosally projecting neurons in the representations of the hand and foot in area 1, and even in area 2 (Fig. 3). Perhaps the callosal transfer of information related to the hand is even further delayed in the somatosensory processing sequence in macaque monkeys.

In both owl and macaque monkeys, callosal terminations related to the earlier stages of the cortical processing sequence tend to avoid layer IV, and thus resemble the feedback type of connection (Fig. 5). In the later stages, especially in areas 2 and 5, callosal terminations are concentrated in layer IV, and projecting cells are supra- and infragranular, as is typical of feedforward connections. Possibly, early stages project callosally to later stages in a feedforward manner, while later stages project callosally to earlier stages in a feedback manner.

Motor Sequences

The evidence for a processing hierarchy is less clear for motor cortex, but the supplementary motor cortex is regarded as "higher" than the primary motor cortex [see Brinkman, 1984], and rostral M-I appears to process different information than the caudal M-I [Wise and Tanji, 1981; Strick and Preston, 1982]. In owl monkeys, both rostral M-I and supplementary motor area (SMA) have denser and more evenly distributed callosal connections than caudal M-I (Fig. 2). The frontal eye fields and premotor cortex also have dense and more evenly distributed callosal connections. Thus, from this limited evidence, it seems that for the motor as well as the somatosensory cortex, "higher-order" cortical areas have more widespread callosal connections.

Visual Sequences

In monkeys, the anatomical evidence for serial processing across subdivisions of the visual cortex is extensive [see Ungerleider and Mishkin, 1982; Maunsell and Van Essen, 1983; Kaas, 1985]. The main feedforward targets of the primary visual cortex (V-I or area 17) are area 18 (V-II) and the middle temporal field (MT) (Fig. 2). These two fields are the first steps in two relatively independent processing sequences [Weller et al., 1984; Kaas, 1985]. Area 18 projects to the dorsolateral field (DL), which then relays to inferotemporal cortex. In humans and monkeys, lesions of inferotemporal cortex interfere with the visual recognition of objects [Ungerleider and Mishkin, 1982]. MT projects densely to the superior temporal field (ST), which then relays to the posterior parietal and temporoparietal cortices [Weller et al., 1984], where lesions produce deficits that suggest that the area 17 to parietal cortex sequence is concerned with spatial localization and visual attention [Ungerleider and Mishkin, 1982].

When the interhemispheric connections of different areas of visual cortex in owl monkeys are compared, each area appears to have its own pattern (Figs. 2,6). In higher areas, connections are found in cortex representing vision well away from the vertical meridian, and while they are associated with the borders of area 17 and MT, they generally do not indicate all the borders of visual areas. Most areas of the extrastriate cortex, with the possible exceptions of dorsomedial (DM) and medial fields (M) [see also

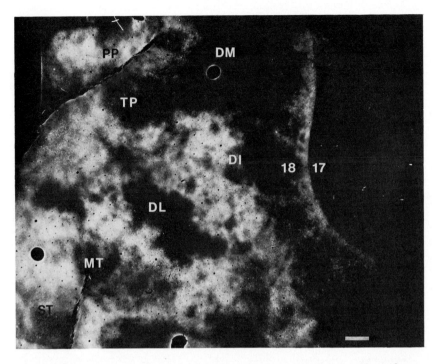

Fig. 6. Distribution of callosal connections in visual cortex of an owl monkey as seen in a darkfield photomicrograph of a single tangential section through flattened cortex. Abbreviations as in Figure 2. Note discontinuous patterns of label in extra-striate areas. Orientation as in previous figures. Scale = 1 mm.

Newsome and Allman, 1980], have at least some connections throughout the visual representation.

The total patterns of callosal connections of the two "second-level" areas in the processing hierarchy, area 18 and the MT, are similar in that large blocks of connections are present near the borders of the two areas where the vertical meridian is represented, and smaller semiperiodic patches are found throughout the fields (Figs. 4,6). The spacing of the smaller foci suggests an uneven distribution of functions and the existence of modular processing units within these fields. The distributions of callosal connections from parts of area 18 are also consistent with this view. In a squirrel monkey brain with injections of wheat germ agglutinin conjugated to HRP (WGA-HRP) in area 18, the contralateral label in area 18 appeared as semiregularly spaced bands (Fig. 7) that corresponded in location to the thin cytochrome oxidase bands [Livingstone and Hubel, 1984]. A similar pattern of connections in area 18 occurred after multiple injections of HRP into the

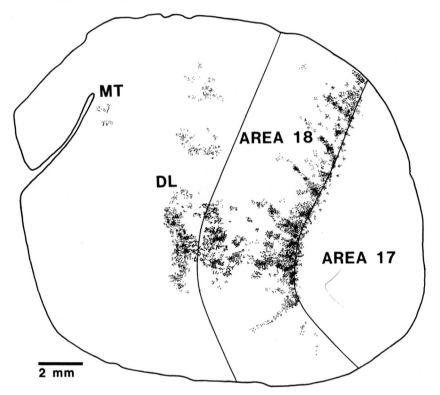

Fig. 7. Distribution of callosally transported anterograde label following a dorso-ventral row of WGA-HRP injections in area 18 of a squirrel monkey. Composite of several tangential sections of flattened cortex. Injections in the opposite hemisphere were largely centered in area 18 away from the 17–18 border, as indicated by displacement of the ipsilateral label into area 17. Callosally transported label was found in area 17 and 18, in a "DL"-like region, and in MT. Orientation as in previous figures.

visual cortex of one hemisphere in an infant macaque monkey [Cusick and Kaas, unpublished].

The callosal connections of areas further in the two parallel processing sequences are, in general, more widespread than for the first- and second-level processing stations. In the ventrally directed sequence, the dorsolateral field (DL) has more widespread connections than area 18. Surprisingly, the dorsal wing of DL has fewer callosal connections in a strip adjacent to the border with MT, where the vertical meridian is represented. In the dorsal sequence, connections of the ST region are more widespread and denser than in MT. However, none of the fields have completely even distributions of connections. In the third-level areas, DL and ST, for example, regions with dense connections generally show patches of terminations in layer IV and dense "columns" of terminations in the supragranular layers. Furthermore, each extrastriate visual area has regions with very dense and regions with very few connections. Thus, even a "higher-order" area such as posterior parietal cortex has zones with only sparse connections. An example of a "higher-order" area with very few connections is the dorsomedial area, DM. DM, like area 17, has callosal connections restricted to its rostral border, where the vertical meridian is represented, and most of the rest of the field has only a few scattered labeled cells.

The laminar patterns of callosal connections also relate to the cortical hierarchies. When the total pattern of callosal connections is considered, at least two, and possibly three, types of laminar patterns occur for the visual cortex in owl monkeys. Area 17 is the only area for which a feedforward pattern of cells and a feedback pattern of terminations has been identified. The cells appear to be exclusively in layer III, and the terminations are dense in layers I–III and VI and are especially concentrated in layer IIIB. In contrast, "higher-order" areas such as the DL and ST send a "feedback" projection from cells in layer V, in addition to cells in layer III, and receive a "feedforward" pattern of input including dense terminations in layer IV. Possibly an "intermediate" pattern of connections exists in the central MT and rostral area 18, where callosally projecting cells are chiefly in layer III, and the rather sparse inputs are mainly to the supragranular layers. In general, the laminar patterns of callosal connections in the first three stages of the two parallel cortical processing sequences correspond to the ipsilateral patterns that define the hierarchical sequences.

TOPOGRAPHIC PATTERNS OF CALLOSAL CONNECTIONS

When the callosal connections of identified portions of sensory and motor representations, rather than the total callosal pattern, are considered, three types of topographic patterns are apparent [see Kaas, '78]. One type relates matched location along the representations of the body midline or zero vertical meridian in the two cerebral hemispheres. These connections are truly homotopic in that they connect neurons with overlapping receptive fields. Direct evidence for such homotopic connections is largely limited to studies of projections of locations along the 17–18 border of cats and monkeys [Tigges et al., 1981; Segraves and Rosenquist, 1982]. In addition, callosal connections for matched sites along the outer border of the MT have been demonstrated [Wall et al., 1982; Maunsell and Van Essen, 1983; Weller et al., 1984], but interhemispheric connections for location along representations of the zero vertical meridian have not yet been demonstrated for other primate visual areas. Likewise, except for parts of S-I of cats [Manzoni et al., 1980] and squirrels [Gould and Kaas, 1980], callosal connections of locations along representation of the body midline have not been specifically determined. Given the clear evidence that cortical regions representing the zero meridian and the body midline have callosal connections, it seems reasonable to suppose that these connections are homotopic. Homotopic callosal connections presumably are functionally similar to local connections within fields, but because neurons with similar receptive field locations are sometimes in opposite hemispheres, interhemispheric connections are needed.

Many callosal connections are between mirror-symmetric locations in the two hemispheres that are not related to the body midline or zero vertical meridian. For example, central parts of MT project callosally to central parts of the MT in the other hemisphere [Spatz and Tigges, 1972; Maunsell and Van Essen, 1983; Wall et al., 1983; Weller et al., 1984]. These mirror-symmetric connections have also been called "homotopic," but they are not really homotopic since central MT on the other hemisphere represents paracentral vision of one hemifield while central MT of the other hemisphere represents paracentral vision of the opposite hemifield. Thus, these callosal connections are not retinotopically matched, are not homotopic, but are homoareal. Mirror-symmetric homoareal callosal connections have been demonstrated for several visual areas in cats [Segraves and Rosenquist, 1982] and for parts of S-I and S-II [Weller and Sur, 1981].

Homoareal callosal connections need not be exclusively mirror-symmetric. For example, injections of tracers made in area 17 away from the area 17–18 border in tree shrews [Sesma et al., 1984a] and rats [Miller and Vogt, 1984] results in dense label at the 17–18 border in the opposite hemisphere. Nonsymmetric homoareal callosal connections also appear to exist for area 18. In the squirrel monkey case shown in Figure 7, the injections were confined to a middle strip of area 18, and yet the callosal label extended caudally to the area 17 border. Thus, homoareal callosal connections may be both symmetric and nonsymmetric for the same field.

Callosal connections from one area to multiple areas in the opposite hemisphere have been demonstrated many times [see Tigges et al., 1981; Segraves and Rosenquist, 1982]. Such heteroareal callosal connections generally follow the same areal patterns as the strongest ipsilateral connections. For example, Figure 7 shows the callosal label in a squirrel monkey resulting from a dorsoventral row of injections of WGA-HRP in area 18. The ipsilateral connections were dense in DL and sparse in MT, and the contralateral connections were similarly dense in DL and sparse in MT. In addition, both ipsilateral and contralateral connections with area 17 were apparent. Thus, the obvious ipsilateral and contralateral cortical connections were with the same visual areas. As a consequence of this typical pattern, processing hierarchies are similarly associated in both the ipsilateral and contralateral hemispheres. Most callosal connections appear to be reciprocal and may follow the laminar patterns (feedforward or feedback) of ipsilateral connections, but such details are presently unknown. Heteroareal callosal connections may connect representations of the body midline or zero vertical meridian, and thereby may be somatotopic or retinotopic, or they may connect other parts of representations, and be nontopographic.

FUNCTIONAL IMPLICATIONS OF CALLOSAL PATTERNS

The complex and widespread patterns of interhemispheric connections, the species differences in patterns, and the different patterns in different areas all have functional implications. First, it is clear that all callosal connections cannot relate to bilateral "midline" receptive fields, such as those for neurons along the 17–18 border. The importance of such connections have been emphasized in the past, but we also need to understand the significance of other callosal connections in sensory fields. Some of these contribute to the large bilateral excitatory receptive fields in the inferotemporal cortex [Rocha-Miranda et al., 1975] and others contribute to the large bilateral antagonistic surrounds of neurons in V-4 (DL) and MT [Moran et al., 1983; Allman, 1985]. Given the callosal patterns of connections, it seems likely that most representations outside the primary sensory fields will have neurons likes those in V-4 and MT with large antagonistic surrounds [see Allman, 1985]. Second, given the uneven distributions of callosal connections within fields, it is likely that functions are unevenly distributed in fields, that fields have some sort of modular organization, and that callosally mediated functions are concentrated in some modules. Possibly some of the subsystems within sensory areas have more callosally mediated functions than others. For example, three types of inputs appear to be related to area 17 of primates over relatively segregated pathways, the X, Y, and W systems [see Norton and Casagrande, 1982; Stone, 1983; Kaas, 1985]. The W-cell system appears to be associated with patchlike regions in area 17 that are revealed by reactions for cytochrome oxidase [see Weber et al., 1983], and in galagos, at least, callosal connections are concentrated in these patches. These patches project ipsilaterally to thin bands of dense cytochrome oxidase in area 18 [Livingstone and Hubel, 1984] and these bands have concentrations of callosal connections. Thus, the W-cell system may be more involved in callosal functions in both areas 17 and 18. The uneven distributions of callosal and other connections have often been referred to as "columnar," but concentrations of callosal label are quite variable in shape from area to area, and this suggests that areas vary in the shapes of the modules they contain. Third, the general increase in the distribution and amount of callosal connections over the first three cortical processing stations in the visual and somatosensory systems of primates suggests that callosal projections favor the transfer of more processed information. In more generalized mammals with fewer sensory representations, it may not be possible to delay such transfer, and thus the primary and secondary fields have more extensive callosal connections.

REFERENCES

Allman J, Miezin F, McGuiness E (1985): Stimulus specific responses from beyond the classical receptive field: Neurophysiological mechanisms for local-global comparisons in visual neurons. Ann Rev Neurosci 8:407–430.

Brinkman C (1984): Supplementary motor area of the monkey's cerebral cortex: Short- and long-term deficits after unilateral ablation and the effects of subsequent callosal section. J Neurosci 4:918–929.

Cusick CG et al. (1984): Interhemispheric connections of visual cortex of owl monkeys (*Aotus trivirgatus*), marmosets (*Callithrix jacchus*) and galagos (*Galago crassicaudatus*). J Comp Neurol 230:311–336.

Cusick CG et al. (1985): Interhemispheric connections of cortical sensory areas in tree shrews. J Comp Neurol 235:111–128.

Cusick CG, Lund RD (1982): Modification of visual callosal projections in rats. J Comp Neurol 212:385–398.

Ebner FF (1969): A comparison of primitive forebrain organization in metatherian and eutherian mammals. Ann NY Acad Sci 167:241–257.

Ebner FF, Myers RE (1965): Distribution of corpus callosum and anterior commissure in cat and raccoon. J Comp Neurol 124:353–366.

Gould HJ, III (1984): Interhemispheric connections of the visual cortex in the grey squirrel (*Sciurus carolinensis*). J Comp Neurol 223:259–301.

Gould HJ, III, Cusick CG, Pons TP, Kaas JH (1983): The relation of callosal connections to microstimulation maps of precentral motor cortex. Soc Neurosci Abstr 9:309.

Gould HJ, III, Kaas JH (1981): The distribution of commissural terminations in somatosensory areas I and II of the grey squirrel. J Comp Neurol 196:489–504.

Kaas JH (1978): Subdivisions and interconnections of the primate visual system. In Cool SJ, Smith EL, III (eds): "Frontiers in Visual Science." Springer Series in Optical Science. New York: Springer Verlag, pp 557–563.

Kaas JH (1982): The segregation of function in the nervous system: Why do sensory systems have so many subdivisions? In Neff WP (ed): "Contributions to Sensory Physiology." New York: Academic Press, Vol 7, pp 201–240.

Kaas JH (1983): What, if anything, is S-I? The organization of the "first somatosensory area" of cortex. Physiol Rev 63:206–231.

Kaas JH (1985): The structural basis for information processing in the primate visual system. In Pettigrew JD et al. (eds): "Visual Neuroscience." Cambridge, MA: Cambridge University Press, in press.

Killackey HP, Gould HJ, III, Cusick CG, Pons TP, Kaas JH (1983): The relationship of corpus callosum connections to architectonic fields and body surface maps in sensorimotor cortex of New and Old World monkeys. J Comp Neurol 219:384–419.

Livingstone MS, Hubel DH (1984): Anatomy and physiology of a color system in the primate visual cortex. J Neurosci 4:309–356.

Manzoni F et al. (1980): Callosal projections from the two body midlines. Exp Brain Res 39:1–9.

Maunsell JHR, Van Essen DC (1983): The connections of the middle temporal visual area (MT) and their relationship to a cortical hierarchy in the macaque monkey. J Neurosci 3:2563–2586.

Miller MW, Vogt BA (1984): Heterotopic and homotopic callosal connections in rat visual cortex. Brain Res 197:75–89.

Moran J, Desimone, R, Schein SJ, Miskin M (1983): Suppression from ipsilateral visual field in Area V4 of the macaque. Soc Neurosci Abstr 9:57.

Mountcastle VB (1984): Central nervous mechanisms in mechanoreceptive sensibility. In: "Handbook of Physiology—The Nervous System III." American Physiological Society, Bethesda, Maryland, pp 789–878.

Myers RE (1962): Commissural connections between occipital lobes of the monkey. J Comp Neurol 118:1–16.

Myers RE, Sperry RW (1953): Interocular transfer of a visual form discrimination in cats after section of the optic chiasma and corpus callosum. Anat Rec 115:351–352.

Newsome WT, Allman JM (1980): Interhemispheric connections of visual cortex in the owl monkey *(Aotus trivirgatus)*, and the bushbaby *(Galago crassicaudatus)*. J Comp Neurol 194:209–233.

Norton TT, Casagrande VA (1982): Laminar organization of receptive field properties in the lateral geniculate nucleus of bushbaby *(Galago crassicaudatus)*. J Neurophysiol 47:714–741.

Pubols BH, Jr, Pubols LM, DiPettc DJ, Sheely JC (1976): Opossum somatic sensory cortex: A microelectrode mapping study. J Comp Neurol 165:229–246.

Rocha-Miranda CE, Bender DB, Gross CG, Mishkin M (1975): Visual activation of neurons in inferotemporal cortex depends on striate cortex and forebrain commissures. J Neurophysiol 38:474–491.

Segraves MA, Rosenquist AC (1982): The afferent and efferent callosal connections of retinotopically defined areas in cat cortex. J Neurosci 2:1090–1107.

Sesma MA Casagrande VA, Kaas JH (1984a): Connections of striate cortex projection zone, Area TD, in tree shrews. Soc Neurosci Abstr 10:933.

Sesma MA, Casagrande VA, Kaas JH (1984b): Cortical connections of Area 17 in tree shrews. J Comp Neurol 230:337–351.

Spatz WB, Kunz B (1984): Area 17 of anthropoid primates does participate in visual callosal connections. Neurosci Lett 48:49–53.

Spatz WB, Tigges J (1972): Experimental-anatomical studies on the "Middle Temporal Visual Area (MT)" in primates: I. Efferent corticocortical connections in the marmoset, *Callithrix jacchus*. J Comp Neurol 146:451–461.

Stone J (1983): "Parallel Processing in the Visual System." New York: Plenum Press.

Strick PL, Preston JB (1982): Two representations of the hand in area 4 of a primate. II. Somatosensory input organization. J Neurophysiol 48:139–149.

Tigges J, Tigges M, Anschel S, Cross NA, Letbetter WD, McBride RL (1981): Areal and laminar distribution of neurons interconnecting the central visual cortical areas 17, 18, 19, and MT in squirrel monkey *(Saimiri)*. J Comp Neurol 202:539–560.

Ungerleider LG, Mishkin M (1982): Two cortical visual systems. In Ingle et al. (eds): "Analysis of Visual Behavior." Cambridge, MA: MIT Press, pp 549–586.

Wall JT, Symonds LL, Kaas JH (1982): Cortical and subcortical projections of the middle temporal area (MT) and adjacent cortex in galagos. J Comp Neurol 211:193–214.

Weber JT, Huerta MF, Kaas JH, Harting JK (1983): The projections of the lateral geniculate nucleus of the squirrel monkey: Studies of the interlaminar zones and the S layers. J Comp Neurol 213:135–145.

Weller RE, Sur M (1981): Some connections of S-I and S-II in the tree shrew, *Tupaia glis*. Anat Rec 199:271A.

Weller RE, Wall JT, Kaas JH (1984): Cortical connections of the middle temporal area (MT) and the superior temporal cortex in owl monkeys. J Comp Neurol 228:81–104.

Weyand TG, Swadlow HA (1980): Interhemispheric striate projections in the prosimian primate, *Galago senegalensis*. Brain Behav Evol 17:473–477.

Wise SP, Tanji J (1981): Supplementary and precentral motor cortex: Contrast in responsiveness to peripheral input in the hindlimb area of the unanesthetized monkey. J Comp Neurol 195:433–451.

Zant D, Strick PL (1978): The cells of origin of interhemispheric connections in the primate motor cortex. Soc Neurosci Abstr 4:308.

Two Hemispheres—One Brain:
Functions of the Corpus Callosum, pages 103–115
© 1986 Alan R. Liss, Inc.

Topography of Cortico-Cortical Connections Related to Tonotopic and Binaural Maps of Cat Auditory Cortex

THOMAS J. IMIG, RICHARD A. REALE, JOHN F. BRUGGE,
ANNE MOREL, AND HUGO O. ADRIAN
*Department of Physiology, Kansas University Medical Center, Kansas City,
Kansas 66103 (T.J.I., A.M.); Department of Neurophysiology, University of
Wisconsin Medical School, Madison, Wisconsin 53706 (R.A.R., J.F.B.);
Department of Physiology and Biophysics, University of Chile, Santiago,
Chile (H.O.A.)*

The cat auditory cortex is a terminus for two major fiber systems. Thalamocortical fibers represent the final link in the synaptic chain connecting the ears with the cerebral cortex. The topographic organization of projections from the tonotopically organized auditory thalamus (ventral nucleus and lateral portion of the posterior group of thalamic nuclei) imposes tonotopic and presumably binaural [Middlebrooks and Zook, 1983] maps upon the auditory cortex. A second system consists of cortical neurons whose axons terminate within the cortex, and these cortico-cortical connections serve to interconnect different areas of the auditory cortex. This report summarizes some features of the topographic organization of auditory cortico-cortical connections in relation to tonotopic and binaural cortical maps in the cat.

Physiological evidence supporting the existence of multiple tonotopic representations within the cat's cerebral cortex has been available for over four decades [Woolsey, 1960,1961]. During the past few years, detailed microelectrode maps of the distribution of neurons' best frequencies in the cortex occupying the exposed gyral surfaces and sulcal walls [Merzenich et al., 1975; Knight, 1977; Reale and Imig, 1980] provide evidence for at least four tonotopically organized fields (A, AI, P, and VP; Fig. 1A). Moving from rostral to caudoventral along the crescent of tissue that the four fields

This work was performed at University of Wisconsin Medical School and Kansas University Medical School.

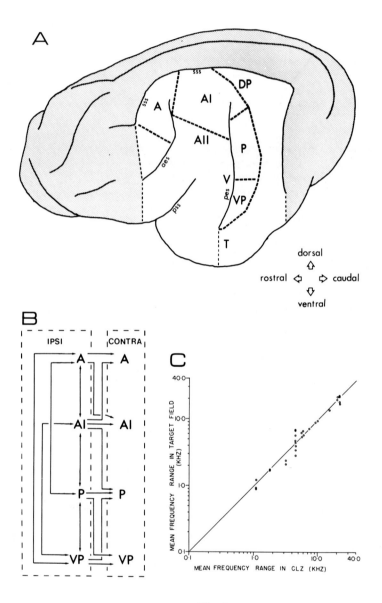

Fig. 1

occupy, best frequencies progress from low-to-high in field A, from high-to-low in field AI, from low-to-high in field P, and from high-to-low in field VP. Borders between the four fields are located in regions where best frequency gradients show reversals. Surrounding the four fields is a belt of cortex containing neurons responsive to acoustic stimulation (e.g., DP, T, V, AII, Fig. 1A). There is some evidence for tonotopic organization within this belt [Woolsey, 1961; Reale and Imig, 1980; Volkov, 1980], although the pattern of tonotopy has not been described in detail.

A complex network of cortico-cortical pathways interconnects various parts of the cat auditory cortex [Diamond et al., 1968a,b; Heath and Jones, 1971; Kawamura, 1973; Paula-Barbosa et al., 1975]. By combining autoradiographic tracing of cortico-cortical pathways using tritiated amino acids, and electrophysiological best frequency mapping in the same brain, it has been possible to closely relate the organization of cortico-cortical pathways to tonotopic maps [Imig and Reale, 1980].

A summary of the known connections between fields A, AI, P, and VP appears in Figure 1B. Each of the four fields is reciprocally connected with the other three located in the same hemisphere (IPSI). Additionally, neurons in each field project to the contralateral hemisphere (CONTRA). Projections have been found from field A to contralateral fields A and AI, from field AI to contralateral fields A, AI, and P, and from each of fields P and VP to both of these fields in the contralateral hemisphere.

Similar portions of the frequency representations in the four fields are interconnected, dissimilar portions are not. A comparison of the range of best frequencies in the heavily labeled region surrounding the site of injection of radioactive amino acid with the range of best frequencies within the region of a target field containing radioactively labeled axon terminals is graphically illustrated in Figure 1C. Each point represents a projection from an injection site to a target field, and these data include both ipsilateral and contralateral cortico-cortical connections between the four tonotopic fields. The abscissa shows the geometric mean of the range of best

---

Fig. 1. Connections among tonotopic auditory cortical fields. A. A lateral view of the left cerebral hemisphere showing the positions of four tonotopically organized fields A, AI, P, and VP [from Imig and Reale, 1980]. B. Pathways interconnecting tonotopic fields are diagrammatically illustrated. All known pathways originating in the fields of one hemisphere (IPSI) are indicated. An arrow represents a pathway originating in one field and terminating in another. This diagram summarizes findings of Imig and Reale [1980] and unpublished results from Imig and Morel [1983] (reproduced, with permission, from the Annual Review of Neuroscience Volume 6, © 1983 by Annual Reviews Inc.). C. Relationship between the geometric mean of best frequencies represented in the dense area of labeling (CLZ) surrounding the site of tritiated amino acid injection (abscissa), and the geometric mean of the range of best frequencies represented in labeled regions of target fields (ordinate) for projections among fields A, AI, P, and VP [from Imig and Reale, 1980].

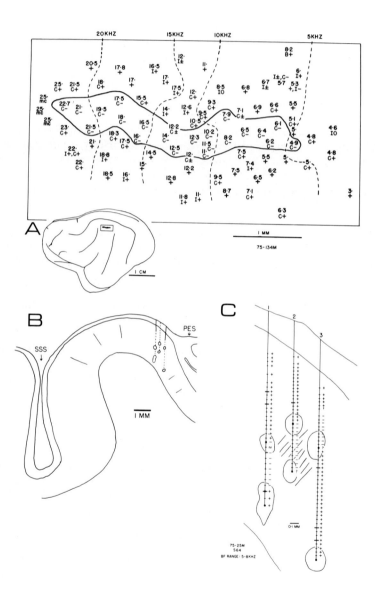

Fig. 2

frequencies represented in the heavily labeled region surrounding the injection site, and the ordinate shows the geometric mean of the range of best frequencies represented in areas of radioactive axon terminal labeling in target fields. Points cluster about the diagonal of the graph indicating that cortico-cortical projections specifically interconnect similar portions of the best frequency representations of the four fields in both hemispheres.

In addition to a tonotopic organization, there is a binaural organization within the high frequency representation of auditory cortex. Most neurons within field AI are sensitive to binaural stimulation [e.g., Hall et al., 1968; Brugge et al., 1969; Kitzes et al., 1980; Phillips and Irvine, 1983], reflecting bilateral convergence of input from the two ears, which occurs initially on auditory brainstem neurons. The most commonly encountered binaural interaction is one in which the response to binaural stimulation is greater than the response to stimulation of either ear alone at the same frequency and sound pressure levels. Such a binaural interaction is referred to as summation [Imig and Adrian, 1977] or as excitatory-excitatory [Middlebrooks et al., 1980]. Other neurons are excited predominantly by stimulation of the contralateral ear, while simultaneous stimulation of both ears at appropriate sound pressure levels is less effective than stimulation of the contralateral ear alone. This type of binaural interaction is referred to as suppression [Imig and Adrian, 1977] or excitatory-inhibitory [Middlebrooks et al., 1980]. A small percentage of neurons display other characteristics.

Neurons displaying similar binaural interactions are often encountered by electrodes oriented perpendicular to the cortical surface. On the other hand, nonperpendicular penetrations generally pass from a zone in which neurons display one type of binaural interaction to a zone in which neurons display a different interaction. The locations of three nonperpendicular electrode penetrations in AI and the distribution of summation (+) and suppression (−) responses encountered along the three penetrations are

Fig. 2. Organization of binaural columns in AI. A. Topography of a suppression column in AI. The hemisphere drawing shows the portion of the auditory cortex that was mapped. Best frequencies and binaural interactions are indicated for each penetration into the cortex. Interrupted lines indicate isofrequency contours. The continuous line surrounds a band in which only suppression (C−) responses were encountered. With the exception of monaural contralateral (mc) responses at the rostral end of the suppression band, most responses in the surrounding region display summation (i.e., +, I+, C+, B+). B, C. Sequences of binaural interactions encountered along three electrode penetrations into AI. Lines near the marking lesions in C indicate the orientation of radial-cell columns. Each depth at which a binaural interaction was assessed is marked by a horizontal bar. Heavy bars indicate locations at which single neurons were studied. Filled circles indicate the positions of marking lesions whose outlines are also shown. With few exceptions, the electrode was advanced 50 μm between successive measurements. PES, posterior ectosylvian sulcus; SSS, suprasylvian sulcus; BF, best frequency; +, summation; −, suppression [from Imig and Adrian, 1977].

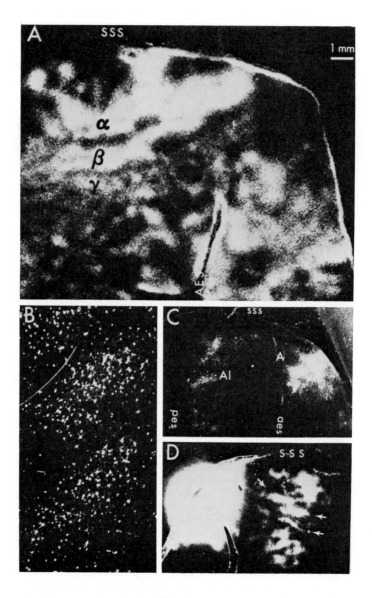

Fig. 3

illustrated in Figure 2B and C, respectively. Each of the three penetrations initially passes through a zone in which neurons display summation into a zone in which neurons display suppression. Two of the penetrations extend further into a second summation zone. Marking lesions placed between sequences of summation and supression responses indicate that the borders between zones containing neurons with different binaural properties are aligned parallel to radial cell columns (indicated by oblique lines). Zones in which neurons display similar binaural responses are referred to as binaural columns. In this experiment, penetrations 1 and 3 passed entirely through a suppression column, which is flanked on both sides by summation columns.

Binaural columns occupy patches or bands of cortex elongated parallel to the frequency gradient in AI [Imig and Adrian, 1977; Imig and Brugge, 1978; Imig and Reale, 1981; Middlebrooks et al., 1980]. A map of the distributions of best frequencies and binaural interactions encountered in many perpendicular electrode penetrations into AI of one brain is illustrated in Figure 2A. Best frequencies in the mapped region range between 3 kHz caudally and 25 kHz rostrally. Neurons displaying suppression responses (indicated by C −) occupy a rostrocaudally oriented strip of cortex. The long axis of the strip is oriented orthogonal to isofrequency contours (indicated by interrupted lines). The strip is about 4 mm long and roughly 0.5 mm in width. Most neurons surrounding the suppression strip display summation, with the exception of monaural contralateral neurons found in three penetrations at the rostral end of the strip (mc, Fig. 2A). Monaural contralateral neurons discharge to stimulation of the contralateral ear and exhibit neither excitation nor inhibition to stimulation of the ipsilateral ear. Bands of summation and suppression neurons alternate across the dorsoventral extent of AI, and at least three bands of each type can been seen in the most complete maps [Imig and Brugge, 1978; Middlebrooks et al., 1980; Imig and Reale, 1981]. Bands are somewhat irregular in shape, running for various distances across the high-frequency representation.

Fig. 3. Topographic patterns of cortico-cortical connections seen in tissue sections cut parallel to the flattened cortical surface of AI. A. Distribution of callosal axon terminals labeled by injecting tritiated proline at multiple sites in the auditory cortex of the left hemisphere [from Imig and Brugge, 1978]. B. Distribution of labeled callosal cell bodies and callosal axon terminals in layer III of AI of the right hemisphere resulting from injections of HRP into three sites in AI of the left hemisphere [from Imig et al., 1982]. C. Distribution of callosal axon terminals in fields A and AI of the right hemisphere resulting from injection of tritiated proline at one site in field A of the left hemisphere [from Imig and Reale, 1980]. D. Distribution of labeled axon terminals in AI resulting from a single injection of tritiated proline into field A [from Imig and Reale, 1980]. sss, suprasylvian sulcus; pes, posterior ectosylvian sulcus; aes, anterior ectosylvian sulcus.

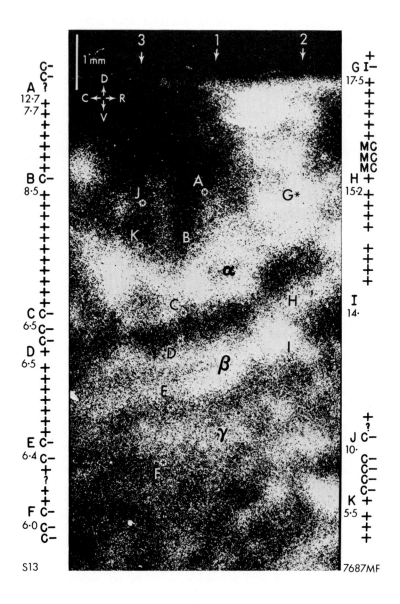

Fig. 4

Axon terminals of callosal projections to field AI occupy patches of the cortex that are elongated in the direction of the low-to-high best-frequency gradient. In tissue sections cut parallel to the flattened cortical surface, this pattern of labeling is particularly apparent (Fig. 3). Aggregates of callosal axon terminals, labeled by injections of tritiated proline at multiple sites in the auditory cortex of the opposite hemisphere, form two irregularly shaped, rostrocaudally elongated bands (α and β, Fig. 3A) that are separated from each other by a more sparsely labeled band. The two bands join together rostrally. Callosal projections originating in both fields A (Fig. 3C) and AI (Fig. 3B) occupy elongated bands in field AI. That this pattern is not an artifact resulting from nonuniform labeling of callosal axon terminals by the multiple injections is suggested by two observations. First, rostrocaudally elongated bands of degenerating axon terminals are seen following section of the corpus callosum, similar to the pattern of callosal axon terminals labeled by injections. Second, single injections of tracers into field A (e.g., Fig. 3C) or field AI [Imig and Brugge, 1978; Imig and Reale, 1980; Imig et al., 1981] produce multiple patches of labeled callosal terminals in AI of the opposite hemisphere that are elongated in a caudal-to-rostral direction.

Experiments in which labeling of cortico-cortical projections is combined with mapping of binaural columns in the same brain reveal a close correspondence between the patterns of cortico-cortical projections and binaural columns within the high-frequency representation of AI. The pattern of callosal terminal labeling in relationship to a map of binaural responses appears in Figure 4. Lesions (A–K) are placed along three electrode penetrations and are used as reference points to align the binaural map with the pattern of labeling. Within densely labeled regions, summation (+) responses are almost invariably encountered. Within the upper densely labeled band (α), i.e., between lesions A and C, dorsal to the monaural contralateral (MC) responses encountered near lesion H, and ventral to lesion K, most neurons display summation. Two electrode penetrations pass through a second band of labeling (β). Between lesions D and E, and between lesions H and I, all neurons exhibit summation. Finally, one penetration passes through a third region of somewhat more dense callosal terminal

---

Fig. 4. Relationship between binaural columns and pattern of callosal terminal labeling in an autoradiograph of a tissue section cut parallel to the flattened surface of AI. This tissue section is also illustrated in Figure 3A. Following injection of tritiated proline in the left hemisphere, responses of neurons were studied at 100-μm intervals along penetrations oriented parallel to the cortical laminae in AI of the right hemisphere. The locations of marking lesions (labeled A through K) placed along three electrode penetrations (labeled 1, 2, and 3) are shown in both the autoradiograph and in the sequences of binaural response symbols. Best frequencies (in kHz) obtained at points where lesions were placed are indicated beneath letters in the symbol sequence [from Imig and Brugge, 1978].

labeling (between lesions E and F), and here summation responses are also found. On the other hand, within regions containing sparse callosal terminations, either suppression or monaural contralateral responses are encountered. Above the α band of labeling, between lesions J and K, suppression (C−) responses are found. More ventrally, two penetrations pass through a sparsely labeled band (between α and β). Suppression responses are found between lesions C and D; and above lesion H, contralateral monaural (MC) responses are encountered. Suppression responses are also found in the more sparsely labeled regions more ventrally (near lesions E and F).

The greatest density of callosal neurons and their axon terminals is found in layer III. The distribution of callosal axon terminals in layer III of AI covaries with the distribution of neurons giving rise to callosal axons, i.e., areas containing high concentrations of callosal axon terminals also contain high concentrations of callosal neurons (Fig. 3B) [Imig et al., 1982]. This observation suggests that the distribution of callosal cell bodies bears the same relationship to the binaural map as the distribution of callosal axon terminals, and experiments combining HRP labeling of callosal neurons and binaural mapping provide confirmation that this is the case [Imig and Brugge, 1978].

Axon terminals of projections from fields A and P to field AI in the same hemisphere often form rostrocaudally elongated bands in AI similar to those formed by callosal projections [Imig and Reale, 1980]. This pattern is related to the binaural map [Imig and Reale, 1981]. The pattern of labeling in AI illustrated in Figure 3D is the result of a single injection of tritiated amino acid in field A. Four of the most prominent patches of dense labeling in AI of this experiment are illustrated in Figure 5, along with the binaural responses of neurons encountered during eight tangential electrode penetrations in the same brain. Marking lesions placed within each penetration are used to align the binaural responses with the pattern of labeling. Summation responses are indicated by open circles and suppression responses are indicated by filled circles. Suppression responses are generally found in areas of dense terminal labeling; summation responses in areas of sparse terminal labeling. This is just opposite to the relationship between summation and suppression responses, and the density of callosal labeling. These findings suggest that there exists within a contiguous territory in field A a population of neurons whose axons provide more dense innervation to suppression columns than to summation columns. Other experiments in which tritiated amino acid was injected into field A reveal more complex relationships between the pattern of terminal labeling and the binaural map in AI. In each experiment, suppression columns correspond with dense labeling, and summation columns correspond with sparse labeling in only a portion of AI. In other regions of AI, however, there is no obvious relationship between the density of labeling in AI and binaural organization. One interpretation of these results is that there may be a territory in field A

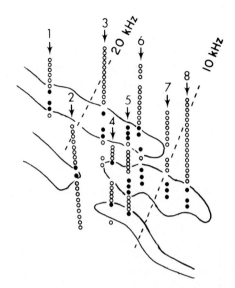

Fig. 5. Relationship of binaural columns to the pattern of axon terminal labeling in AI resulting from an injection of tritiated proline into ipsilateral field A. Outlines of patches of heavy labeling in Figure 3D are represented by continous lines. Binaural responses of neurons were studied along eight penetrations directed tangentially through the cortex. The orientation of the penetrations is indicated by the arrows. Interrupted lines indicate 10- and 20-kHz isofrequency contours. Filled circles represent suppression responses, open circles represent summation responses. Suppression responses are found in more densely labeled regions than those in which summation responses are found [from Imig and Reale, 1981].

containing neurons whose projections are systematically related to the binaural map in AI, and this territory is flanked by one or more territories containing neurons whose projections bear a different relationship to the binaural map.

The directional sensitivities of neurons in the high-frequency representation in field AI of the cat auditory cortex have recently been described [Middlebrooks and Pettigrew, 1981]. Two classes of units, hemifield and axial, have directional sensitivities restricted to contralateral sound space. Omnidirectional units, on the other hand, respond to sound regardless of its direction. Middlebrooks and Pettigrew suggest that axial and hemifield units correspond to units that display suppression (excitatory-inhibitory binaural interactions), and that omnidirectional units may correspond to units that display summation (excitatory-excitatory interactions). If so, then areas of sparse callosal connections appear to correspond to cortical areas devoted solely to the representation of contralateral sound space, whereas areas of dense callosal connections correspond to regions in which neurons are nonselective for sound direction. Sparse callosal connectivity of the representation of contralateral sound space parallels the lack of callosal connections with the representation of the peripheral visual field in the visual cortex, and portions of the representation of distal body parts in the somatosensory cortex as described in other chapters in this volume.

REFERENCES

Brugge JF, Dubrovsky NA, Aitkin LM, Andersen DJ (1969): Sensitivity of single neurons in auditory cortex of cat to binaural tonal stimulation: Effects of varying interaural time and intensity. J Neurophysiol 32:1005–1024.

Diamond IT, Jones EG, Powell TPS (1968a): Interhemispheric fiber connections of the auditory cortex of the cat. Brain Res 11:177–193.

Diamond IT, Jones EG, Powell TPS (1968b): The association connections of the auditory cortex of the cat. Brain Res 11:560–579.

Hall JL, Goldstein MH (1968): Representation of binaural stimuli by single units in primary auditory cortex of unanesthetized cats. J Acoust Soc Am 43:456–461.

Heath CJ, Jones EG (1971): The anatomical organization of the suprasylvian gyrus of the cat. Ergeb Anat Entwicklung Gesch 45:1–64.

Imig TJ, Adrian HO (1977): Binaural columns in the primary field (AI) of cat auditory cortex. Brain Res 138:241–257.

Imig TJ, Brugge JF (1978): Sources and terminations of callosal axons related to binaural and frequency maps in primary auditory cortex of the cat. J Comp Neurol 182:637–660.

Imig TJ, Morel A (1983): Organization of the thalamocortical auditory system in the cat. Ann Rev Neurosci 6:95–120.

Imig TJ, Morel A, Kauer CD (1982): Covariation of distributions of callosal cell bodies and callosal axon terminals in layer III of cat primary auditory cortex. Brain Res 251:157–159.

Imig TJ, Reale RA (1980): Patterns of cortico-cortical connections related to tonotopic maps in cat auditory cortex. J Comp Neurol 192:293–332.

Imig TJ, Reale RA (1981): Ipsilateral cortico-cortical projections related to binaural columns in cat primary auditory cortex. J Comp Neurol 203:1–14.

Kawamura K (1973): Corticocortical fiber connections of the cat cerebrum. I. The temporal region. Brain Res 51:1–21.

Kitzes LM, Wrege KS, Cassady JM (1980): Patterns of responses of cortical cells to binaural stimulation. J Comp Neurol 192:455–472.

Knight PL (1977): Representation of the cochlea within the anterior auditory field (AAF) of the cat. Brain Res 130:447–467.

Merzenich MM, Knight PL, Roth GL (1975): Representation of the cochlea within primary auditory cortex in the cat. J Neurophysiol 38:231–249.

Middlebrooks JC, Dykes RW, Merzenich MM (1980): Binaural response-specific bands in primary auditory cortex (AI) of the cat: Topographical organization orthogonal to isofrequency contours. Brain Res 181:31–48.

Middlebrooks JC, Pettigrew JD (1981): Functional classes of neurons in primary auditory cortex of the cat distinguished by sensitivity to sound location. J Neurosci 1:107–120.

Middlebrooks JC, Zook JM (1983): Intrinsic organization of the cat's medial geniculate body identified by projections to binaural response-specific bands in the primary auditory cortex. J Neurosci 3:203–224.

Paula-Barbosa MM, Feyo PB, Sousa-Pinto A (1975): The association connections of the suprasylvian fringe (SF) and other areas of the cat auditory cortex. Exp Brain Res 23:535–554.

Phillips DP, Irvine DRF (1983): Some features of binaural input to single neurons in physiologically defined AI of cat cerebral cortex. J Neurophysiol 49:383–395.

Reale RA, Imig TJ (1980): Tonotopic organization of auditory cortex in the cat. J Comp Neurol 192:265–291.

Volkov IO (1980): The cochleotopic organization of the cat second auditory cortex. Neirofiziologiya 12:18–26 (in Russian).

Woolsey CN (1960): Organization of cortical auditory system: A review and a synthesis. In Rasmussen GL, Windle, WF (eds): "Neural Mechanisms of the Auditory and Vestibular Systems." Springfield: Charles C. Thomas, pp 165–180.

Woolsey CN (1961): Organization of the cortical auditory system. In Rosenblith WA (ed): "Sensory Communication." Cambridge: The MIT Press, pp 235–257.

Two Hemispheres—One Brain:
Functions of the Corpus Callosum, pages 117–137
© 1986 Alan R. Liss, Inc.

Wires of the Mind: Anatomical Variation in the Corpus Callosum in Relation to Hemispheric Specialization and Integration

SANDRA F. WITELSON

*Departments of Psychiatry, Psychology, and Neurosciences, McMaster
University, Hamilton, Ontario, L8N 3Z5, Canada*

INTRODUCTION

Functional differentiation of the two hemispheres of the human brain is now a well established fact, although it was only in the mid-19th century that Marc Dax and then Paul Broca noted the relationship between right-sided hemiplegia and speech difficulties and recorded their seminal inference that the left hemisphere must play some special role in speech and language functions. It was recorded over 2,000 years ago that forms of speech loss or aphasia followed brain damage, but no inference about neural localization was made [see Benton, 1964]. Such 18th century writers as Benjamin Rush and Franz Joseph Gall, and later, A.L. Wigan [1884] began to focus attention on the existence of the two hemispheres in subserving mind and consciousness, but they conceptualized them as having duplicate functions [see Harrington, 1985]. Even Morgagni, who did extensive human neuropathological study correlated with disease symptoms in the mid-18th century, apparently did not deduce the concept of cerebral dominance. In this historical context, the insight that led to the concept of functional asymmetry seems even more remarkable. Now books by the dozens [e.g., Beaumont, 1982; Bryden, 1982; Bradshaw and Nettleton, 1983; Corballis, 1983; Corballis and Beale, 1983; Hellige, 1983; Perecman, 1983; Young, 1983 Geschwind and Galaburda, 1984; Heilman and Valenstein, 1985; Kolb and Whishaw, 1985, in just the last few years] and journal articles by the thousands attest to the phenomenon of cerebral dominance and to the extensive attention given it.

More recently, however, a movement against this intense focus on hemispheric differences, the concept of hemisphericity, and the implicit assumption of a separateness in the function of the hemispheres has arisen. The concept of integrated functioning of the two hemispheres within one brain has gained prominence—not the earlier notion of an undifferentiated homogeneous organ, but one of an integrated system of functionally distinct regions or modules within and between hemispheres [see e.g., Dimond, 1972; Gazzaniga and Ledoux, 1978; Best, 1985].

The observation of the behavioral consequences of sectioning the interhemispheric commissures has underlined not only the functional specialization of the hemispheres but also the importance of the integration of their functioning in the intact brain. The remarkable and dramatic isolation phenomena that can be demonstrated in artificial laboratory situations in split-brain individuals are well known. These phenomena clearly indicate that the mental processing of lateralized input, which is predominantly transmitted to only one hemisphere, is, in commissurotomized individuals, unavailable to and therefore cannot be acted upon by the other hemisphere [Sperry, 1974]. Also of particular relevance here are the less obvious and less well understood deficits in these patients in mnemonic functions, in regulatory and arousal factors for perception and cognition, in perseverence, and in mental capacity [Sperry, 1974; Levy, 1985]. These deficits in commissurotomized individuals led not only to the issue of a united versus a divided brain, but also to the issue of the unity of mind versus a divided mind or two streams of consciousness, as initially presented by Sperry [e.g., Sperry, 1966] and further considered by cognitive philosophers [e.g., Marks, 1981].

The main structure directly connecting the cortex of the two hemispheres is the corpus callosum. This structure has an interesting history of hypothesized function or lack thereof [see Colonnier, this volume; Ettlinger et al., 1965; Russell and Russell, 1979]. The early clinical reports of individuals with forebrain commissurotomy indicated no behavioral or cognitive deficits [Akelaitis, 1944]. Interestingly, the Zeitgeist in the early sixties may have facilitated the recognition of the functional role of the callosum. Two reports appeared almost simultaneously that described hemispheric isolation phenomena and clearly attributed behavioral and cognitive functions to the forebrain commissures. These reports were based on two patients, operated on and tested psychologically within months of each other, on opposite sides of the American continent. One patient (W.J.) in Los Angeles underwent a single-staged complete commissurotomy for the relief of intractable epilepsy in February, 1962 [Gazzaniga et al., 1962]. The other patient (P.J.K.) in Boston underwent surgery for removal of a tumor in the left frontal lobe in March, 1961. Postmortem examination of P.J.K. in June, 1962 revealed marked thinning of at least the anterior callosum [Geschwind and Kaplan, 1962]. The study of P.J.K. resulted in Geschwind's (1965) seminal papers describing the disconnexion syndrome, the phenomenon of behavioral deficits resulting from lesions of cortico-cortical connexions. The psychological studies of the series of patients who underwent therapeutic commissurotomy following W. J., led to a clearer understanding of the specialized cognitive functions and limitations of each hemisphere, and to consideration of the "unity of mind" in relation to neurobiological findings by Sperry and colleagues.

CORPUS CALLOSUM AND HAND PREFERENCE

The callosum is obviously important for the integrated functioning of the two hemispheres. It may also play a role in functional specialization of the hemispheres—perhaps in maintaining the functional asymmetry that appears to be present from birth [Witelson, 1985a]. There are individual differences in the pattern of hemispheric functional specialization, particularly for right versus left handers [Bryden, 1982]. Moreover, the hemispheres show anatomical right-left asymmetry in gyral and sulcal morphology, such as a greater expanse of the posterior part of the superior temporal gyrus, a wider breadth of the occipital lobe, and a longer, more horizontally positioned Sylvian fissure on the left [see reviews in Witelson, 1977a, 1985b]. These morphological asymmetries are beginning to be documented as a physical substrate of functional asymmetry [Witelson, 1983]. In this context, and as part of a larger study attempting to investigate the possible relation between anatomical asymmetry and functional asymmetry, the opportunity arose to study the anatomy of the corpus callosum in relation to one index of functional asymmetry—namely, hand preference [Bryden, 1982].

Method

Both anatomical and psychological data were available for 42 individuals. The subjects were cancer patients with metastatic disease who agreed to neuropsychological testing and, in the event of death, to a clinical autopsy which would allow anatomical study of the brain. Psychological testing included, in addition to hand preference, tests of auditory and tactual perception of stimuli presented in the lateral sensory fields, which are considered to be indices of cerebral dominance, and tests of the level of various cognitive skills including linguistic, spatial, musical, and motoric functions. Anatomical measures included extensive caliper measurements of gyri and sulci, ventricular size, area measurements, and histological analysis of posterior and frontal language regions, as well as measures of the corpus callosum [Witelson, 1983]. This paper reports the association of two of the methodologically more simple measures: callosal area with hand preference.

Handedness may be defined by preference or performance on a group of skilled manual tasks. In this study, handedness was determined by direct observation of the subject's demonstrated hand preference on 12 unimanual tasks adopted from Annett's [1967] questionnaire. The subjects were classified into hand preference categories following the categories used by Annett [1967]. A stringent criterion of right hand preference was used. Those individuals having only right and no left hand preferences were classified as consistent-right handers, and those having some right but also some left hand preferences, regardless of which hand was preferred for writing, were classified as nonconsistent-right handers or mixed handers. Consistent-left handers, individuals who show only left and no right hand preferences, were not available in the present sample of 42 cases. In large samples, the distribution of consistent-right, mixed, and consistent-left handers is approximately 66, 30, and 4%, respectively [Annett, 1972]. In addition to classifying the subjects into groups, a quantitative score was calculated for each subject. The test was scored such that each item having a right hand preference was assigned a score of +1; each item having a left hand preference was assigned a score of −1; and any item with no preference (i.e., either hand was used) was assigned a score of 0. The possible range of scores on the test was thus +12 to −12. Table 1 presents descriptive data for the two hand preference groups available in the present study: consistent-right handers and nonconsistent-right or mixed handers. The groups did not differ significantly in age at death or brain weight [t (40) = 0.51, 0.34; P = .6, .7, respectively].

The brains were obtained from clinical autopsies and fixed immediately in 10% formalin. Each specimen was bisected in the midsagittal plane, photographs (magnification ×1) of the medial view of each hemisphere were taken, and the area of the corpus callosum was measured via a computerized digitizer and Bioquant II Digitizing Morphometry Program A5-1A2. In addition to total midsagittal area, measures were obtained for the anterior and posterior halves, the posterior fifth and, additionally, for the posterior third. The subdivisions were defined as shown in Figure 1.

Results

The total area of the corpus callosum was found to be significantly larger for the mixed handers than for the consistent-right handers by 11% [732 vs. 659 mm^2, t (40) = 2.6, P = .01]. Such a difference could represent as many as 25 million fibers [Blinkov and Glezer, 1968]. The mixed handers also had significantly larger anterior and posterior halves [t (40) = 2.5, 2.1; P = .02, .04, respectively]. No significant difference was observed for the posterior fifth section, which roughly corresponds to the splenium [t (40) = 1.3; P =

TABLE 1. Description of the Consistent-Right and Nonconsistent-Right (Mixed) Handed Groups

	Consistent-right handers	Nonconsistent-right handers
N	27	15
Sex		
Female	20	10
Male	7	5
	Mean ± standard error of measurement	
Age (yr)	50.3 ± 1.8	48.7 ± 2.3
Brain weight (gm)	1,314 ± 20.6	1,328 ± 43.3
Hand score	+11.4 ± 0.3	+4.9 ± 1.5

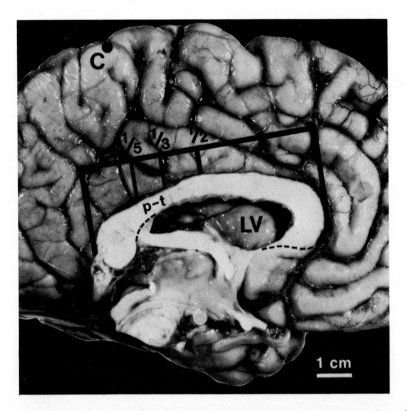

Fig. 1. The human corpus callosum is shown in midsagittal section with its bound-aries indicated by dashed lines. The line joining the most anterior and posterior points of the callosum is used as the axis to define the subdivisions as indicated. The posterior fifth is roughly congruent with the splenium. The midposterior region (the posterior third minus the posterior fifth region) is approximately the area of the callosum that connects the right and left posterior parietotemporal regions. Abbreviations: C, central sulcus at the dorsomedial aspect; LV, lateral ventricle exposed by removal of the septum pellucidum; p-t, parietotemporal region of the callosum.

.2]. These results are presented in Figure 2 and are reported in more detail elsewhere [Witelson, 1985c].

Parietotemporal callosal region.

The posterior third was subsequently measured and found to be larger in the group of mixed handers [t (40) = 1.9, P = .06]. The fact that the area of the posterior fifth, which did not differ between the hand groups, makes up

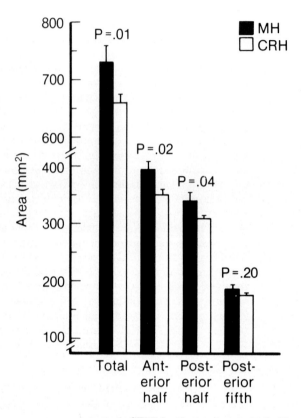

Fig. 2. Mean area measurements ($\pm$ SEM) for the total, anterior half, posterior half, and posterior fifth of the corpus callosum for consistent-right handers (CRH) (N = 27) and for mixed handers (MH) (N = 15). Each score is the mean of the right- and left-hemisphere measurements, and each hemisphere score is the mean of two measurements whose difference was less than 2%. Two-tailed t-tests (df = 40) were used. (Reprinted with permission from Witelson [1985c]. Copyright 1985 by the AAAS.)

approximately 75% of the posterior third suggests that the region constituting the difference between these two subdivisions may be particularly different between the two hand groups. This region, the midsection of the posterior half (labeled p-t in Fig. 1), is of particular functional interest as it likely carries the fibers connecting the posterior parietal and temporal regions of the two hemispheres [see Pandya, this volume; Seltzer and Pandya, 1983], in other words, the posterior language and praxis regions [Heilman and Valenstein, 1985]. Figure 3 shows the results for the posterior callosal subsections. The parietotemporal region of the callosum is signifi-

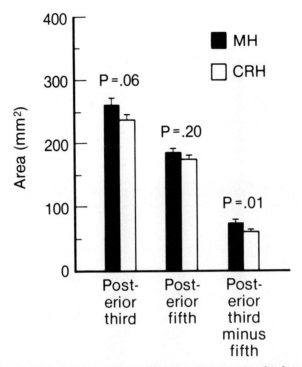

Fig. 3. Mean area measurements (±SEM) for the posterior third, posterior fifth, and the midposterior region (the parietotemporal region) of the corpus callosum for consistent-right handers (CRH) (N = 27) and for mixed handers (MH) (N = 15). Two-tailed t-tests (df = 40) were used.

cantly larger in mixed handers (74.1 vs. 62.3 mm^2) [$t(40)$ = 2.4, P = .01)] by 19%, which is the largest difference observed.

Sex and callosal size.

Callosal size was also examined in relation to sex. Males have larger brains, both in weight and volume [Holloway, 1980]. Accordingly, at least some parts must be larger and it was thought worthwhile to check whether this was so for the callosum. An analysis of possible sexual dimorphism in the callosum was also of interest because, although sex differences were not documented in older anatomical reports [e.g., Bean, 1906], a recent study has reported that in a sample of five female and nine male brains, the females showed a larger posterior fifth region [de Lacoste-Utamsing and Holloway, 1982]. Figure 4 shows a comparison of the sexes within each hand group for the callosal measurements. Analyses of variance (hand-by-sex)

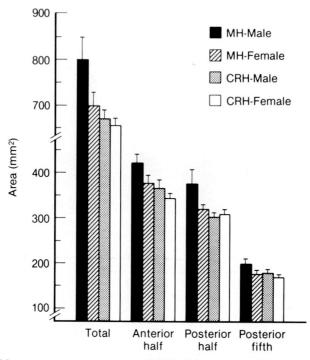

Fig. 4. Mean area measurements (±SEM) of the corpus callosum regions for the four hand-sex subgroups. Abbreviations: CRH, consistent-right handers; MH, mixed handers.

indicated that hand was a significant factor for size of the callosal regions as before, but that neither sex nor the hand-by-sex interactions were significant factors. These results indicate that in contrast to the significant effect of hand preference, there were no anatomical differences observed between the total sex groups or between the sexes within each hand group. The posterior fifth region was not found to be larger in females; in fact, males tended to have a larger area, but not significantly.

Since females have smaller brains than males and, in the present sample, total callosal area was observed to correlate with brain weight ($r = 0.46$, $df = 40$, P < .001) and with cerebrum weight (cerebrum defined as that part of the brain above the pons) ($r = 0.51$, $df = 40$, P < .001), further analyses were done to compare the sexes for callosal size with the factor of cerebrum weight partialed out (two-way analyses of covariance for hand-by-sex with cerebrum weight as the covariate). Again, hand was a significant factor, but neither sex nor the hand-by-sex interaction was significant for total area, anterior half, posterior half, or posterior fifth measures. One further analysis of the relative size of the posterior fifth region between the sexes was done in which the ratio score of the posterior fifth to total callosal area was used. The mean ratio scores for the two total sex groups (n = 30 females, n = 12 males) were identical: 0.26 for each sex. These analyses for sex differences are presented in greater detail elsewhere [Witelson, 1985c].

Consistent-right versus nonconsistent-right handedness.

Consistent-right handers were found to differ in callosal morphology from the nonconsistent-right or mixed handers. Various classifications of hand preference other than this dichotomy exist, but it is not known which is the most biologically valid one. Following one frequently used classification, the heterogeneous group of mixed handers was further subdivided into right- and left-mixed handers, defined on the basis of the hand used for writing. Table 2 describes the two subgroups of mixed handers.

If the essential characteristic of right hand preference were writing with the right hand, then it would be expected that the subgroup of right-mixed handers would not differ from the consistent-right handers in callosal anatomy, but would differ from the subgroup of left-mixed handers. Figure 5 presents the anatomical comparisons for these two subgroups. The mean total callosal area for the right- and left-mixed subgroups was 722 and 746 mm^2, respectively, in contrast to the mean score of 659 mm^2 for the consistent-right handers. There was no indication in t-tests ($df = 13$) of significant differences between the mixed subgroups in callosal size for total or any partial areas. Since the mixed subgroups differed in their sex distributions, comparison of total callosal area was also evaluated with one-way analyses of covariance, with the factor of cerebrum weight partialed out. Again, the two mixed subgroups did not differ from each other (F = 0.1, P = .8). In contrast, the right-mixed group did differ significantly from the consistent-right group (F = 4.8, P = .04). These results suggest that unless an individual is a consistent-right hander, preferred writing hand is *not* a factor in callosal morphology. In other words, the main dichotomy may not be between right and left writers, but between consistent-right handers and

TABLE 2. Description of the Right- and Left-Mixed Handed Subgroups

	Right-mixed handers		Left-mixed handers	
n	9		6	
Sex				
Female	5		5	
Male	4		1	
	Mean	Range	Mean	Range
Age (yr)	48.8	36 – 65	48.7	41 – 60
Brain weight (gm)	1,318	1,119 – 1,606	1,343	1,148 – 1,602
Hand score	+8.4	+10 – +7	−4	+6 – −6

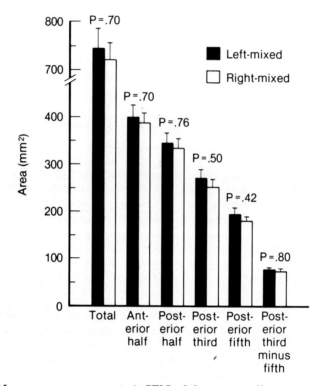

Fig. 5. Mean area measurements (±SEM) of the corpus callosum regions for the right-mixed (N = 9) and left-mixed (N = 6) subgroups. Two-tailed *t*-tests (*df* = 13) were used.

everyone else. It is noted that in terms of magnitude of hand preference score, the right-mixed individuals not only write with their right hand as do the consistent-right handers, but are closer in hand score to them (+8.4 vs. +11.4, respectively) than to the left-mixed handers (whose mean hand score is −4). Yet the right-mixed handers differ anatomically from the former, but not the latter. This point will be further discussed in a later section.

It could be argued that the difference between the consistent-right handers and the mixed handers is related to the factor of consistency rather than directionality of preference. No consistent-left handers were available in the postmortem sample to help evaluate these alternative possibilities. However, two normal male volunteers with consistent-left hand preference were available for magnetic resonance imaging (MRI) scans. Coronal scans were initially done in order to determine the true midsagittal plane for each subject for the subsequent midsagittal scan that was used for callosal measurement. A ruler was included in the scans to allow determination of absolute size of measurements. Although such scans (which used 1-cm slices) do not provide measurements completely comparable with postmortem measurements based on two-dimensional midsagittal sections, the results clearly showed that for each consistent-left hander, callosal area measured from the MRI scan was well above the mean of the male consistent-right group, at least by three standard deviations. In other words, consistent-left handers appear to differ from consistent-right handers in callosal anatomy in the same manner as do mixed handers. These results suggest that the group differences in callosal size are not due to a difference in consistency per se, but rather to the consistent-right versus nonconsistent-right classification.

To test further the possibility that callosal morphology may be more subtly related to hand preference than by a dichotomous classification, correlations were calculated between callosal area and the magnitude of hand preference, as measured by the numerical scores from $+12$ to -12. Since the 27 consistent-right handers had almost identical hand scores, correlations could only be calculated for the 15 mixed handers whose hand scores ranged from $+10$ to -6. Since the mixed group involved both sexes, in an attempt to control for any contribution of brain size, partial correlations were determined with the variable of cerebrum weight factored out. The partial correlation for total callosal area and hand score, which reflects both direction and magnitude, was not significant ($r = -0.03$; $df = 12$, $P = .9$); nor was the partial correlation for absolute hand score, which reflects only degree of hand preference ($r = 0.26$; $df = 12$, $P = .4$). Therefore there is no evidence that callosal size is associated with degree of hand preference.

CALLOSAL SIZE AND FUNCTIONAL ASYMMETRY

The fact that handedness is associated, although imperfectly, with the pattern of functional asymmetry, combined with the finding that handedness is correlated with callosal size, suggests that a correlation may exist between callosal morphology and hemispheric functional specialization. Numerous psychological studies indicate that left handers have greater bihemispheric representation of function. For example, left handers with unilateral brain damage show a higher incidence of aphasia, but show less severe deficits or greater recovery in language than right handers [e.g., Hécaen et al., 1981; Kimura, 1983]. Neurologically intact left handers show less behavioral asymmetry on numerous lateralized perceptual tasks [e.g., Bryden, 1982]. It may be hypothesized, specifically, that the larger callosum of left handers is part of a neural substrate that provides relatively greater interhemispheric communication for a brain in which the functions of the two hemispheres are less lateralized.

Greater bihemispheric representaton in left handers could mean that each hemisphere operates independently and provides a duplication of function, or that the hemispheres form an integrated system with neither being able to maintain speech and language on its own. The data from intracarotid Amytal testing support the latter situation. Duplication of speech functions would be expected to lead to no speech loss regardless of the hemisphere injected. This does not happen. What does happen, and what is used to infer bilateral speech representation is the observation of loss of speech functions with injections on either side, which indicates that neither remaining intact hemisphere was functionally sufficient to maintain speech normally. Such an interhemispheric functional organization for speech processes might be expected to require more fibers for more communication.

Thus, the larger callosum may be part of a neurobiological substrate of a less lateralized or less focused brain organization. Analyses of further psychological data from the current project may help test this hypothesis of the association between callosal anatomy and cerebral dominance. The relative ease and safety of MRI scanning in normal individuals lends itself to further studies evaluating the association between callosal size and hand preference. Such gross variation in a very visible structure that may be related to aspects of brain organization makes it a potential marker for use in MRI studies of clinical populations, such as dyslexics, who are suspect for atypical patterns of functional asymmetry [e.g., Witelson, 1977b].

The finding that callosal size is related to direction but not degree of hand preference lends support to the biological validity of the dichotomous classification of consistent-right handers versus all others. In this framework, the biological characteristic of left handedness would have a broad range of manifestation, from predominantly right hand preference, even including right-hand writing, to consistent-left hand preference. This anatomically derived classification, having a biologically based or bottom-up approach [Dennett, 1978], is congruent with the model of the inheritance of hand preference proposed by Annett [1972, 1981]. In her "right-shift" hypothesis, she proposes the existence of a single allele, the presence of which leads to left hemisphere speech and, in most cases, to consistent-right handedness as a by-product. In the absence of this allele, there is no systematic biological bias for neural organization and hand preference. In these cases, hand preference is determined by chance and environmental factors and manifests mainly as mixed and only infrequently as consistent-left.

To date, few studies of hand preference in relation to functional asymmetry and cognitive skills have used such a dichotomous classification. Kinsbourne [1986] has used this dichotomy in a recent replication of Geschwind and Behan's [1982] study of an association between left handedness and immune diseases, and found the highest correlations with the use of this dichotomy—that is, with a broad rather than a stringent definition of left hand preference. The genetics of hand preference has been a difficult issue to study, as the definition of the phenotype is not clear. Moreover, hand preference is subject to many factors, including social pressure and environmental situations, which may render the resulting phenotype an inaccurate representation of the underlying genotype. If callosal anatomy proves to be associated with hand preference and functional asymmetry, anatomical imaging techniques may be useful in studying the genetics of hand preference and cerebral dominance. If Annett's model is correct in that it is not handedness, but hemispheric laterality that is inherited, then family studies of cerebral dominance patterns may be a key issue.

CALLOSAL SUBDIVISIONS: DIFFERENTIAL VARIATION AND FUNCTIONAL IMPLICATIONS

Total area and area of all the subdivisions measured, except for the posterior fifth, were observed to vary with hand preference classification. Of all the callosal regions studied to date, the midposterior region, which is considered to house predominantly the fibers connecting the posterior parietotemporal regions, showed the greatest size difference between the two hand groups. This finding is interesting in that it occurs in a region that is particularly relevant for cognitive functions for which brain functional organization differs in right and left handers.

That the region of the splenium, which connects the occipital and inferior temporal visual regions, is not similarly correlated with hand preference raises interesting neuroembryological and psychological considerations. It may be noteworthy that the splenium, the one subdivision not correlated with hand preference, is also the callosal region that undergoes the greatest rate of growth in overall size after birth [Rakic and Yakovlev, 1968]. Some functional information about this region is provided by the psychological test results of the more recent commissurotomy cases in which partial rather than complete sectioning was done. With the aim of sectioning the commissures extensively enough to reduce seizure activity and transmission while preserving sufficient interhemispheric communication to avoid some of the hemispheric isolation symptoms, P.J. Vogel and J.E. Bogen treated two patients in whom only the anterior commissure and a major portion of the anterior end of the corpus callosum were cut, and what was described alternatively as "the posterior third" or the "splenium" was spared. Surprisingly, few isolation deficits were manifested, and interhemispheric integration was observed for verbal and nonverbal information in the visual and tactual modalities [Gordon et al., 1971].

The more recent cases studied by Gazzaniga and colleagues and operated on by D.H. Wilson, who carried out staged sectioning of the anterior and posterior halves of the forebrain commissures, yielded similar results. Sectioning of the posterior half, but not the anterior half, resulted in the full manifestation of the isolation deficits, suggesting that the posterior end serves as a "sensory window" between the hemispheres. The interhemispheric functions of the anterior regions are less obvious, but appear to be involved in higher level mental processes [Sperry, 1974] and in the interaction between cognitive rather than sensory systems [Sidtis et al., 1981].

It is interesting to note the parallel between the functional and the anatomical variation for different callosal regions. The splenium serves to integrate sensory information and this region *does not* vary anatomically with hand preference. The callosum anterior to the splenium may be involved in higher cognitive processing, that is, the later stages of information processing in which functional asymmetry comes into play [Moscovitch, 1983], and this part of the callosum *does* vary anatomically between groups of individuals known to vary in patterns of functional asymmetry. Doty et al. [1979] also have suggested a different functional role in the interhemispheric production and access to memory traces for different parts of the forebrain commissure in monkeys: the splenium acts to produce unilateral engrams and the anterior commissure produces bilateral traces.

If this hypothesis is to be considered, it becomes important to determine whether the parietotemporal region of the callosum, which shows a marked size difference between right and left handers, was in fact sectioned as part of the anterior section in the cases reported by Gordon et al. [1971]. The anatomy of the operation done on the cases studied by Sidtis et al. [1981] cannot provide information about this issue. Gordon et al. [1971] reported that a 5-cm anteroposterior section of the callosum was cut. Since the average maximum length of the callosum is 7.2 cm (Witelson [1985d]; 6.2 cm according to Rakic and Yakovlev [1968]), this leaves approximately the posterior 2 cm of the callosum intact. The posterior fifth region (by definition, 20% of the length) is about 1.5 cm in length. Since the callosum arches and the precise maximum anteroposterior length is likely difficult to ascertain from above, the 5-cm cut may well have extended sufficiently posteriorly so that the parietotemporal region was severed and the cut extended to the neck of the splenium. This suggests that the isolation phenomena may be produced without sectioning of the parietotemporal region. Of course, MRI scans on these patients could empirically test such speculation.

It seems worthwhile to study the anatomical variation of different anterior subdivisions. This is currently being done. In addition, the anterior commissure will be studied for anatomical variation, particularly since there is now evidence in monkeys that the anterior commissure transmits fibers from temporal lobe regions that extend quite posteriorly and that even include part of the superior temporal gyrus [Jouandet and Gazzaniga, 1979].

CALLOSAL HISTOLOGY

If the larger callosum of left handers is a substrate of their greater bihemispheric representation of cognitive functions and serves to provide greater interhemispheric transfer of information, then it might be predicted that the total number of callosal fibers is greater in left handers. If this were so, then one might question whether left handers also have more neurons, or at least more callosal neurons such as the pyramidal cells of lamina III. Such histological investigation is underway in the present project in collaboration with M. Colonnier. A recent finding employing functional imaging techniques provides some support of this hypothesis. Measurement of isotope clearance rates in regional cerebral blood flow studies in right and left handers revealed that left handers had a greater percentage of grey matter than did right handers [Gur et al., 1982].

The larger callosum could of course reflect other histological differences, such as more myelin, a different distribution of thick and thin fibers, or a lower packing density of axons. Unfortunately, there are no data pertaining to this issue. In fact relatively little data on any aspect of the histology of the callosum are available for humans. Some information regarding fiber counts at different fetal and neonatal stages [Luttenburg, 1965] and at maturity [Tomasch, 1954], and the developmental course of myelination [Yakovlev and Lecours, 1967] has been reported. But clearly this is an area requiring further research. As an extension of the work reported here, an analysis of at least the number of myelinated fibers per unit area in different regions of the callosum in individuals with different hand preference is underway.

Whatever histological variation may accompany the gross difference in callosal size between individuals, it remains to be determined what functional or physiological differences may be associated with the anatomical difference. For example, does the larger callosum result in more excitatory or inhibitory transmission; what is the direction of any extra information flow; and is there a difference in the rate of interhemispheric transmission? For such issues, electrophysiological studies of interhemispheric transmission times and of latency and amplitude of some components of cortical evoked potentials in right and left handers may be appropriate [e.g., Hellige, 1983].

EARLY NEURAL REGRESSIVE EVENTS

The phenomenon of regressive events in neural development involving both neuronal cell death and axonal elimination [Cowan et al., 1984] may be relevant here. For example, the number of fibers has been shown to be greater before birth than at maturity in the callosum in the cat [Koppel and Innocenti, 1983] and in the optic nerve in monkeys [Rakic and Riley, 1983]. In humans, the only data available are from a relatively older study [Luttenberg, 1965] which reported a decrease in the density of axons (number per unit area) after 7 months gestation, but an overall increase in total number of fibers associated with the increase in total callosal area. However, the small, nonmyelinated fibers may not have been visible with the light microscopy technique used [Innocenti, 1985]. Clearly, developmental studies of callosal histology using electronmicroscopy are needed. Axonal elimination is thought to be completed soon after birth, by about the time myelination begins [Cowan et al., 1984], which appears to be about 3 months of age in humans [Yakovlev and Lecours, 1967].

If it were found that there are more callosal fibers in left handers, then the early regressive phenomena of neuronal degeneration and axonal elimination may be one mechanism responsible for this difference. Perhaps in the minority of people, the approximately one-third of the population who are nonconsistent-right handers, less fine sculpting of the nervous system occurs early in life, which results in a greater total number of fibers remaining. If heterotopic fibers are among those that are eliminated by early regressive events, then perhaps left handers have more heterotopic connections than do right handers. At an even more speculative level, perhaps such an anatomical feature may in part underlie the greater incidence of certain cognitive developmental disorders, such as dyslexia, dysphasia, and stuttering, in mixed and left handers then in right handers [Corballis, 1983].

Consistent-right handers and mixed handers vary in the unimanual versus bimanual nature of their sensorimotor experience, and accordingly, one might raise the hypothesis that callosal size is determined by differential environmental or learning factors. For example, perhaps bimanual experience itself or the neural organization of left hemisphere representation of language combined with right-sided primary motor control for left-hand writing results in differential development of callosal connections. The current neurobiological information, however, is not compatible with a change in the number of axons at the stage of development when such differential manual experience could occur. The early neural regressive phenomena are thought to be completed before differential hand experience becomes a factor. Moreover, the anatomical and psychological correlations found in the present study do not support any major environmental influence. Consistent-left handers are as strongly directionally biased as are consistent-right handers. Yet the consistent-left handers were found to have larger callosa than the consistent-right handers, and callosa similar in size to the mixed handers. Also, magnitude of hand preference was not correlated with callosal size. Finally, the analysis of the two mixed-hand subgroups is relevant to the issue of the role of experience. The mixed subgroups differed in the nature of their manual experience, but not in callosal anatomy. The right-mixed group had a mean hand preference score of +8.4, indicating a relatively strong bias for the right side, whereas the left-mixed group had a mean hand score of −4, reflecting a more ambidextrous hand usage. If bimanual experience were a factor in determining callosal size, one might predict that the more strongly lateralized mixed group (the right-mixed group) would differ little, if at all, from the consistent-right group, but would differ from the more ambidextrous group (the left-mixed group). But such was not the case. The two mixed groups did not differ, and the two more strongly lateralized groups did differ from each other. These results do not support an environmental determinant of callosal size. However, even in the proposed framework of a preprogrammed developmental neurobiological basis for anatomical variation in the callosum, environmental factors could have a modifying role, perhaps in maintaining fiber connections or in influencing myelin development.

CALLOSAL VARIATION AND COGNITION

One of the psychological questions raised by the current findings concerns the effects that the different anatomy of the corpus callosum could have on cognition. If the callosal difference between different hand groups proves to be reliable, then it surely must be just one aspect of a more complex picture of concomitant morphological differences. If so, then left handedness in its broad definition could well be associated with a different type of mental processing or cognition, and not merely motoric behavior with a different laterality bias. The anatomical differences may be related to the level of performance on some cognitive tasks or to the degree of integration possible between lateralized information processing. Here too there is little information. Several findings that may be related to the differences in callosal anatomy are of particular interest here. In some visuospatial and nonverbal auditory tasks, left handers are superior to dextrals. Moreover, left handers appear to be overrepresented in certain occupations, such as art, architecture, music, engineering, and some sports [Bradshaw and Nettleton, 1983]. Left handers also appear to have greater cognitive variability than right handers; that is, they have more extreme scores at both the high and low ends of the continuum [e.g., Levy and Reid, 1978] and they have a higher incidence of some neurocognitive disorders, such as epilepsy, dyslexia, and speech difficulties [Bradshaw and Nettleton, 1983]. The developmental period during which children show mirror-image reversals in perception and in writing is purported to be of longer duration in left handed children, and such reversals are a particularly marked symptom in some developmental dyslexics who have a relatively high frequency of nonright-hand preference and possibly atypical patterns of cerebral dominance [Orton, 1937]. Peters [1983a] has suggested that young children who subsequently grow up to be left handed may show later development in certain speech production skills and in bimanual coordination. There is in fact some evidence that mirror-writing is easier for adults who write with their left hand than with their right hand [Schott, 1980; Jung, 1981; Peters, 1983b].

As Professor Sperry queried [see Levy, this volume]: why does such an apparently inefficient neural organization exist in some individuals such that oral language is represented in one hemisphere and writing is mediated by the other? The different gross anatomy of the corpus callosum and possibly other associated neuronal differences in nonconsistent-right handers may offer an initial clue to the neurobiological substrate that results in such individual variation. In summary, there may be variation in the biological mechanisms underlying neurogenesis that results in individual differences in brain morphology and that influences or has implications for functional organization of the brain and for individual differences in behavior and cognition.

ACKNOWLEDGMENTS

The research reported in this chapter was supported by NIH-NINCDS contract N01-NS-6-2344, NINCDS grant R01-NS 18954, and Ontario Mental Health Foundation research grant 803. I thank the administrative and clinical staffs of McMaster University and affiliated Hospitals, including Drs. P.B. McCulloch, A.T. Figueredo, and D.A. Clark for referring patients; Drs. G. Frank, J.T. Groves, F. Cole, T.J. Muckle, V.B. Fowler, and R.A. Haggar for doing the postmortem examinations; the patients and their families for participating in this project; Debra Kigar for excellent anatomical technical assistance; and Drs. S. Black, T. Carr, D. Drost, and A. Kertesz of St. Joseph's Hospital, London, Ontario for doing the MRI scans. I thank Dr. M. Colonnier for initiating my participation in this symposium.

REFERENCES

Akelaitis AJ (1944): A study of gnosis, praxis and language following section of the corpus callosum and anterior commissure. J Neurosurg 1:94–102.

Annett M (1967): The binomial distribution of right, mixed and left handedness. Q J Exp Psychol 19:327–333.

Annett M (1972): The distribution of manual asymmetry. Br. J. Psychol. 63:343–358.

Annett M (1981): The genetics of handedness. Trends. Neurosci 4:256–258.

Bean RB (1906): Some racial peculiarities of the negro brain. Am J Anat 5:353–432.

Beaumont JG (1982): Divided Visual Field Studies of Cerebral Organization. Toronto: Academic Press.

Benton AL (1964): Contributions to aphasia before Broca. Cortex 1:314–327.

Best C (1985): "Hemispheric Function and Collaboration in the Child." New York: Academic Press.

Blinkov SM, Glezer II (1968): "The Human Brain in Figures and Tables." New York: Plenum Press.

Bradshaw JL, Nettleton NC (1983): "Human Cerebral Asymmetry." Englewood Cliffs, New Jersey: Prentice-Hall.

Bryden MP (1982): "Laterality, Functional Asymmetry in the Intact Brain." Toronto: Academic Press.

Corballis MC (1983): "Human Laterality." New York: Academic Press.

Corballis MC, and Beale IL (1983): "The Ambivalent Mind: The Neuropsychology of Left and Right." Chicago: Nelson-Hall.

Cowan WM, Fawcett JW, O'Leary DDM, Stanfield BB (1984): Regressive events in neurogenesis. Science 225:1258–1265.

de Lacoste-Utamsing C, Holloway RL (1982): Sexual dimorphism in the human corpus callosum. Science 216:1431–1432.

Dennett DC (1978): "Brainstorms: Philosophical Essays on Mind and Psychology." Cambridge, Massachusetts: MIT Press.

Dimond S (1972): "The Double, Brain." London: Churchill Livingstone.

Doty RW, Overman WH, Jr. Negrão N (1979): Role of forebrain commissures in hemispheric specialisation and memory in macaques. In Russell IS, Van Hof MW, Berlucchi G (eds): "Structure and Function of Cerebral Commissures." Baltimore: University Park Press, pp 333–342.

Ettlinger EG, De Reuck AVS, Porter R (1965): "Functions of the Corpus Callosum." Ciba Foundation Study Group No. 20. London: JA Churchill.

Gazzaniga MS, Bogen JE, Sperry RW (1962): Some functional effects of sectioning the cerebral commissures in man. Proc Natl Acad Sci. USA 48:1765–1769.

Gazzaniga MS, LeDoux JE (1978): "The Integrated Mind." New York: Plenum Press.

Geschwind N (1965): Disconnexion syndromes in animals and man. Brain 88: Part I 237–294, Part II 585–644.

Geschwind N, Kaplan E (1962): A human cerebral deconnection syndrome. Neurology, (N.Y.) 12: 675–685.

Geschwind N, Galaburda AM (1984): "Cerebral Dominance, The Biological Foundations." Cambridge: Harvard University Press.

Geschwind N, Behan P (1982): Left-handedness: Association with immune disease, migraine, and developmental learning disorder. Proc Natl Acad Sci USA 79: 5097–5100.

Gordon HW, Bogen JE, Sperry RW (1971): Absence of deconnexion syndrome in two patients with partial section of the neocommissures. Brain 94:327–336.

Gur RC, Gur RE, Orbist WD, Hungerbuhler JP, Younkin D, Rosen AD, Skolnick BE, Reivich M (1982): Sex and handedness differences in cerebral blood flow during rest and cognitive activity. Science 217:659–661.

Harrington A (1985): Nineteenth century ideas on hemisphere differences and "duality of mind." Behav Brain Sci, 8:617–659.

Hécaen H, de Agostini M, Monzon-Montes A (1981): Cerebral organization in left-handers. Brain Lang 12:261–284.

Heilman KM, Valenstein E (1985): "Clinical Neuropsychology," 2nd Ed. New York: Oxford University Press.

Hellige JB (1983): "Cerebral Hemisphere Asymmetry. Method, Theory, and Application." New York: Praeger.

Holloway RL (1980): Within-species brain-body weight variability: A reexamination of the Danish data and other primate species. Am J Phys Anthropol 53:109–121.

Innocenti, GM 1985 (Personal communication, Oct. 1985). I thank G.M.I. for clarification of my discussion of this study.

Jouandet ML, Gazzaniga MS (1979): Cortical field of origin of the anterior commissure of the Rhesus monkey. Exp Neurol 66:381–397.

Jung R (1981): Perception and action. In Szentagothai J, Palkovitz M, and Hamori J (eds): "Regulatory Functions of the CNS, Principles of Motion and Organization." Oxford: Pergamon Press.

Kimura D (1983): Speech representation in an unbiased sample of left-handers. Hum Neurobiol 2:147–154.

Kinsbourne M (1986): Relationships between nonright-handedness and diseases of the immune systems. Abstract. To be presented at the 14th annual meeting of the Internat Neurospsychol Soc, Denver.

Kolb B, Whishaw IQ (1985): "Fundamentals of Human Neuropsychology," 2nd Ed. New York: WH Freeman.

Koppel H, Innocenti GM (1983): Is there a genuine exuberancy of callosal projections in development? A quantitative electron microscopic study in the cat. Neurosc Lett 41:33–40.

Levy J (1985): Interhemispheric collaboration: Single-mindedness in the asymmetric brain. C Best (Ed) "Hemispheric Function and Collaboration in the Child." New York: Academic Press.

Levy J, Reid, M (1978): Variations in cerebral organization as a function of handedness, hand posture in writing, and sex. J Exp Psychol: Gen 107:119–144.

Luttenberg J (1965): Contribution to the fetal ontogenesis of the corpus callosum in man. II. Folia Morphologica (Warsaw) (Engl Transl) 13:136–144.

Marks CE (1981): "Commissurotomy, Consciousness and Unity of Mind." Cambridge, Mass: MIT Press.

Moscovitch M (1983): Stages of processing and hemispheric differences in language in the normal subject. In Studdert-Kennedy M (ed): "Psychobiology of Language." Cambridge, Mass: MIT Press, pp 88–104.

Orton ST (1937): "Reading, Writing and Speech Problems in Children." New York: Norton.

Perecman E (1983): "Cognitive Processing in the Right Hemisphere." Toronto: Academic Press.

Peters M (1983a): Differentiation and lateral specialization in motor development. In Young G, Segalowtiz, SJ, Corter CM, and Trehub SE (eds): "Manual Specialization and the Developing Brain." New York: Academic Press pp 141–159.

Peters M (1983b): Inverted and noninverted left handers compared on the basis of motor performance and measures related to the act of writing. Aust J Psychol 35:405–416.

Rakic P, Yakovlev PI (1968): Development of the corpus callosum and cavum septi in man. J Comp Neurol 132:45–72.

Rakic P, Riley KP (1983): Overproduction and elimination of retinal axons in the fetal Rhesus monkey. Science 219:1441–1444.

Russell GA, Russell IS (1979): Introduction to the beginnings of commissure research. In Russell IS, Van Hof MW, and Berlucchi G (eds): "Structure and Function of Cerebral Commissures." Baltimore: University Park Press pp xii–xviii.

Schott GD (1980): Mirror movements of the left arm following peripheral damage to the preferred right arm. J Neurol Neurosurg Psychiatry 43:768–773.

Seltzer B, Pandya DN (1983): The distribution of posterior parietal fibers in the corpus callosum of the Rhesus monkey. Exp Brain Res 49:147–150.

Sidtis JJ, Volpe BT, Holtzman JE, Wilson DH, Gazzaniga MS (1981): Cognitive interaction after staged callosal section: Evidence for transfer of semantic activation. Science 212:344–346.

Sperry RW (1966): Brain bisection and consciousness. In Eccles JC (ed): "Brain and Conscious Experience." New York: Springer-Verlag pp 298–313.

Sperry RW (1974): Lateral specialization in the surgically separated hemispheres. In Schmitt FO, and Worden FG (eds): "The Neurosciences Third Study Program." Cambridge, Mass: MIT Press pp 5–19.

Tomasch J (1954): Size, distributions, and number of fibres in the human corpus callosum. Anat Rec 119:119–135.

Wigan AL (1844): "A New View of Insanity: The Duality of the Mind." London: Longman, Brown, Green, and Longmans. Reprinted (1985) Malibu, California: J. Simon.

Witelson SF (1977a): Anatomic asymmetry in the temporal lobes: Its documentation, phylogenesis and relationship to functional asymmetry. Ann NY Acad Sci 299:328–354.

Witelson SF (1977b): Developmental dyslexia: Two right hemispheres and none left. Science 195:309–311.

Witelson SF (1983): Bumps on the brain: Right-left anatomic asymmetry as a key to functional asymmetry. Segalowitz S (ed): "Language Functions and Brain Organization." New York: Academic Press pp 117–143.

Witelson SF (1985a): On hemisphere specialization and cerebral plasticity from birth. Mark II. Best C (ed): "Hemispheric Function and Collaboration in the Child." New York: Academic Press pp 33–85.

Witelson SF (1985b): Brain asymmetry, functional aspects. Adelman G (ed): "Encyclopedia of Neuroscience." Boston: Birkhäuser (in press).

Witelson SF (1985c): The brain connection: The corpus callosum is larger in left handers. Science 229:665–668.

Witelson SF (1985d): Unpublished data.

Yakovlev PI, Lecours A (1967): The myelogenetic cycles of regional maturation of the brain. In Minkowski A (ed): "Regional Development of the Brain in Early Life." London: Blackwell pp 3–65.

Young AW (1983): "Functions of the Right Cerebral Hemisphere." Toronto: Academic Press.

Two Hemispheres—One Brain:
Functions of the Corpus Callosum, pages 139–148
© 1986 Alan R. Liss, Inc.

The Anatomical Organization of Interhemispheric Connections of the Anterior Ectosylvian Visual Area in the Cat

D. MICELI, F. LEPORÉ, R. WARD, AND M. PTITO

Group de Recherche en Neuropsychologie Expérimentale, Université du Québec, Trois-Rivières, Québec G9A 5H7 (D.M., R.W., M.P.) and Département de Psychologie, Université de Montréal, Montréal, Québec H3C 3J7 (F.L.) Canada

Numerous visual cortical areas have been identified in the cat that are situated in the caudal portion of the cerebral hemisphere [for review, see Sprague et al., 1977]. More recently, however, a specific visual area has been described rostrally within a ventral bank of the anterior ectosylvian sulcus [Olsen and Graybiel, 1981, 1983; Mucke et al., 1982]. This region, referred to as the anterior ectosylvian visual area (AEV), has been shown to receive direct input from the tecto-recipient zone of the thalamic lateral posterior nucleus and the lateral suprasylvian visual area (LSS) [Olsen and Graybiel, 1981; Mucke et al., 1982]. In addition, reciprocal projections of the AEV upon the LSS as well as more extensive connections between the AEV and area 20, regions of the posterior suprasylvian gyrus including area 21, and both the AEV and LSS of the opposite hemisphere have been reported [Olsen and Graybiel, 1981, 1983; Miceli et al., 1984, 1985]. At present, there is little available information regarding the commissural pathway(s) involved in the interhemispheric connections of the AEV. In view of its rostrallocation within the hemisphere and its topographical isolation from the more classical visual cortical areas, it is conceivable that the AEV contralateral projections are routed differently than those of the other visual areas. This suggestion is partly based upon the generally accepted notion that the interhemispheric transfer of visual information associated with the latter areas, in the cat, is channeled through the posterior third, or splenium, of the corpus callosum.

The aim of the present study was to examine the organization of AEV afferent and efferent connections with the opposite hemisphere using different neuroanatomical techniques. (1) Horseradish peroxidase (HRP): The cells of origin of AEV callosal projections were revealed by charting the somatic labeling in AEV resulting from the uptake and retrograde transport of the enzyme from sectioned callosal fibers. (2) Fluorescence: The callosal

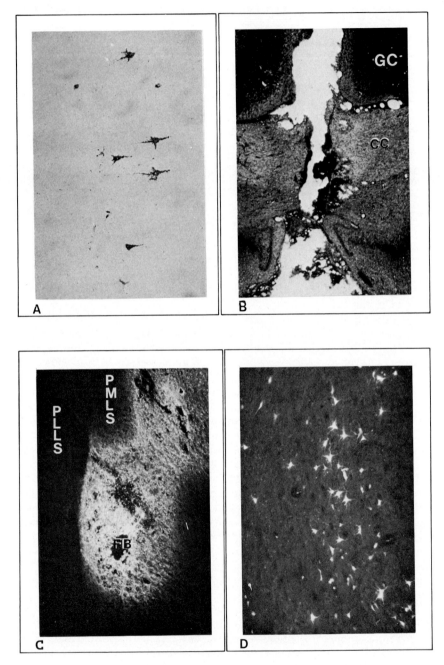

Fig. 1

and/or extracallosal projection neurons in the AEV and LSS were identified using the retrograde fluorescence double-labeling method [Van der Kooy et al., 1979; Bentivoglio et al., 1980; Kuypers et al., 1980]. In these experiments, sequential injections of different fluorescent tracers (fast blue [FB], Evans blue [EB], nuclear yellow [NY]) were made into either the AEV or the LSS prior to and following a complete transection of the callosum, and the cell labeling in these same areas of the contralateral hemisphere was compared.

MATERIALS AND METHODS
HRP

Under Rompun/ketamine anesthesia, six adult cats underwent a partial transection of the corpus callosum extending from its caudal extremity to different levels rostrally. A Gelfoam sponge soaked in a 30% (W/V) solution of HRP (Sigma Type VI) was then placed along the midline between the cut ends of the callosal fibers. Following survival periods of 2–4 days, the animals were deeply anesthetized and perfused transcardially with 0.1 M phosphate-buffered saline (pH 7.4) followed by a 25% Karnovsky solution. The brains were sectioned at 40 μm in the frontal plane on a freezing microtome. The sections were processed according to the tetramethylbenzidine (TMB) method [Mesulam, 1978] and counterstained with neutral red.

Fluorescence

Five animals received unilateral injections of 0.1–0.3 μl of FB (5% wt/vol) or EB (10% solution containing 1% poly-L-ornithine) either into the AEV or within the posterior lateral (PLLS) and/or the posterior medial (PMLS, Fig. 1C) subdivisions of the LSS [Palmer et al., 1978]. The dyes were injected through glass micropipettes having tip diameters of 60–85 μm, which were adapted to a 1.0-μl-capacity Hamilton microsyringe. The LSS injections were performed using a direct dorsal approach into the respective banks of the PMLS and PLLS. In the case of AEV injections, a direct lateral approach was employed involving oblique penetrations parallel to the sulcus (Fig. 2B). The latter were restricted to the caudal aspect of the anterior ectosylvian sulcus at the level where it arches dorsocaudally toward the LSS sulcus.

Fig. 1. A. HRP-labeled cells in layer III of AEV observed following the application of the enzyme to sectioned callosal fibers. ×93. B. A frontal section showing the cut corpus callosum (CC) GC, gyrus cinguli. ×16. The section was performed in the interval between injections of different fluorescent tracers into AEV. C. An FB injection site within the PMLS subregion of LSS. ×38. D. Retrogradely labeled cells in PMLS on the side contralateral to the initial injection of EB into the corresponding region of LSS and performed before sectioning the corpus callosum. ×93.

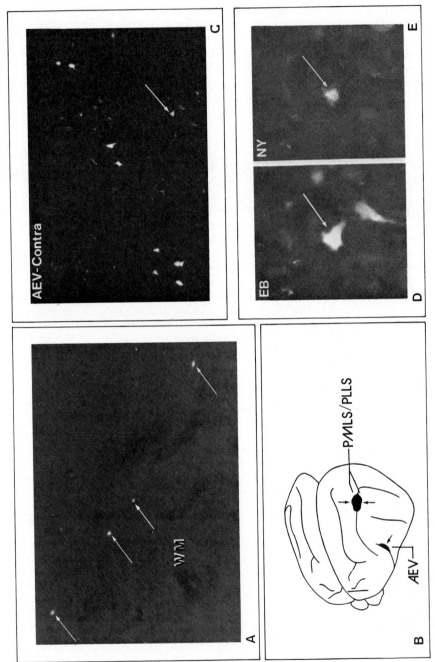

Fig. 2

Four to five days later, the corpus callosum was completely sectioned and a second tracer NY (3%) was injected into either AEV or LSS using the same pre-section coordinates. Following a 2–3-day survival period, the cats were perfused transcardially with saline, then with 10% formol, and finally with a 30% sucrose solution. The brains were removed and 40-μm-thick frozen sections were obtained and were immediately mounted on glass slides. Alternate sections were coverslipped using a low-fluorescence mounting medium.

The labeling was viewed using a Leitz Ploemopack fluorescence microscope equipped with filter-mirror systems A (360 nm) and N2 (550 nm) for revealing either FB or NY and EB fluorescence, respectively. The HRP- and fluorescent-labeled cells were mapped using either a camera lucida or on a monitor screen using a video camera. The laminar distributions of the fluorescent neurons were determined by (1) comparing maps of labeling with the cytoarchitecture in alternate sections stained with cresyl violet, (2) charting labeled neurons in unmounted sections that were subsequently counterstained, and (3) viewing the sections with a D (390 nm) filter-mirror system, which reveals background autofluorescence. The areal boundaries and laminar organization of the AEV and LSS followed various electrophysiological maps and cytoarthitectonic descriptions [Gurewitsch and Chatschaturian, 1928; Palmer et al., 1978; Mucke et al., 1982; Seagraves and Rosenquist, 1982, 1982a; Olsen and Graybiel, 1983].

RESULTS
HRP

After applying HRP to the cut ends of the callosal fibers, retrogradely labeled cells were found bilaterally within various visual cortical areas and their distribution, for the most part, was comparable to that reported in a previous HRP study employing a similar procedure [Seagraves and Rosenquist, 1982]. Furthermore, in the experimental animals where the section

---

Fig. 2. A. Low-power view ($\times$86) of AEV cells (arrows) labeled with NY, which was injected into the corresponding region of the opposite hemisphere after a complete transection of the corpus callosum. WM, white matter. B. Schematic dorsolateral view of the cat brain showing the extent of the AEV and LSS (PMLS/PLLS) regions sampled (shaded areas). First, EB or FB and then the NY tracers were injected sequentially into either area, respectively, prior to and following a complete callosal section. The injections were performed deep within the respective banks and parallel to the sulci (arrows). C. EB-labeled cells in AEV contralateral to the pre-section injection of the tracer into AEV. $\times$96. D. A higher-power view ($\times$385) of the EB cell indicated by the arrow in C as observed with the N2 (550 nm) filter. E. The same cell as viewed with the A (360 nm) filter is shown to be double labeled with NY. The latter dye was injected into AEV after the callosal section and using the same pre-section EB injection coordinates.

of the corpus callosum was the most extensive and rostrally attained levels corresponding to intermediate portions of the claustrum (Ant: 12.5–14 mm), labeled neurons were identified in the AEV (Fig. 1A). They were predominantly concentrated within layer III and many were clearly pyramidal, although some smaller polymorphic cells were also labeled in layers V and VI. In four of the animals, in which HRP was applied to a more restricted posterior segment of the callosum, a marked reduction in the AEV labeling was noted. Only occasional labeled cells were detected in the caudal most regions of the AEV. Histological reconstructions of the corpus callosum showed that the commissure had been sectioned rostrally to levels corresponding approximately to the anterior aspect of the dorsal lateral geniculate nucleus (Ant: 6.5–8 mm). In none of the HRP experiments was there sufficient orthograde labeling of callosal fibers to allow the tracing of afferents to their cortical target areas.

Fluorescence

The initial tracer injection EB or FB into the AEV made prior to the callosal section resulted in the labeling of cell bodies bilaterally in the LSS and in the contralateral AEV. In both of these areas contralaterally, the fluorescent neurons were found mainly in layer III and to a lesser extent in layers V and VI. In the LSS injection experiments, retrogradely labeled cells were observed in the LSS of the opposite hemisphere (layers III, V, and VI) and in the AEV bilaterally (layers V and VI) (Figs. 1D, 3A, B).

In comparison to the latter distribution of label, the second tracer (NY) injected into the AEV immediately following the complete transection of the callosum failed to label neurons in the contralateral LSS and layer III of the AEV entirely. However, some NY labeling of cells was still observed in layers V and VI of the AEV (Figs. 2A,C–E, 3). In individual sections, the proportions of post-/pre-section-labeled neurons in these deeper layers attained values as high as 36%. Furthermore, virtually all of the NY cells were found to be double labeled, also containing the fluorescent dye injected into the AEV prior to the callosal section. In the LSS injection preparations, the contralateral LSS and AEV labeling could no longer be obtained with the NY tracer injected after sectioning the callosum. In all of the experiments, the distribution of ipsilateral label observed in either the LSS or the AEV with both of the dyes injected sequentially was consistent, and the majority of the cells were double labeled.

DISCUSSION

The HRP results indicate that the corpus callosum is involved in AEV projections to the contralateral hemisphere and that the cells of origin are located in layers III, V, and VI. Furthermore, the relative reduction of

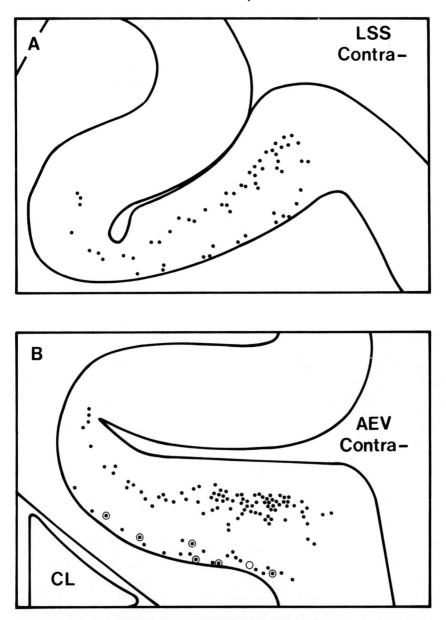

Fig. 3. Maps of the distribution of EB-labeled (dots) and NY-labeled (open circles) neurons in contralateral (A) LSS (PMLS/PLLS) and (B) AEV, obtained in different animals after injections of the two tracers into the corresponding regions of the opposite hemisphere. The EB and NY tracers were injected, respectively, prior to and following a complete section of the callosum. The circled dots indicate double labeling.

retrograde labeling in the AEV observed in those cases where the uptake of the enzyme was restricted to more caudal portions of the callosum suggests that rostral regions of this commissure also receive axons from the AEV. This is compatible with the previously reported orthograde labeling of fibers within the rostral callosum obtained following the injection of different fluorescent tracers into the AEV [Miceli et al., 1985].

The present results derived using the fluorescence method showed that the reciprocal interhemispheric LSS homotopic projections and LSS-AEV interconnections are exclusively callosal. This was demonstrated by the fact that the retrograde labeling in either the contralateral LSS or AEV observed after injections of the tracers into the AEV and LSS, respectively, was completely abolished after sectioning the callosum. In contrast, the contralateral AEV homotopic projections have a dual trajectory; layer III neurons, which compose a major part of this projection system, send axons through the corpus callosum, whereas the efferent pathways arising from layers V and VI are both callosal and extra-callosal.

The data suggest that, unlike the more classical visual areas, which transfer visual information to the opposite hemisphere through the posterior third (splenium) of the corpus callosum, the visual input from the AEV may in addition crossover within its rostral portions as well as via an extra-callosal route. At present the latter pathway remains to be clearly elucidated, although there is evidence suggesting that the anterior commissure may be involved. Employing the HRP technique, it has been shown that cells in layers V and VI of the anterior ectosylvian region send axons through this commissure [Jouandet, 1982]. These same layers of the AEV were here observed to provide extracallosal homotopic projections upon the contralateral AEV. Moreover, some preliminary results using the Fink-Heimer method have shown degenerating fibers in the anterior commissure following lesions of the ventral bank of the anterior ectosylvian sulcus that involved extensive portions of the AEV [Miceli, Ward and Leporé, unpublished observations]. More studies will be required to verify the existence of an AEV projection through the anterior commissure and particularly using complementary anatomical tracing methods such as orthograde auto-radiography.

The AEV extra-callosal and callosal projections through extensive regions of the rostrocaudal plane of the commissure represent additional paths by which visual information may be transferred to the opposite hemisphere. Such an organization may explain some of the behavioral data that have shown interhemispheric communication to be maintained after sections of the corpus callosum [Sechzer, 1963]. On the basis of the receptive field properties of its component neurons, retinotopic organization, as well as its topographical and connectional distance from area 17, the AEV resembles higher-order visual areas of primates such as the inferior temporal cortex

[Olsen and Graybiel, 1983], which is known to play an important role in interhemispheric transfer [Seacord et al., 1979]. The present findings suggest a further parallel between the latter and the AEV in that both receive converging callosal and extra-callosal input from the opposite hemipshere [Pandya et al., 1971; Zeki, 1973]. Further physiological and behavioral studies of the AEV should provide a better understanding of the nature of the interhemispheric input and the role of this area in processing visual information.

REFERENCES

Bentivoglio M, Kuypers HGJM, Catsman-Berrevoetz CE, Loewe H, Dann O (1980): Two new fluorescent retrograde neuronal tracers which are transported over long distances. Neurosci Lett 18:25–30.

Gurewitsch M, Chatschaturian A (1928): Zur Cytoarchitectonik der Grosshirnrinde der Feliden. Z Anat Entwicklungsgesch 87:100–138.

Jouandet ML (1982): Neocortical and basal telencephalic origins of the anterior commissure of the cat. Neuroscience 7:1731–1752.

Kuypers HGJM, Bentivoglio M, Catsman-Berrevoetz CE, Bharos AT (1980): Double retrograde neuronal labeling through divergent axon collaterals, using two fluorescent tracers with the same excitation wave-length which label differnt features of the cell. Exp Brain Res 40:383–392.

Mesulam MM (1978): Tetramethyl benzidine for horseradish peroxidase neurohistochemistry: A non-carcinogenic blue reaction-product with superior sensitivity for visualizing neural afferents and efferents. J Histochem Cytochem 26:106–117.

Miceli D, Ptito M, Leporé F, Repérant J (1984): Interhemispheric connections of the anterior ectosylvian visual area in the cat. ARVO Abstr 25:212.

Miceli D, Repérant J, Ptito M (In Press) Intracortical connections of the anterior ectosylvian and lateral suprasylvian visual areas in the cat. Brain Res.

Mucke L, Norita M, Benedek G, Creutzfeld O (1982): Physiologic and anatomic investigation of a visual cortical area situated in the ventral bank of the anterior ectosylvian sulcus in the cat. Exp Brain Res 46:1–11.

Olsen CR, Graybiel AM (1981): A visual area in the anterior ectosylvian sulcus of the cat. Neurosci Abstr p 831.

Olsen CR, Graybiel AM (1983): An outlying visual area in the cerebral cortex of the cat. Prog Brain Res 58:239–245.

Palmer LA, Rosenquist AC, Tusa RJ (1978): The retinotopic organization of the suprasylvian visual areas in the cat. J Comp Neurol 177:237–256.

Pandya DN, Karol EA, Heilbronn D (1971): The topographical distribution of interhemispheric projections in the corpus callosum of the rhesus monkey. Brain Res 32:31–43.

Seacord L, Gross CG, Mishkin M (1979): Role of inferior temporal cortex in interhemispheric transfer. Brain Res 167:259–272.

Seagraves MA, Rosenquist AC (1982): The distribution of the cells of origin of callosal projections in cat visual cortex. J Neurosci 2:1079–1089.

Seagraves MA, Rosenquist AC (1982a): The afferent and efferent callosal connections of retinotopically defined areas in cat cortex. J Neurosci 2:1090–1107.

Sechzer JA (1963): Successful interocular transfer of pattern discrimination in split-brain cats with shock avoidance motivation. J Comp Physiol Psychol 58:76–83.

Sprague JM, Levy J, DiBerardino A, Berlucchi G (1977): Visual cortical areas mediating form discrimination in the cat. J Comp Neurol 172:441–488.

Van der Kooy D, Kuypers HGJM, Catsman-Berrevoetz CE (1979): Single mammillary body cells with divergent axon collaterals. Demonstration by a simple, fluorescent retrograde labeling technique in the rat. Brain Res 158:189–196.

Zeki SM (1973): Comparison of the cortical degeneration in the visual regions of the temporal lobe of the monkey following section of the anterior commissure and the splenium. J Comp Neurol 148:167–176.

Two Hemispheres—One Brain:
Functions of the Corpus Callosum, pages 149–164
© 1986 Alan R. Liss, Inc.

Corpus Callosum—One System, Two Approaches

E.G. JONES

*Department of Anatomy, University of California at Irvine, Irvine, California
92717*

INTRODUCTION

Roger Sperry's contributions in two major areas of neuroscience are well
exemplified by the presentations made at this meeting on "Two Hemispheres—One Brain?" In one area, several examples of callosal organization, function, and dysfunction were presented, while, in another, the
specification of callosal connections during development formed the subject.
Obviously, neither of these aspects of study is entirely independent of the
other in any area of the nervous system for it is the establishment and
stabilization of synapses and of connectional topography during development that determines the ultimate patterns of organization and function
that we see in the adult. Sperry is obviously well aware of the close associations between his two seemingly disparate areas of research when he
writes in "Science and Moral Priority" [1983]: "The tremendously intricate
patterning of the brain circuits for behavior was found to be mainly achieved
by growth processes, prefunctionally under genetic control, and carried out
with great precision, involving an enormously complex system of preprogrammed cell-to-cell chemical affinities."

SPECIFICITY IN CALLOSAL CONNECTIVITY

Much that is known about callosal connectivity pertains to the organization of the system, and many details of this organization, ranging from the
topography in the corpus callosum of fibers emanating from different lobes
of the cerebral hemisphere [Pandya, this volume] to the distribution of
callosal axon terminations in relation to particular cortical fields [Kaas and
Cusick, this volume; Imig, this volume], were presented at the symposium.
Although some degree of variability in this organization is suggested by
Kaas, the overall impression is one of the considerable specificity with
which fibers emanating from the same lobe associate with one another and
of the constancy with which terminal distribution maps are formed in
relation to representation maps (Fig. 1). If we couple this impression with

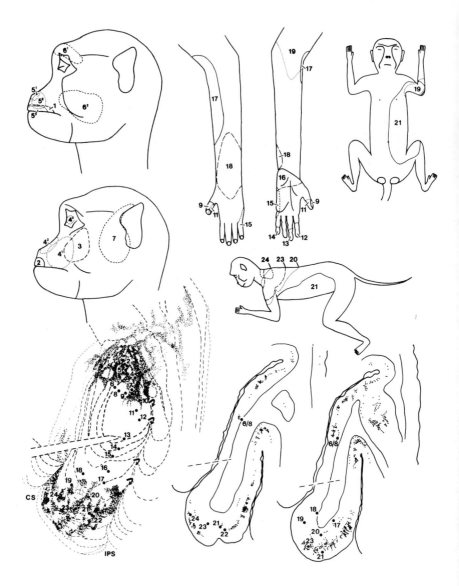

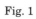
Fig. 1

the clear evidence from Imig's work that callosal fibers seek out only binaurally excited columns in the auditory cortex (even though the binaurality does not depend on the callosal fibers), together with the evidence showing the constancy with which heterotopic and homotopic connections are formed by callosal fibers emanating from a particular cortical area (Fig. 3), as well as the precise reciprocity in the callosal connection (Fig. 2), then the overwhelming evaluation must be one of great connectional specificity.

The regional specificity of callosal fiber terminations (and because of the reciprocity in the connection, of the callosally projecting neurons), is carried

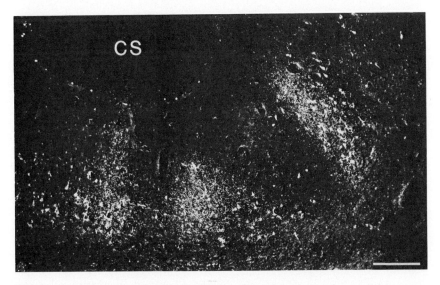

Fig. 2. Superimposed columns of callosal cells and axons in the somatic sensory cortex of a monkey [from Jones et al., 1979]. CS, central sulcus.

Fig. 1. Lower left: reconstruction made by stacking camera lucida tracings of a series of sections (lower right) cut parallel to surface of right postcentral gyrus. From a brain in which recordings were made 2 days after injecting a large amount of horseradish peroxidase (HRP) in the contralateral SI cortex. Stipple indicates retrogradely labeled callosal cells and anterogradely labeled callosal axonal ramifications. Numbered dots indicate electrode penetrations. Curved arrows indicate label in depths of intraparietal sulcus (IPS). Interrupted line indicates cut made in brain as a reference point for reconstruction. Upper: receptive fields of units recorded in vicinity of layer IV in penetrations illustrated on left. Note the representation of distal aspects of the digits well posteriorly in SI (in areas 1 and 2) and the distribution of callosal cells and axons only in relation to units with receptive fields proximal to the elbow. Tracks for which sequential receptive fields are illustrated descended posterior bank of central sulcus in layer IV of area 3b. Units in track 10 were activated by movement of shoulder [from Jones and Hendry, 1980].

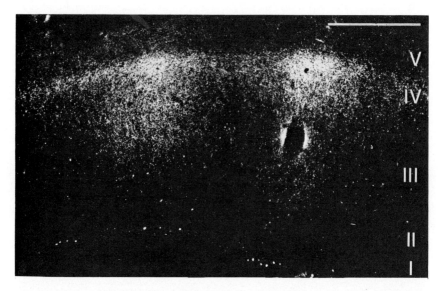

Fig. 3. Anterograde labeling of callosal axons in SII cortex of a monkey following an injection of tracer in the contralateral SI. In contrast to Figure 2, no cells are retrogradely labeled [from Jones et al., 1979].

to a much finer level of resolution. Within an area of callosal fiber terminations, there is a clear fractionation of the terminal pattern into columnar zones of termination (Fig. 2) that may well alternate with comparable columnar zones of termination of ipsilateral cortical association fibers [Goldman-Rakic and Schwarz, 1981], though in the areas that I have studied, this alternation is by no means a clear-cut one (Fig. 4). Nevertheless, at the heart of each callosal column is a bundle of vertical callosal axons with dense masses of boutons through the granular and supragranular layers of the primate cortex (Fig. 5), where they terminate on pyramidal and other neurons [Jones and Powell, 1970; Sloper and Powell, 1979; Hendry and Jones, 1983] (Fig. 5), including those that also receive monosynaptic thalamic inputs (Fig. 6).

The precision with which callosal fibers are distributed and with which they terminate in the adult is also reflected in the predictability regarding their origin. At one level is the evidence that in a reciprocally connected area, wherever callosal fibers terminate, callosally projecting neurons are situated (Fig. 2), though it has sometimes been contested that this is an absolute rule. There is also the evidence for consistency in the callosal connectional patterns of different cortical areas. The first somatic sensory area, for example, projects to the opposite first (SI) and second (SII) somatic sensory areas, while the SII area projects only to its counterpart [Jones and

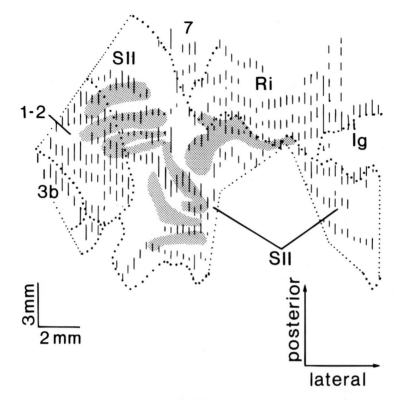

Fig. 4. Flattened-out map of monkey SII cortex showing terminations of callosal fibers (lines), labeled by degeneration, and of cortico-cortical fibers (stipple) from ipsilateral SI, labeled by autoradiography [from Jones et al., 1979].

Powell 1968, 1969] (Fig. 3). Similarly, in the SI area of the monkey, the somata of most callosally projecting cells lie in layer III [Jones et al., 1979], while in the motor area substantial numbers are also found in layer VI [Zant and Strick, 1979].

Callosally-projecting neurons are all pyramidal neurons (Fig. 6). I consider that occasional reports of non-pyramidal neurons projecting axons into the corpus callosum result from incomplete retrograde labeling of pyramidal neurons or from failure to recognize that layer VI projecting neurons are a modified form of pyramidal cell [Peters and Jones, 1984]. This too, speaks for the specificity of callosal connectivity, a specificity that is additionally reflected in the facts that in cortical transplants and in portions of the cortex malplaced by interference with their development (Fig. 7), only pyramidal cells, even though distorted morphologically, project across the midline [Floeter and Jones, 1984, 1985; Yurkewicz et al., 1984]. In these

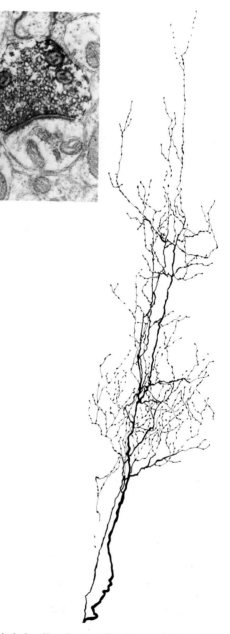

Fig. 5. Anterogradely labeled callosal axon [Hendry and Jones, 1983] and one of its terminations (inset) on a dendritic spine in the monkey somatic sensory cortex.

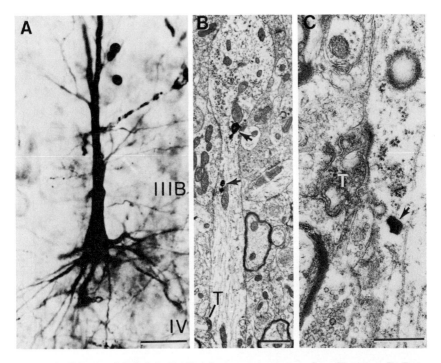

Fig. 6. A. Retrogradely labeled callosal neuron in the monkey SI cortex. B. Dendrite of a similar labeled neuron showing horseradish peroxidase label (arrows) and a degenerating thalamic axon terminal (T). C. The same degenerating terminal in an adjacent section. Bars = 50 μm (A); 5 μm (B); 1 μm (C) [from Hendry and Jones, 1983].

observations there is food for further thought; this subject will be taken up again below. Apart from being pyramidal cells with somata situated in particular layers of a given cortical area, callosally projecting cells seem largely independent of ipsilaterally projecting cortico-cortical neurons with somata in the same layers [Jones and Wise, 1977]. It would not have been surprising to have found that a significant number of callosally projecting pyramidal neurons possessed collateral axon branches projecting ipsilaterally. This, however, has not proven to be the case in the adult primate; the number of doubly projecting cells shown in any area to date has not exceeded about 5% of the projecting population [Schwartz and Goldman-Rakic, 1982; Andersen et al., 1982]. The number of callosally projecting cells with subcortical collaterals is zero [Jones and Wise, 1977; Catsman-Berrevoets et al., 1980].

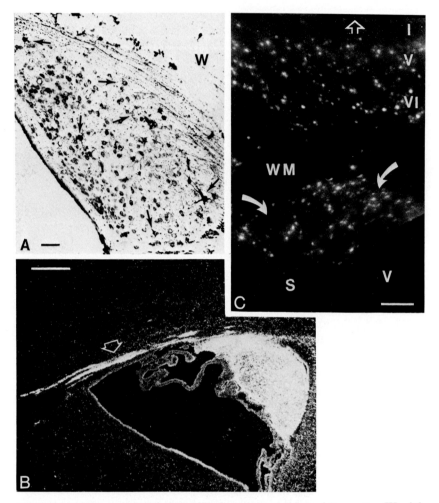

Fig. 7. A. Anterogradely labeled callosal axons traversing white matter (W) of the cerebral cortex in vicinity of a graft of fetal cortex made to a newborn rat permitted to survive to maturity. Arrows indicate retrogradely labeled callosal neurons in graft [from Floeter and Jones, 1984]. Bar = 50 μm. B. Growing axons (arrowheads) leaving a graft similar to that seen in A and entering the corpus callosum. The graft was soaked in tritiated amino acids prior to insertion in the host rat 7 days previously [from Floeter and Jones, 1985b]. Bar = 100 μm. C. Retrogradely labeled callosal cells (curved arrows) in a group of neurons that failed to migrate to the cortex during development on account of treatment of fetus with a cytotoxic drug. WM, white matter; V, ventricle; S, striatum [from Yurkewicz et al., 1984]. Bar = 250 μm.

DEVELOPMENT OF CALLOSAL CONNECTIVITY

The precision of callosal connectivity seen in the adult brain raises many questions about the development of such orderliness. These include the factors that govern the specificity of interareal connections and the columnar patterns within them as well as the general developmental biological questions of axon guidance, axon-target cell recognition, synapse formation, and synaptic stabilization. Perhaps underlying all of these, and certainly the fundamental prerequisite for all of them, is the question of how the callosal axons find their way across the midline.

Recent experiments in rats [Floeter and Jones, 1985a] support the long-suspected view that callosal fiber outgrowth toward the midline is internally programmed. Callosal axon outgrowth from pyramidal neurons occurs soon after these cells reach the cortical plate, and as might be expected, outgrowth from future layer V and VI cells precedes that from future layer III cells. This results in two waves of axons growing toward the midline, one reaching the midline on the eighteenth day of gestation, and the second on the day of birth (21 days of gestation). The programming is more complicated than this, however, for in the sensory motor regions the earliest growing axons of each wave arise from medially and laterally placed groups of cells (Fig. 8), while axons growing from intervening cells lag behind by approximately 1 day. This lag correlates with the slightly later birthdate of the intervening cells.

In the rat the earliest callosal fibers reach the midline at the 18th day of gestation and make the first crossing approximately 12 hours later [Valentino and Jones, 1982]. There are, as yet, no comparable data in other species. At the midline, growing callosal fibers exhibit typical growth cones (Figs. 9, 10) and grow through a meshwork of astrocytic processes (Fig. 10) attached to the posterodorsal surface of the commisure of the fornix. My colleagues and I have not been able to detect any preferentially oriented neuroglial substrate in this region [Valentino and Jones, 1982; Valentino et al., 1983] and feel that the callosal axons are probably seeking molecular cues to the guidance of their growth on the surfaces of the astrocytes. However, a more morphologically oriented theory of guidance across the midline has also been proposed [Silver et al., 1982]. It still remains a mystery, nevertheless, how axons growing from the right and left sides can meet, as they do, and grow along one another in opposite directions. Mechanisms of guidance operating here, as at the optic chiasm and pyramidal decussation, surely cannot simply be temporal or based upon local "signposts" for the growing axons but must involve very complicated associations between axons and substrate and between axons and axons.

It is evident that the developing cortex produces an excess of callosal axons and then "prunes" them as development proceeds. Perhaps it is a differential pruning that accounts for reports of sex differences in the size of the corpus callosum in man? The first indications of an excessive produc-

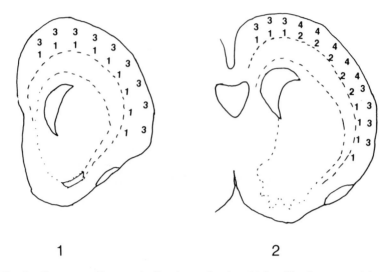

Fig. 8. Summary diagram indicating order in which callosal axons arising from the rat frontoparietal cortex cross the midline. Axons from cells in a deeper lamina cross first (1,2), and those arising from cells in medial and lateral areas of the sensory motor region (1) precede those arising from intervening cells (2). Axons from a superficial stratum of cells cross next (3,4), with a similar lag between those from medial and lateral (3) and intervening cells (4) [from Floeter and Jones, 1985a].

tion of callosal fibers came in studies indicating an unusually widespread distribution of callosally projecting cells in comparison with the adult distribution in the somatic sensory and visual areas of the cortex in cats and rats [Wise and Jones, 1976; Innocenti et al., 1977; Ivy and Killackey, 1981; Jones, 1981]. Now more direct evidence is becoming available indicating that the fetal corpus callosum may contain five or more times as many axons as in the adult [LaMantia and Rakic, 1985]. It has been suggested that the extra axons die owing to a failure to establish contralateral synapses but that the parent cells survive owing to their possession of an ipsilateral axon branch [Innocenti, 1981; O'Leary et al., 1982]. Loss of an early callosal axon undoubtedly, however, leaves some parts of many cortical areas significantly devoid of callosally projecting cells and is one factor in the establishment of the unique patterns of callosal connectivity seen in relation to motor and sensory representations in the mature cortex.

The factors that influence the regression of some callosal axons are not known. It has been shown that changes in the cortical visual field representation, ocurring in the Siamese cat [Shatz, 1977] or in the common domestic cat after the introduction of a squint in kittens [Lund, et al., 1978], are associated with a change in callosal axon terminations that occurs in a manner that follows the changed representation of visual space close to the

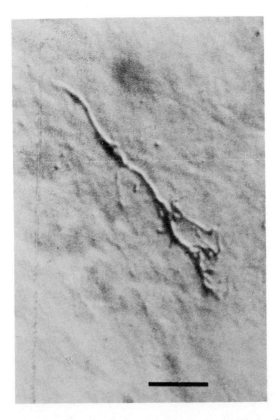

Fig. 9. Anterogradely labeled growth cone at the tip of a growing callosal fiber in an 18.5-day rat fetus. Nomarski photomicrograph [from Floeter and Jones, 1985a].

vertical meridian. This suggests that growing callosal axons are influenced by cues regarding the topographic representation in their target cortical area.

Growth of callosal axons across the midline and their innervation of the cortex is a two-stage process. Although in the rat, by birth the corpus callosum is fully formed and all callosal fibers appear to have crossed the midline (Fig. 1), the axons have not entered the cortex. Instead, they accumulate for some 5 days beneath the cortical plate before a second growth spurt carries them into the cortex [Wise and Jones, 1976; Wise et al., 1977]. The nature of the signal inducing this second growth spurt is not known, but it seems to be independent of that which influences the innervation of the cortex by thalamocortical fibers, since after a comparable period of waiting, they make their second growth spurt 4–5 days prior to the callosal fibers [Wise et al., 1977; Wise and Jones, 1978]. Perhaps it is here, beneath

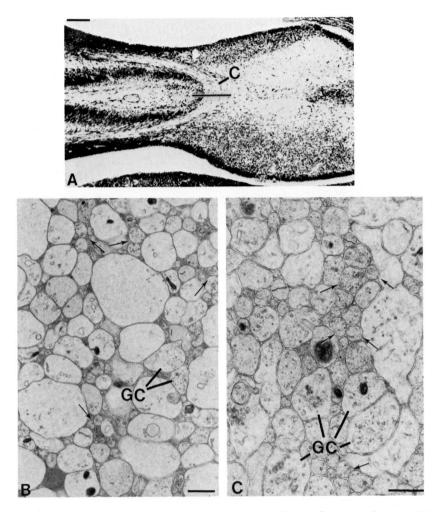

Fig. 10. A. The earliest appearance of the corpus callosum (C) in a rat fetus at 18.5 days of gestation. Horizontal section. Bar = 100 μm. B,C. Electron micrographs in plane indicated in (A) showing large astrocytic processes and penetrating callosal axons (arrows) at 18.5 (B) and 19 (C) days of gestation. GC, growth cones. Bars = 1μm [from Valentino and Jones, 1982].

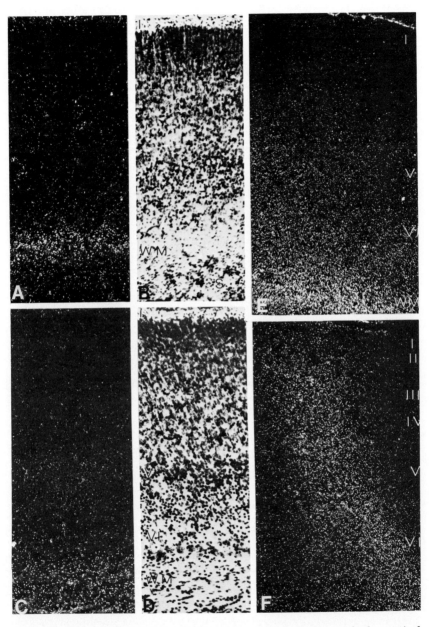

Fig. 11. Anterogradely labeled callosal axons accumulating beneath the cortical plate in rats at 1 (A,B) and 3 (C,D) days of age, and entering and colonizing the somatic sensory cortex at 5 (E) and 7 (F) days of age [from Wise and Jones, 1977].

the cortex, that callosal axons become topographically targeted on cortical areas and on particular parts of these areas and perhaps it is here that those destined to regress are culled. Alternatively, of course, those destined to be lost may meet their fate through ineffectual competition for synaptic space in the cortex itself, after making an entry into it.

CONCLUSIONS

Callosal connectivity is a highly structured thing and it is difficult to see how this structure could arise except under a series of very powerful developmental constraints. Working out the nature of these constraints should not only lead to a more complete understanding of the corpus callosum and possibly to methods of influencing its structure and function in disease but should also lead to an understanding of those developmental mechanisms that regulate axon growth and target finding and synaptogenesis in general. In this there is the further hope of union between what Sperry [1983] called "the functional plasticity of brain organization and . . . of behavior and . . . human nature in general."

ACKNOWLEDGMENTS

Personal work reported in the text was supported by grants NS10526 and NS15070 from the National Institutes of Health, United States Public Health Service.

REFERENCES

Andersen, RA, Asanuma C, Cowan WM (1982): Observations on the callosal and associational cortico-cortical connections of area 7a of the macaque monkey. Neurosci Abstr 8:210.

Catsman-Berrovoets CE, Lemon RN, Verburgh CA, Bentivoglio M, Kuypers HGJM (1980): Absence of callosal collaterals derived from rat corticospinal neurons. Exp Brain Res 39:433–440.

Floeter MK, Jones EG (1984): Connections made by transplants to the cerebral cortex of rat brains damaged *in utero.* J Neurosci 4:141–150.

Floeter MK, Jones EG (1985a): The morphology and phased outgrowth of callosal axons in the fetal rat. Dev Brain Res (in press).

Floeter MK, Jones EG (1985b): Transplantation of fetal postmitotic neurons: Early pathway choices and long term projections of outgrowing axons. Dev Brain Res (in press).

Goldman-Rakic PS, Schwartz ML (1982): Interdigitation of contralateral and ipsilateral columnar projections to frontal association cortex in primates. Science 216:755–757.

Hendry SHC, Jones EG (1980): Electron microscopic demonstration of thalamic axon terminations on identified commisural neurons in monkey somatic sensory cortex. Brain Res 196:253–257.

Hendry SHC, Jones EG (1983): Thalamic inputs to identified commissural neurons in the monkey somatic sensory cortex. J Neurocytol 12:299–316.

Innocenti GM (1981): Growth and reshaping of axons in the establishment of visual callosal connections. Science 212:824–827.

Innocenti GM, Fiore L, Caminiti R (1977): Exuberant projection into the corpus callosum from the visual cortex of newborn cats. Neurosci Lett 4:237–242.

Ivy GO, Killackey HP (1981): The ontogeny of the distribution of callosal projection neurons in the rat parietal cortex. J Comp Neurol 195:367–389.

Jones EG (1981): Development of connectivity in the cerebral cortex. In: Cowan WM (ed): Studies in Developmental Neurobiology in Honor of Victor Hamburger. New York: Oxford University Press.

Jones EG, Coulter JD, Wise SP (1979): Commissural columns in the sensory-motor cortex of monkeys. J Comp Neurol 188:113–136.

Jones EG, Hendry SHC (1980): Distribution of callosal fibers around the hand representations in monkey somatic sensory cortex. Neurosci Lett 19:167–172.

Jones EG, Powell TPS (1968): The commissural connexions of the somatic sensory cortex in the cat. J Anat (Lond) 103:433–455.

Jones EG, Powell TPS (1969): Connexions of the somatic sensory cortex of the rhesus monkey. II. Contralateral cortical connexions. Brain 92:717–730.

Jones EG, Powell TPS (1970): An electron microscopic study of the laminar pattern and mode of termination of the afferent fibre pathways to the somatic sensory cortex. Philos Trans R Soc Lond [Biol] 257:45–62.

Jones EG, Wise SP (1977): Size, laminar and columnar distribution of efferent cells in the sensory-motor cortex of monkeys. J Comp Neurol 175:391–438.

LaMantia A-S., Rakic P (1984): The number, size, myelination, and regional variation of axons in the corpus callosum and anterior commissure of the developing rhesus monkey. Neurosci Abstr 10:1081.

Lund RD, Mitchell DE, Hendry GH (1978): Squint-induced modification of callosal connections in cats. Brain Res 144:169–172.

O'Leary DDM, Stanfield BB, Cowan WM (1981): Evidence that the early postnatal restriction of the cells of origin of the callosal projection is due to the elimination of axonal collaterals rather than to the death of neurons. Dev Brain Res 1:607–617.

Peters A, Jones EG (1984): Classification of cortical neurons. In: Peters A, Jones EG, Cerebral Cortex Vol. 1 (eds) New York: Plenum Press, pp 107–122.

Schwartz ML, Goldman-Rakic PS (1982): Single cortical neurons have axon collaterals to ipsilateral and contralateral cortex in fetal and adult primates. Nature 299:154–156.

Shatz C (1977): Abnormal interhemispheric connections in the visual system of Boston Siamese cats: A physiological study. J Comp Neurol 171:229–246.

Silver J, Lorenz SE, Wahlstein D, Coughlin J (1982): Axonal guidance during development of the great cerebral commissures: Descriptive and experimental studies, in vivo, on the role of performed glial pathways. J Comp Neurol 210:10–29.

Sloper JJ, Powell TPS (1979): An experimental electron microscopic study of afferent connections to the primate motor and somatic sensory cortices. Philos Trans R Soc Lond [Biol] 285:199–226.

Sperry RW (1983): "Science and Moral Priority." Oxford: Blackwell.

Valentino KL, Jones EG (1982): The early formation of the corpus callosum: A light and electron microscopic study in fetal and neonatal rats. J Neurocytol 11:583–609.

Valentino KL, Jones EG, Kane SA (1983): Expression of GFAP immunoreactivity during development of long fiber tracts in the rat CNS. Dev Brain Res 9:317–336.

Wise SP, Jones EG (1976): The organization and postnatal development of the commissural projection of the rat somatic sensory cortex. J Comp Neurol 163:313–343.

Wise SP, Jones EG (1978): Developmental studies of thalamocortical and commissural connections in the rat somatic sensory cortex. J Comp Neurol 178:187–208.

Wise SP, Hendry SHC, Jones EG (1977): Prenatal development of sensorimotor cortical projections in cats. Brain Res 138:538–544.

Yurkewicz L, Valentino KL, Floeter MK, Fleshman JW Jr, Jones EG (1984): Effects of cytotoxic deletions of somatic sensory cortex in fetal rats. Somatosensory Res 1:303–327.

Zant JD, Strick PL (1978): The cells of origin of interhemispheric connections in the primate motor cortex. Neurosci Abstr 4:308.

SECTION III
ELECTROPHYSIOLOGY

Two Hemispheres—One Brain:
Functions of the Corpus Callosum, pages 167–169
© 1986 Alan R. Liss, Inc.

Introductory Comments

D. HUBEL

Department of Neurobiology, Harvard Medical School, Boston, Massachusetts 02115

It is a great honor for me to be speaking to you at a meeting celebrating Roger Sperry, because I think that to all of us, and to me not least, he has represented an enormously important example in the field of neurobiology. I met Ronald Myers long before I met Roger Sperry, because I started my research at Walter Reed Army Medical Center in Washington and there found myself put in a laboratory consisting of three little cubicles, the person in the next cubicle being Ronald Myers, who had also been caught in the American doctors' draft of the 1950s. We worked at very close quarters for a couple of years. We didn't collaborate, but I became well indoctrinated into the mysteries of the corpus callosum.

Myers was certainly a very important figure in the field, the importance being of course derived in some measure from Roger Sperry, since he had been Roger Sperry's graduate student and co-worker in the early corpus callosum work. They were the first to show, in an animal, that the corpus callosum did something besides holding the two hemispheres together. I didn't meet Roger Sperry for some years, but I went out West once in the early 1960s to give a seminar at Caltech, and to my surprise, he saw fit to come to the seminar. He was a formidable, very well known figure at that point, and I was just an infant in research. So I was very impressed at meeting him.

I got to know him much better later, especially in 1981, when we were both in Sweden together. My family roomed next to his at the Grand Hotel in Stockholm. I had never met any of his family. But on the evening of the first banquet, my wife, our three boys, and I were in our room trying to get our clothing assembled—for these formal occasions in Sweden, the men wear tails and a white tie—when there came a knock on our door and it was Roger Sperry's son, holding a white tie, saying, "Does anybody know what to do with these things?" Probably none of us had an apraxia for dressing, but when it comes to white ties, I suspect everybody has an apraxia. I wear the kind that is already tied, and by making it look messy enough I can make it resemble a real one. The only person in our family who could help was our youngest boy, who plays the trumpet and has to turn up at concerts in such an outfit. So he knew very well how to tie a black tie (a white tie isn't that different) and was able to get all of our ties tied, including Sperry's and his son's.

It's impressive to think of Roger Sperry and what he did for the field of brain research. On the subject of corpus callosum, of course I have no credentials, other than having roomed next to Sperry once (and Ronald Myers another time). I have done some research that has to do with the corpus callosum, but always in a somewhat secondary way. Yet in the context of today's talks I think the visual cortex (which is my home ground) is an important region—ironically, in a way, because, as you have heard and you will hear many more times, of all the areas in the cerebral cortex, the primary visual cortex is perhaps the one that is least corpus-callosally connected. It should, I suppose, have been obvious all along, from Talbot and Marshall and any of the cortical localizationists, that the primary visual cortex is not strongly callosally connected. Why would the creator see fit to connect the part of area 17 that has to do with one region of the visual field with a part of 17 that has to do with the mirror-image region in the opposite visual field? Area 17 does, however, have some callosal connections, and these have been useful in understanding corpus callosum function. The reason that the primary visual cortex looms rather large in studies of the corpus callosum is that, at the single-cell level, this region is far better known in detail than any other region of the cortex. One can ask rather precise questions about what, if any, role the corpus callosum plays in vision. Let us suppose that we had been called on to design a brain and were told that we had to have a region, which we are going to call area 17, onto which the visual fields should be mapped. Since the visual fields are more-or-less hemispherical, we design a visual cortex that is more or less hemi-spherical and we map the visual fields onto it. Now some wet blanket, such as a classical embryologist, comes along and says, "Look, after all, we're vertebrates, we're bilaterally symmetric, you can't do this unless you want to go back to Descartes and think that there are really midline organs like the pineal—you've got to put half of this cortex on one side and half on the other." Of course, our immediate reaction would be absolute outrage, be-cause for the fovea, the region where vision is most precise, we are asked to move half the cells to one side and the other half to the other: on the face of it, an outrageous assignment. But that is what is done, obviously. It is as though you drew a line and said, "Every cell to the left, go to the left hemisphere; every cell to the right, go to the right hemisphere: it doesn't matter if you are all locally richly connected, you just have to drag your connections along. You must pull them out and make a big band of fibers doing what the local connections would do." Those fibers, of course, become a large part of the population of the splenium of the corpus callosum.

Of course, the visual part of the corpus callosum forms only a small fraction of this huge commissure, but if its function—that of cementing together the cortical regions subserving the two half-fields of vision—is at all representative, we can expect that the remainder of this structure—still largely not understood—will similarly consist of countless very specialized components.

For the rest of this small disquisition I want to discuss a very different kind of thing, and now I'm going to allow myself to become cosmic and philosophical, or if you prefer, woolly and vague. It seems to me, thinking about Roger Sperry's contributions, that they represent a revolution in science comparable to the Copernican revolution or the Darwinian revolution. The word "revolution" obviously has to be used loosely, but Sperry certainly originated a different way of thinking about consciousness. Suddenly it became compellingly clear that if you bisect the brain, you end up with something that you can't think of any longer, in any sensible way, as a single mind, since thought processes are now going on simultaneously and independently in the two separate hemispheres. The same thing happened when Galileo turned his telescope on the sky and discovered that Jupiter had satellites, and that it no longer made sense to talk about the "sky" as if it were some concrete thing. "Sky" is still a good poetic term, and we still know what we mean when we use the word, but if we use it in the same sentence with words that we understand with a different kind of reality, such as "galaxy" or "globular cluster," we are in danger of not making sense. Darwin perhaps did the same thing with the word "creation." Each of these revolutionaries had trouble convincing the rest of the world, and particularly religious groups, of the validity of their ideas. But time seems to take care of such things (except perhaps in the minds of a few people—like our present American president). So I suspect time will also settle the problem of the mind, and when we discuss the questions of whether the brain informs the mind and how the brain interacts with the mind, we will come to realize that we're not making semantic sense. Sooner or later, I would guess, the mind will be retired to the same position of poetry and lay speech as the sky, a very useful term but not one that we can make valid statements about if we try to reify it. This is something that the work of Roger Sperry has brought about. Now ironically, many of the giants in central nervous system neurobiology—Sherrington, Penfield, Eccles, and also Sperry—have all been to some extent and in different ways dualists, or at least mystic in their feelings about the brain, even though each, in his own way, has helped lay the groundwork for a demystification of the brain. It seems that the mind, when fragmented, splits along surprising lines of cleavage and becomes impossible to sustain as any kind of unitary concept. Intuitively, this may be a hard thing to swallow, and it may not be easy for us to do so emotionally—but how salutory a medicine for our scientific health!

Two Hemispheres—One Brain:
Functions of the Corpus Callosum, pages 171–188
© 1986 Alan R. Liss, Inc.

The Organization of the Callosal Connections According to Sperry's Principle of Supplemental Complementarity

GIOVANNI BERLUCCHI, GIANCARLO TASSINARI, AND
ANTONELLA ANTONINI
Istituto di Fisiologia umana, Universita' di Verona, Verona, Italy

The classical studies of Sperry and his collaborators on interhemispheric communication are rightly credited with providing the first direct demonstration of the functional significance of the forebrain commissures for the control of behavioral and mental activities. Given that the corpus callosum and the anterior commissure constitute the largest connection system of the neocortex, the discovery that they are essential for the bihemispheric utilization of sensory information initially confined to one hemisphere was no small feat, particularly if one considers that so many previous investigators had failed to present an interpretation supported by any convincing evidence regarding the role of the interhemispheric connections in cerebral organization. By the late sixties, the work performed in Sperry's laboratory on cat [Myers, 1961], monkey [Sperry, 1968], and man [Sperry et al., 1969] had made it clear that after section of the forebrain commissures, sensory information restricted to one hemisphere is usually available only to that hemisphere, in sharp contrast to the constant bilateral processing of information that occurs in the intact brain. The corpus callosum and anterior commissure were thus proven to be indispensable for the unification and coordination of cognitive processes that take place separately and independently in the two hemispheres.

Subsequent attempts to establish neural counterparts to these striking behavioral findings have disclosed several important features of the morphological and functional organization of the commissural connections, but our understanding of the nervous substrates of hemispheric interaction is still very fragmentary. The major weakness of current approaches to the analysis of commissural function is the lack of a general theory of cortical organization that can incorporate the anatomical and physiological data on interhemispheric connections into an appropriate framework of neurobehavioral significance. Sperry himself has always been keenly aware of this problem [Sperry, 1962a,b]. Convinced that the apparent anatomical sym-

metry of the callosal system, with its prevailing pattern of homotopic interconnections between the two hemispheres, makes little sense from a
physiological point of view, he suggested that a "principle of supplemental
complementarity" would be better suited for grasping the main functional
purpose of the interhemispheric pathways. In his words, the corpus callosum
is primarily "a means of supplementing the activity of each hemisphere
with different and complementary information about what is happening on
the other side" [Sperry, 1962b].

Although at first sight (and according to Sperry) the principle of supplemental complementarity would seem to require a heterotopic patterning of
callosal connections to link up non-corresponding cortical sites of the two
hemispheres, subsequent research showed that such a principle is by no
means incompatible with the fundamentally homotopic distribution of the
callosal fibers [see Berlucchi and Antonini, in press]. This review will
consider current ideas and controversies related to this concept and indicate
some possible avenues for future research.

SUPPLEMENTAL COMPLEMENTARITY AND THE MIDLINE RULE

The meaning of the principle of supplemental complementarity is best
illustrated in relation to the visual system. A large portion of the neocortex
of carnivores and primates contains neurons that respond to visual stimulation. Visually responsive cortex in the occipital, temporal, and parietal
lobes of cat and monkey has been subdivided into several areas, each of
which contains a more-or-less complete and continuous representation of
visual space [Tusa, 1982]. In keeping with the basic plan of organization of
the optic pathways, the various visual cortical areas receive information
chiefly from the contralateral half of the visual field; however, owing to the
corpus callosum, they may also be reached by visual information from the
ipsilateral hemifield. Since the pioneering work in anatomy by Myers [1965]
and in physiology by Whitteridge [1965], it has been shown repeatedly that
callosal fibers running between areas 17 and 18 of the two sides are endowed
with visual fields on the vertical meridian, and distribute themselves to
cortical neurons that are also concerned with the vertical midline of the
visual field [for recent reviews, see Berlucchi, 1981; Elberger, 1982; Innocenti, 1985]

Sperry's principle of supplemental complementarity is clearly applicable
to the callosal connections of areas 17 and 18. The intrahemispheric input
from the contralateral visual field and the interhemispheric input from the
ipsilateral visual field converge onto single neurons of these areas in a very
orderly way, because the inputs that participate in the convergence are
spatially matched at the vertical meridian of the visual field [Berlucchi and
Rizzolatti, 1968; Lepore and Guillemot, 1982; Antonini et al., 1985]. More
precisely, visual receptive fields built up by the convergence of intra- and
interhemispheric inputs extend in a continuous fashion across the vertical

midline of the visual field. If callosal connections were supplied or received by cortical neurons outside of the representation of the vertical meridian, the receptive fields resulting from the convergence of these callosal connections with intrahemispheric connections would be formed by two disjoint portions lying in opposite hemifields. Such receptive fields have been observed very rarely and only in areas 17 and 18 of Siamese cats; their existence in these animals is accounted for by a genetic abnormality of the visual pathways rather than by the action of a callosal input unrelated to the vertical meridian [Hubel and Wiesel, 1970].

In the normal brain it appears that afferent and efferent callosal projections are indeed limited to those cortical neurons that have receptive fields on or near the vertical meridian, and that this limitation is the necessary and sufficient condition for ensuring a continuous representation of the visual field over the cortex, notwithstanding the wide separation of the direct representations of the right and left hemifields in different hemispheres. As envisaged by Sperry, the visual information conveyed by the callosal connections and that supplied by the direct input to the cortex are, thus, both supplementary, because they make an addition to one another, and complementary, because this mutual addition results in a homogeneous whole.

This pattern of organization appears to apply not only to areas 17 and 18 but to the other visual cortical areas as well, as seen most clearly in the split-chiasm preparation. A critical determinant of the successful demonstration of the behavioral effects of hemispheric disconnection in Sperry's laboratory was the rigorous and systematic lateralization of the sensory input to one side of the brain. In the experiments on animals this was best obtained for the visual modality by a mid-sagittal splitting of the optic chiasm, which destroys the crossed projections of the retinae but spares the uncrossed ones [Myers, 1955]. We found this preparation very suitable for physiological studies of the corpus callosum in the cat. Since the neural outflow from each retina is restricted to the ipsilateral cerebral hemisphere, responses of cortical neurons to visual stimuli presented to the opposite eye are mediated exclusively through the corpus callosum, whereas the responses of the same neurons to stimuli presented to the ipsilateral eye are mediated exclusively by uncrossed thalamocortical afferents. One can thus distinguish callosal receptive fields, mapped through the eye contralateral to the side of recording, and thalamocortical receptive fields, which are mapped through the eye ipsilateral to the side of recording.

Two recent experiments using this technique [Antonini et al., 1983, 1985] have explored four cortical visual areas of the cat: areas 17, 18, 19, and a visual lateral suprasylvian area named posteromedial lateral suprasylvian (PMLS) by Palmer et al. [1978]. The percentage of neurons responding to stimulation of either eye after chiasm splitting was about 50% at the 17/18 border, about 31% in area 19 [Antonini et al., 1985], and about 57% in

PMLS [Antonini et al., 1983]. The other neurons responded solely to stimulation of the ipsilateral eye. The interhemispheric nature of the response to stimulation of the contralateral eye was proven by its disappearance following a callosal section and/or indicated by the fact that the receptive field was ipsilateral to the side of recording.

The observed efficacy of the transcallosal visual input is in accord with previous works [Berlucchi and Rizzolatti, 1968; Cynader et al., 1981; Lepore and Guillemot, 1982] but at variance with other reports of an almost total unresponsiveness of visual cortex neurons to contralateral eye stimulation after chiasm splitting [Yinon and Hammer, 1981; Milleret and Buser, 1984]. Perhaps the latter results may be accounted for by an unintentional deafferentation of the visual cortex by sectioning many uncrossed fibers along with the crossed fibers, as suggested by the strong reduction of the reactivity of the cortex to stimulation of the ipsilateral as well as contralateral eye.

The common property of the callosal connections of all visual cortical areas investigated in the experiments of Antonini et al. [1983, 1985] was that the intrahemispheric and interhemispheric receptive fields of each binocular neuron matched each other at the vertical meridian, forming a combined bilateral receptive field that was continuous across the midline. This obviously does not mean that the callosal connections of all visual cortical areas serve the same function; the neuronal circuitry of interhemispheric connections may be the same in all cortical areas, and in fact Innocenti [1985] believes that in principle it does not differ from the circuitry for intrahemispheric cortical interconnection. However, we maintain that in each cortical area callosal connections become part of the neural substrate of the function served by that particular area. For example, in the cat, callosal connections of areas 17/18 may be involved in binocular stereopsis, while callosal connections of visual suprasylvian areas may be involved in visual learning [Berlucchi et al., 1979].

The matching at the midline of intra- and interhemispheric connections requires that callosal connections selectively come from and impinge upon neurons whose direct, intrahemispheric visual input originates from visual field regions overlapping or adjoining the vertical meridian. However, because of the different average size of receptive fields in the different cortical areas, the amount of visual field represented in each area through the corpus callosum varied considerably from area to area. For example, the maximal width of callosal receptive fields was about 12–13° both at the 17/18 border and in area 19, whereas it was about 35° in area PMLS. (Larger callosal receptive fields have been described in area 18 by Sanides and Albus, [1980] and Lepore and Guillemot [1982]).

Since callosal receptive fields systematically adjoined the vertical meridian, the width of the largest of these receptive fields indicated the amount of visual field represented in each area through the corpus callosum. In keeping with conclusions drawn from anatomical studies [see, e.g., Segraves and Rosenquist, 1982a,b], the physiological evidence of Antonini et al. [1983, 1985] supports the hypothesis that in visual cortical areas other than 17 the corpus callosum can transmit information from visual field zones which are quite distant from the vertical meridian. However, this occurs not because in these areas callosal connections invade the cortical representations of visual field areas unrelated to the vertical meridian, but simply because of the increased size of the receptive fields (Fig. 1).

Receptive fields that include the vertical meridian and, thus, may belong to neurons projecting to or receiving from the corpus callosum may be so large as to extend toward the extreme periphery of the visual field along the horizontal meridian. Further, the seemingly diffuse anatomical character of the callosal connections of areas 19 and PMLS [see Segraves and Rosenquist, 1982a,b] is not incompatible with the selective relation of these connections with the vertical meridian if one considers that visuotopic maps in these areas are so irregular as to allow the intermingling at the same cortical sites of neurons with receptive fields on the vertical meridian and neurons with receptive fields near one end of the horizontal meridian [Hubel and Wiesel, 1969; Albus and Beckmann, 1980]. It is our contention that in these sites of intermingling of cortical neurons with receptive fields in different locations, callosal connections are restricted to at least some of those neurons whose receptive field, whether large or small, is in contact or in close proximity with the vertical meridian. This limitation has been observed also in some "ectopic" islands of visual field representation in area 18 [Sanides and Albus, 1980].

BINOCULAR INTERACTIONS AND CORPUS CALLOSUM

In the experiments on split-chiasm cats, the corpus callosum has been shown to be essential both for forming receptive fields across the vertical midline, in accordance with the principle of supplemental complementarity, and for maintaining binocular interaction in the cortex, in spite of the surgical separation of the inputs from the two eyes. How does the interhemispheric visual input to the cortex interact with the intrahemispheric input when the optic pathways are intact?

In theory this question can be answered by assessing the extension of visual receptive fields of cortical neurons into the hemifield ipsilateral to the side of recording. The ipsilateral extension may be due not only to the callosal input, but also to the contingent of crossed projections from the temporal hemiretina. These two possibilities can be distinguished experimentally in two ways: (a) by cutting the corpus callosum, which obviously eliminates the callosal but not the retinal ipsilateral representation, and (b) by assessing the cortical representation of the ipsilateral hemifield in the eye ipsilateral to the side of recording. Such ipsilateral representation is transmitted through the nasal hemiretina and, thus, can be mediated only through the corpus callosum.

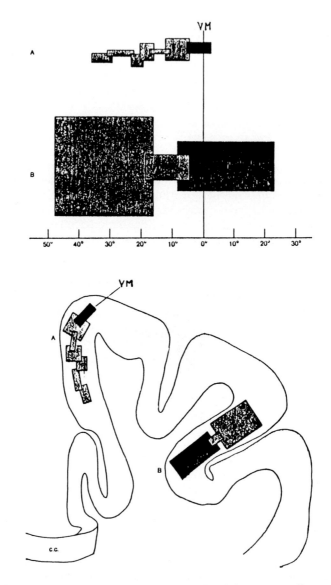

Fig. 1. Schematic illustration of the participation of the corpus callosum (c.c.) to the representation of the visual field in areas 17/18 (A) and in the lateral suprasylvian areas (B). In both cases the corpus callosum is necessary for extending receptive fields in the central visual field across the vertical meridian (VM) into the ipsilateral hemifield (darker rectangles). Owing to the larger size of receptive fields in the lateral suprasylvian areas, the callosal representation of the ipsilateral hemifield in these areas is much more extensive than in areas 17/18.

In practice, in those cortical areas where the representation of the ipsilateral visual field is limited to a few degrees from the vertical meridian, these experimental approaches suffer from the difficulty in defining the precise position of the vertical meridian itself [for a discussion, see Antonini et al., 1985]. By contrast, in those areas where the representation of the ipsilateral visual field is very extensive, the results have been unequivocal. Recording from the crown of the middle suprasylvian gyrus in the cat, Dow and Dubner [1971] described neurons that responded to visual targets moving across large portions of both contralateral and ipsilateral hemifields. Cutting the corpus callosum or destroying the cortex in the opposite hemisphere abolished the response in the ipsilateral but not in the contralateral visual field. Similarly Marzi et al. [1982] found that the extensive representation of the ipsilateral visual field in area PMLS of normal cats was lost in the eye ipsilateral to the side of recording and reduced in the other eye following section of the posterior half of the corpus callosum. As a result of this section receptive fields of PMLS neurons in the vertical meridian region were significantly reduced in width compared to the receptive fields recorded before the section, as though a portion of these receptive fields had been suppressed by callosotomy. In the inferotemporal cortex of the macaque, neurons are usually endowed with large binocular and bilateral visual receptive fields, but after section of the corpus callosum and anterior commissure, they respond only to stimuli in the hemifield contralateral to the side of recording [Rocha-Miranda et al., 1975; Gross et al., 1977]. The following common conclusions can be drawn from the above experiments on cats and monkeys: (1) The callosal visual input is quite effective in driving cortical neurons. (2) The supplementary and complementary interactions between intrahemispheric and interhemispheric visual inputs to the cortex that can be shown to occur across the eyes of the split-chiasm cat are manifest also in each eye of cats and monkeys with intact visual pathways, independent of binocular interaction. (3) At least in suprasylvian visual areas of the cat and in the inferotemporal cortex in the monkey, the main function of the interhemispheric connections is to provide a representation of the ipsilateral visual field that is continuous with that of the contralateral visual field.

These conclusions do not rule out the possibility that callosal connections may also be involved in binocular interactions. This possibility is relevant to binocular stereopsis, since, as originally discussed by Blakemore [1969, 1970], cortical neurons that code for large binocular disparities in the central visual field must have a receptive field in one eye and one hemifield paired with a receptive field in the other eye and the other hemifield. The problem of the effect of callosotomy on binocular interactions in areas 17 and 18 of the cat is discussed in this volume by Elberger and Payne and in recent papers by Blakemore et al. [1983], Payne et al. [1984], and Elberger and Smith [1985]. In our laboratory Minciacchi and Antonini [1984] recorded from single neurons of the visual cortex of awake, unanesthetized adult cats with acute or chronic callosal sections. In their experiments the interhemispheric disconnection, whether acute or chronic, did not disrupt binocularity in areas 17 and 18; moreover, the analysis of the ocular dominance for binocular neurons did not reveal any imbalance between the inputs from the two eyes that could be attributed to the callosal section (see Fig. 2). These findings agree with those of Elberger and Smith [1985], who reported that a reduction of binocular interaction in the cat visual cortex could be observed after a callosal section performed before, but not after, 19 days of age.

The suggestion by Minciacchi and Antonini [1984] that the observation of a loss of binocular cortical neurons in the visual cortex of cats callosotomized when adult may require the presence of general anesthesia is not incompatible with the hypothesis of a subliminal facilitatory role of the corpus callosum in binocular interaction [Payne et al., 1984]. It should be noted, however, that the latter authors indirectly infer the facilitatory action of the corpus callosum in binocular interaction from a rather peculiar transitory intrahemispheric effect which they attribute to recurrent ipsilateral collaterals of callosal projecting neurons. In addition, their hypothesis completely ignores the inhibitory effects ultimately exerted on the cortex by intrahemispheric recurrent collaterals of callosal fibers [Feeney and Orem, 1971].

Whatever the role of the corpus callosum in the organization of the visual cortex, it appears that in normal cats the overwhelming majority of visual cortical neurons can be activated from both eyes independent of interhemispheric connections. Interhemispheric connections may become important for binocular interactions in those cats that owing to genetic abnormalities have an in-built lateralization of the optic input. This has been shown in Siamese cats [see Marzi et al., 1982; and this volume] and in albino rats [Diao et al., 1983].

FUNCTIONAL SIGNIFICANCE AND POSSIBLE ONTOGENESIS OF SUPPLEMENTAL COMPLEMENTARITY

Intensive work by several groups, especially by Innocenti and his colleagues [see Innocenti and Clarke, 1984; Innocenti, 1985; and this volume], has shown that the organization of the callosal connections typical of the adult brain is achieved through an exorbitant prenatal formation of interhemispheric fibers followed by a postnatal elimination of many presumably useless elements. Genetic and experiential factors appear to cooperate in these processes [see, e.g., Rhoades and Fish, 1983; Mooney et al., 1984]. It has been suggested that the patterning of the callosal connections of the visual cortex may come about as a result of the elimination of inappropriate combinations of thalamocortical and callosal afferents to the cortex that would generate receptive fields in disagreement with the principle of supplemental complementarity [Berlucchi, 1981].

Figure 3 illustrates a number of hypothetical combinations of callosal and thalamocortical visual inputs that can be predicted to lead to the maintenance or the elimination of interaction between the two inputs. The basic assumption is that cortical neurons reject one of the two inputs (possibly the weaker callosal input) if during a critical postnatal period the two inputs do not convey synchronous and congruent visual information. A right-left mirror symmetrical object positioned on the vertical meridian is apt to provide such synchronous and congruent stimulation through both the direct and the interhemispheric inputs to the visual cortex, and most targets in the natural visual field of an animal possess these properties. On the contrary, the natural simultaneous occurrence of identical stimulus configurations in the far peripheries of the right and left visual fields is most probably exceptional if not downright impossible. The supplemental complementarity ensured by the interhemispheric connections may thus be seen as a selective link between neurons that are widely separated in the two hemispheres, but that nonetheless must cooperate for allowing the organism to deal with perceived objects as unified wholes [see Sperry, 1952]. Neurons in the two hemispheres that are not functionally conjoint in such unitary patterns of brain organization do not require interhemispheric connections.

In vision, given that the two halves of the visual field are projected to different hemispheres, the principle of supplemental complementarity is indissociable from the midline rule. An exception may be represented by albino mammals, which suffer from an abnormality of the optic pathways and of the representation of the visual field over the cortex. In these animals the combination of intrahemispheric and interhemispheric visual inputs may take place within each half field and across eyes [see Antonini et al., 1981; Marzi et al., 1982; Diao et al., 1983]. In normally pigmented animals the matching of intrahemispheric and interhemispheric visual inputs necessary for the integrated perception of an object whose right and left halves are projected to different hemispheres, or for perceptual generalization between the right and left visual fields, occurs consistently at the vertical meridian [see also Gross and Mishkin, 1977; Mishkin, 1979].

In somatoesthesis, however, supplemental complementarity is not necessarily bound to cross-midline interactions. Sperry's original figure on supplemental complementarity (Fig. 4) did, in fact, stress that interhemispheric cooperation is mostly needed for cross-integration of cutaneous information between the two hands in stereognosis. Sensory receptors in the two hands are very far from the midline, but contrary to the far peripheries of the two visual hemifields, they are often submitted to synchronous and congruous stimulation, as in bimanual exploration and handling of the same object. While it is true that in the primary somatic sensory cortex of the monkey

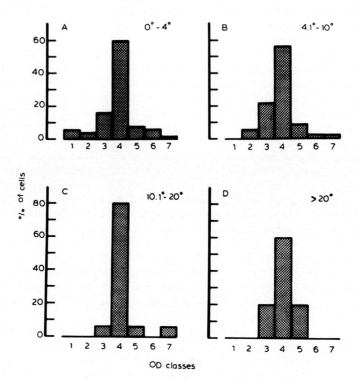

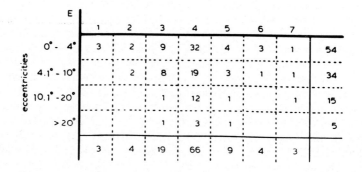

Fig. 2

(S1, including citoarchitectonic areas 3a, 3b, 2, and 1), the representations of the distal parts of the limbs have few interhemispheric connections compared to the proximal and axial regions, which are closer to the body midline and are strongly interconnected through the corpus callosum [see, e.g., Killackey et al., 1983; Shanks et al., 1985], dense callosal connections join the hand representations in area S2 of the two sides [see Manzoni et al., 1984]. Thus substrates for orderly interhemispheric interactions exist for somesthetic receptors both near the midline and away from it. It remains to be determined why interhemispheric connections for the distal extremities are so more numerous in S2 than in S1. Further, it is possible that in S1 callosal connections unite cortical zones that already receive bilateral information through their thalamic inputs [see, e.g., Barbaresi et al., 1984; Shanks et al., 1985], and therefore are not indispensable for generating bilaterality. On the contrary, the callosal connections of the hand representations in S2 would seem essential for the establishment of bimanual receptive fields by providing the input from the ipsilateral hand [Manzoni et al., 1984].

Shanks et al. [1985] maintain that "a common and fundamental principle of the callosal connexions of all the sensory areas . . . is that they pass between those parts of the two hemispheres that are concurrently activated by a peripheral stimulus . . ."; further, they consider that bilateral activation is consistently associated with stimuli near the midline both in vision and in somatoethesis. Their proposal is akin to that of Berlucchi [1981] in many respects; however, in stressing the similarities between the callosal connections of the visual system and those of the somesthetic system, Shanks et al. [1985] underestimate the functional need for supplemental complementarity between the two hands. Cortical neurons with widely disjoint bimanual receptive fields, partly mediated through the corpus callosum, would seem necessary for intermanual transfer of tactual learning [see Mishkin, 1979; Manzoni et al., 1984]. Lesions of S2 do indeed interfere with interlimb transfer in the cat [Teitelbaum et al., 1968] and with intermanual transfer in the monkey [Garcha and Ettlinger, 1980].

Fig. 2. Binocular interactions in areas 17 and 18 of callosotomized cats. The upper part of the figure (bar histograms) shows the percentages of neurons falling into different classes of ocular dominance. Classes 1 and 7 contain neurons driven only from the contralateral or ipsilateral eye, respectively. Neurons in class 4 are driven equally from both eyes. Neurons in classes 2 and 3 are binocular but show a preference for stimuli presented to the contralateral eye, this preference being relatively greater in class 2. Conversely, neurons in classes 5 and 6 show a preference for the ipsilateral eye. The four histograms show the breakdown for ocular dominance of neurons with receptive fields at different distances from the vertical meridian. The lower part of the figure shows the actual number of neurons in each class and at each level of excentricity [from Minciacchi and Antonini, 1984].

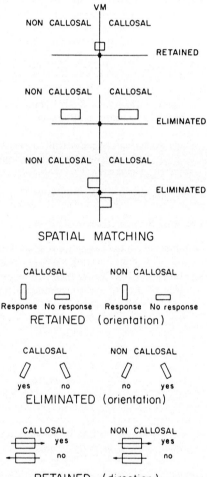

Fig. 3. Hypothetical combinations of thalamocortical and callosal visual inputs during the maturation period. A cortical neuron receiving a thalamocortical visual input and a callosal visual input would retain both inputs if they transmit synchronous and congruous visual information: that is, if the two inputs are spatially matched at the vertical meridian, and if the thalamocortical and callosal receptive fields have the same orientation and directional selectivity. Absence of correspondence between the two inputs on one or more of these features is assumed to cause the elimination of the weaker callosal input [from Berlucchi, 1981].

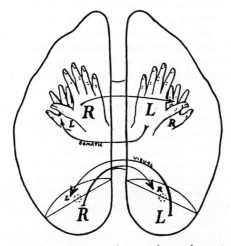

Fig. 4. Sperry's diagram of the supplemental complementarity needed for inter-manual (interhemispheric) cooperation in stereognosis [from Sperry, 1962a].

That the relation of the callosal connections to sensory maps is different for the visual and somesthetic systems is clearly shown by physiological studies of the information transmitted by these connections in cats. In the visual modality, among more than 100 visual receptive fields of callosal fibers described in three independent studies [Berlucchi et al., 1967; Hubel and Wiesel, 1967; Shatz, 1977], only one lay more than 4° from the vertical meridian. In the somatoesthetic modalities, almost 20% of the receptive fields had a distal location on a forepaw [Spidalieri et al., 1985]. This is a most convincing direct demonstration of the fact that visual callosal connections entertain a systematic relation with the midline while somatic callosal connections do not.

PRESENT ADVANCES AND POSSIBLE FUTURE DEVELOPMENTS

Quite recently there have been a large number of anatomical investigations on the callosal connections of various cortical areas in primates. Many of these studies have dealt with visual cortical areas [see, e.g., Weyand and Swadlow, 1980; Newsome and Allman, 1980; Van Essen et al., 1982; Cusick et al., 1984]. While the findings lend general support to the notion that in all visual areas callosal projection neurons and terminals are concentrated in the representations of the vertical meridian, other aspects of the results provide material for new hypotheses and considerations, and possibly for a reevaluation of the functional significance of the callosal connections.

First, there is considerable variability in the anatomical appearance of visual callosal connections among different species and among different individuals of the same species. The term "callosal fingerprint" has been used to express the possibility that each individual animal can have its own unique pattern of callosal interconnections [Van Essen et al., 1982]. This interspecies and interindividual variability is important in its own right both for the general purposes of comparative neuroscience [Bullock, 1984] and, possibly, for the interpretation of the differential function of various cortical areas in vision [Zeki, 1978; Merzenich and Kaas, 1980]. However, since it appears that there is a great deal of variability in the topographic properties of the cortical areas themselves [see, e.g., Van Essen et al., 1984], variations in the pattern of callosal interconnections need not be taken to imply that such a pattern does not follow a common principle. The fact that a gross anatomical landmark, such as a sulcus or gyrus, is found to be endowed with callosal connections in one animal and devoid of them in another may be accounted for by a different relation of such anatomical landmark to functional maps in the two animals. However, the relation between the callosal connections and the functional map could be constant in the two animals. Combined anatomical and physiological experiments are the tool of choice for solving these problems. For example, by using this combination of methods, Sanides and Albus [1980] were able to show that the individual anatomical variability of the callosal connections of area 18 of cats is in no way incompatible with the restriction of these connections to the vertical meridian representation.

The second point that has been raised on the basis of the new anatomical findings has more serious implications for general concepts about the physiological organization of the callosal connections. There have been reports of histological evidence for the presence of callosal elements well outside the vertical meridian representation in visual areas such as areas 17 and 18 of the tree shrew [Sesma et al., 1984], owl monkey, marmoset, and galago [Cusick et al., 1984]. Also in this case, physiological studies could help the assessment of the functional significance of these anatomical findings. Do the callosal connections unrelated to the vertical meridian representation transmit visual information? This question could be answered directly by recording visual responses from single fibers in the corpus callosum of these animals, as has been done in the cat [Berlucchi et al., 1967; Hubel and Wiesel, 1967; Shatz, 1977]. The hypothesis that some callosal fibers transmit visual information unrelated to the vertical meridian must be corroborated by the finding of at least some visual callosal receptive fields away from the midline.

The third point regarding the anatomy of the callosal connections is the undisputed fact that in some retinotopically organized areas these connections appear so diffuse as to render unlikely the hypothesis of a selective relation with the visuotopic map. However, this generally occurs in cortical areas where the retinotopic organization is so crude that adjacent neurons can be connected to quite different portions of the visual field, and some receptive fields can be so large as to occupy most of the visual field. Physiological analysis at the neuronal level suggests the preservation of the prevalent relation of the callosal connections with the vertical meridian even in these areas [Antonini et al., 1983, 1985].

On balance, it seems that at present there is no valid alternative to Sperry's principle of supplemental complementarity for providing a basic conceptual plan for the interpretation of the anatomical, physiological, and behavioral evidence on interhemispheric connections. Suggestions that the corpus callosum may be generically involved in diffuse hemispheric facilitation and inhibition, energizing effects or "extra-receptive field" influences smack of the way of thinking of the pre-Sperry era, when wild interpretations of the functional significance of the corpus callosum ranged from the purely mechanical ones—e.g., the corpus callosum keeps the two hemispheres from sagging—to rather implausible functional analogies—e.g., the corpus callosum mediates arousal of the cortex horizontally, as opposed to the vertical ascending action of the reticular activating system. We are far from understanding the general rules of the anatomofunctional organization of the interhemispheric connections, but whatever interpretation we propose, we must consider that Sperry's work on split-brain animals and people leaves no doubt that the corpus callosum is an incredibly complex system for the transmission of very specific information within the brain.

REFERENCES

Albus K, Beckmann R (1980): Second and third visual areas of the cat: Interindividual variability in retinotopic arrangement and cortical location. J Physiol (Lond) 299:247–266.

Antonini A, Berlucchi G, Di Stefano M, Marzi CA (1981): Differences in binocular interactions between cortical areas 17 and 18 and superior colliculus of Siamese cats. J Comp Neurol 200:597–611.

Antonini A, Berlucchi G, Lepore F (1983): Physiological organization of callosal connections of a visual lateral suprasylvian cortical area in the cat. J Neurophysiol 49:902–921.

Antonini A, Di Stefano M, Minciacchi D, Tassinari G (1985): Interhemispheric influences on area 19 of the cat. Exp Brain Res 59:179–186.

Barbaresi P, Conti F, Manzoni T (1984): Topography and receptive field organization of the body midline representation in the ventrobasal complex of the cat. Exp. Brain Res 54:327–336.

Berlucchi G (1981): Recent advances in the analysis of the neural substrates of interhemispheric communication. In Pompeiano O, Ajmone-Marsan CA (eds): "Brain Mechanisms of Perceptual Awareness and Purposeful Behavior." New York: Raven Press, pp 133–152.

Berlucchi G, Antonini A (1985): The role of the corpus callosum in the representation of the visual field in cortical areas. In Trevarthen C (ed): "Brain Circuits and Functions of the Mind." Cambridge: Cambridge University Press, (in press).

Berlucchi G, Gazzaniga MS, Rizzolatti G (1967): Microelectrode analysis of transfer of visual information by the corpus callosum. Arch Ital Biol 105:583–596.

Berlucchi G, Rizzolatti G (1968): Binocularly driven neurons in visual cortex of split-chiasm cats. Science 159:308–310.

Berlucchi G, Sprague JM, Antonini A, Simoni A (1979): Learning and interhemispheric transfer of visual pattern discriminations following unilateral suprasylvian lesions in split-chiasm cats. Exp Brain Res 34:551–574.

Blakemore C (1969): Binocular depth discrimination and the nasotemporal division. J Physiol (Lond) 205:471–497.

Blakemore C (1970): Binocular depth perception and the optic chiasm. Vision Res 10:43–47.

Blakemore C, Diao Y, Pu M, Wang Y, Xiao Y (1983): Possible functions of the interhemispheric connexions between visual cortical areas in the cat. J Physiol (Lond) 337:331–349.

Bullock TH (1984): Comparative neuroscience holds promise for quiet revolutions. Science 225:473–478.

Cusick CG, Could HJ III, Kaas JH (1984): Interhemispheric connections of visual cortex of owl monkeys (Aotus trivirgatus), marmosets (Callitrix jacchus), and galagos (Galago crassicaudatus). J Comp Neurol 230:311–336.

Cynader M, Lepore F, Guillemot JP (1981): Interhemispheric competition during postnatal development. Nature 290:139–140.

Diao YG, Wang YK, Pu ML (1983): Binocular responses of cortical cells and callosal projections in the albino rat. Exp Brain Res 49:410–418.

Dow BM, Dubner R (1971): Single-unit responses to moving stimuli in middle suprasylvian gyrus of the cat. J Neurophysiol 34:47–55.

Elberger AJ (1982): The functional role of the corpus callosum in the developing visual system: A review. Prog Neurobiol 18:15–79.

Elberger AJ, Smith EL (1985): The critical period of corpus callosum section to affect cortical binocularity. Exp Brain Res 57:213–223.

Feeney DM, Orem JM (1971): Influence of antidromic callosal volleys on single unit in visual cortex. Exp Neurol 33:310–321.

Garcha HS, Ettlinger G (1980): Tactile discrimination learning in the monkey: The effects of unilateral or bilateral removals of the second somatosensory cortex (area S2). Cortex 16:397–412.

Gross CG, Bender DB, Mishkin M (1977): Contributions of the corpus callosum and the anterior commissure to visual activation of inferior temporal neurons. Brain Res 131:227–239.

Gross CG, Mishkin M (1977): The neural basis of stimulus equivalence across retinal translations. In Harnad S, Doty RW, Goldstein L, Jaynes J and Krauthamer G. (eds): "Lateralization of the Nervous System." New York: Academic Press, pp 109–122.

Hubel DH, Wiesel TN (1967): Cortical and callosal connections concerned with the vertical meridian of visual fields in the cat. J Neurophysiol 30:1561–1573.

Hubel DH, Wiesel TN (1969): Visual area of the lateral suprasylvian gyrus of the cat. J Physiol (Lond) 202:251–260.

Hubel DH, Wiesel TN (1971): Aberrant visual projections in the Siamese cat. J Physiol (Lond) 218:33–62.

Innocenti GM (1985): The general organization of callosal connections. In Peters A, Jones EG (eds): "Areas and Connections of the Cortex." New York: Plenum Publishing Corp. (In press).

Innocenti GM, Clarke S (1984): The organization of immature callosal connections. J Comp Neurol 230:287–309.

Killackey HP, Gould HJ III, Cusick CG, Pons TP, Kaas JH (1983): The relation of corpus callosum connections to architectonic fields and body surface maps in sensorimotor cortex of New and Old World monkeys. J Comp Neurol 219:389–419.

Lepore F, Guillemot JP (1982): Visual receptive fields properties of cells innervated through the corpus callosum. Exp Brain Res 46:413–424.

Manzoni T, Barbaresi P, Conti F (1984): Callosal mechanism for the interhemispheric transfer of hand somatosensory information in the monkey. Behav Brain Res 11:155–170.

Marzi CA, Antonini A, Di Stefano M, Legg CR (1982): The contribution of the corpus callosum to receptive fields in the lateral suprasylvian visual area of the cat. Behav Brain Res 4:155–176.

Merzenich MM, Kaas JH (1980): Principles of organization of sensory-perceptual systems in mammals. Prog Psychobiol Physiol Psychol 9:1–42.

Milleret C, Buser P (1984): Receptive field sizes and responsiveness to light in area 18 of the cat after chiasmotomy. Postoperative evolution: Role of visual experience. Exp Brain Res 57:73–81.

Minciacchi D, Antonini A (1984): Binocularity in the visual cortex of the adult cat does not depend on the integrity of the corpus callosum. Behav Brain Res 13:183–192.

Mishkin M (1979): Analogous visual models for tactual and visual learning. Neuropsychologia 17:139–151.

Mooney RD, Rhoades RW, Fish SE (1984): Neonatal superior colliculus lesions alter visual callosal development in hamster. Exp Brain Res 55:9–25.

Myers RE (1955): Interocular transfer of pattern discrimination in cats following section of crossed optic fibers. J Comp Physiol Psychol 48:470–473.

Myers RE (1961): Corpus callosum and visual gnosis. In Delafresnaye JF (ed): "Brain Mechanisms and Learning." Oxford: Blackwell, pp 481–505.

Myers RE (1965): Organization of visual pathways. In Ettlinger G (ed): "Functions of the Corpus Callosum." London: Churchill, pp. 133–143.

Newsome WT, Allman JM (1980): Interhemispheric connections in the owl monkey, Aotus trivirgatus, and the bushbaby, Galago senegalensis. J Comp Neurol 194:209–233.

Palmer LA, Rosenquist AC, Tusa RJ (1978): The retinotopic organization of the lateral suprasylvian visual areas in the cat. J Comp Neurol 177:237–256.

Payne BR, Pearson HE, Berman N (1984): Role of corpus callosum in functional organization of cat striate cortex. J Neurophysiol 52:570–594.

Rhoades RW, Fish SE (1983): Bilateral enucleation alters visual callosal but not corticotectal or corticogeniculate projections in hamster. Exp Brain Res 51:451–462.

Rocha-Miranda CE, Bender DB, Gross CG, Mishkin M (1975): Visual activation of neurons in inferotemporal cortex depends on striate cortex and forebrain commissures. J Neurophysiol 38:475–491.

Sanides D, Albus K (1980): The distribution of interhemispheric projections in area 18 of the cat. Coincidence with discontinuities of the representation of the visual field in the second visual area (V2). Exp Brain Res 38:237–240.

Segraves MA, Rosenquist AC (1982a): The distribution of the cells of origin of callosal projections in cat visual cortex. J Neurosci 2:1079–1089.

Segraves MA, Rosenquist AC (1982b): The afferent and efferent callosal connections of retinotopically defined areas in cat visual cortex. J Neurosci 2:1090–1107.

Sesma MA, Casagrande VA, Kaas JH (1984): Cortical connections of area 17 in tree shrews. J Comp Neurol 230:337–351.

Shanks MF, Pearson RCA, Powell TPS (1985): The callosal connexions of the primary somatic sensory cortex in the monkey. Brain Res Rev 9:43–65.

Shatz C (1977): Abnormal interhemispheric connections in the visual system of Boston Siamese cats: A physiological study. J Comp Neurol 171:229–246.

Sperry RW (1952): Neurology and the mind-brain problem. Am Sci 40:291–312.

Sperry RW (1962a): Orderly function with disordered structure. In Foerster HV, Zopt GW (eds): "Principles of Self-Organization." New York: Pergamon Press, pp 279–290.

Sperry RW (1962b): Some general aspects of interhemispheric integration. In Mountcastle VB (ed): "Interhemispheric Relations and Cerebral Dominance." Baltimore: The Johns Hopkins Press, pp 43–49.

Sperry RW (1968): Mental unity following disconnection of the cerebral hemispheres. Harvey Lect 62:293–323.

Sperry RW, Gazzaniga MS, Bogen JE (1969): Interhemispheric relationships: The neocortical commissures; syndromes of hemisphere disconnection. In Vinken PJ, Bruyn GW (eds): "Handbook of Clinical Neurology." Amsterdam: North-Holland, Vol 4, pp 273–290.

Spidalieri G, Franchi G, Guandalini P (1985): Somatic receptive-field properties of single fibers in the rostral portion of the corpus callosum in awake cats. Exp Brain Res 58:75–81.

Teitelbaum H, Sharpless SK, Byck R (1968): Role of somatosensory cortex in interhemispheric transfer of tactile habits. J Comp Physiol Psychol 66:623–632.

Tusa RJ (1982): Visual cortex: Multiple areas and multiple functions. In Morrison AR, Strick PL (eds): "Changing Concepts of the Nervous System." New York: Academic Press, pp 235–259.

Van Essen DC, Newsome WT, Bixby JL (1982): The pattern of interhemispheric connections and its relationship to extrastriate visual areas in the macaque monkey. J Neurosci 2:265–283.

Van Essen DC, Newsome WT, Maunsell JHR (1984): The visual field representation in striate cortex of the macaque monkey: Asymmetries, anisotropies, and individual variability. Vision Res 24:429–448.

Weyand TG, Swadlow HA (1980): Interhemispheric striate projections in the prosimian primate, Galago senegalensis. Brain Behav Evol 17:473–477.

Whitteridge D (1965): Area 18 and the vertical meridian of the visual field. In Ettlinger EG (ed): "Functions of the Corpus Callosum." London: Churchill, pp 115–120.

Yinon U, Hammer A (1981): Physiological mechanisms underlying responsiveness of visual cortex neurons following optic chiasm section. In Flohr H, Precht W (eds): "Lesion Induced Neuronal Plasticity in Sensorimotor Systems." Berlin: Springer, pp 360–368.

Zeki S (1978): Functional specialization in the visual cortex of the rhesus monkey. Nature 274:423–428.

Two Hemispheres—One Brain:
Functions of the Corpus Callosum, pages 189–209
© 1986 Alan R. Liss, Inc.

Interhemispheric Communication and Binocular Vision: Functional and Developmental Aspects

M. CYNADER, J. GARDNER, A. DOBBINS, F. LEPORÉ, AND
J.P. GUILLEMOT

*Departments of Psychology and Physiology, Dalhousie University, Halifax, Nova
Scotia B3H 4J1 (M.C., A.D., A.G.), Département du Psychologie, Université de
Montréal (F.L.), Département du Kinanthropologie, Université du Québec à
Montréal (J.P.G.), Montréal, Canada*

It has long been known that the representation of each half of the visual
field is projected onto the visual cortical surface of the opposite hemisphere.
This arrangement useful, for it enables visual stimuli in the right visual
hemifield to interact with motor pathways on the same side of the brain
concerned with the right arm or leg. Yet this projection pattern raises
questions about the representation of the visual field along the vertical
midline, and poses special problems for mechanisms of stereoscopic binocular vision at the midline. Interhemispheric connectivity mediated by the
corpus callosum provides a mechanism for the unification of the two halves
of the visual field. Since it interconnects the two halves of visual space, with
special emphasis on the vertical meridian (midline) representation, the
corpus callosum has been implicated in processes like interhemispheric
transfer of learned visual discriminations [Sperry, 1961; Myers, 1962; Berlucchi, 1972], the fusion of the two hemifields [Berlucci, 1980], and midline
stereopsis [Mitchell and Blakemore, 1970]. This report focuses on the possible role of the corpus callosum in stereoscopic binocular vision, the process
by which the slight differences in the angle of view of the two eyes are
converted to useful information about an object's location and trajectory in
depth.

Figure 1 reminds the reader of the essential geometry of stereopsis. With
each eye looking at a fixation point, the image of an object beyond the

J. Gardner's current address is Research Lab of Electronics, Building 36-873, MIT,
Cambridge, MA 02139.

We thank GLAXO Labs for their generous donation of Alfathesin and MRC grant
PG-29 for support.

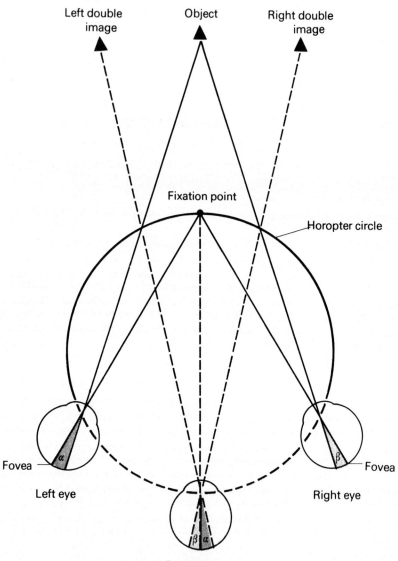

Fig. 1. The perspective of this figure is from above. It shows the two eyes aligned on a fixation point. An object located directly beyond the fixation point is projected to the right of the fovea in the left eye and to the left of the fovea in the right eye (i.e., onto the nasal retina in each eye). The opportunity for binocular fusion in a "cyclopean eye" cannot exist unless the nasotemporal line of decussation is imprecise or callosal projections allow the two images to be combined within a single hemisphere. This figure is redrawn from Grusser and Grusser-Cornehls [1978].

fixation plane falls on the nasal retina of each eye (nasal retina is that part of the retina closer to the nose than the fovea). Since, in general, fibers from the nasal retina project to the opposite side of the brain, the image of this object would be projected to the left and right hemispheres via the right and left eye, respectively, with no opportunity to combine the two images on the same side of the brain. A similar situation would obtain with an object located directly in front of the fixation point (not illustrated). The image of such an object would be projected onto the temporal retina of each eye. (The temporal retina is that part of the retina located further from the nose than the fovea.) Again, images of such a point would be projected to two different hemispheres with no opportunity for binocular combination in a single hemisphere.

This situation described above does not occur, since we *are* able to use stereoscopic disparity in a most effective way at the midline of our visual field. There are two obvious mechanisms that could allow for the binocular integration of visual information originating from both temporal or both nasal retinae. First, the process of partial decussation at the optic chiasm whereby fibers from nasal retina cross to the opposite side of the brain and those from temporal retina remain uncrossed need not be precise. Indeed, there is good evidence, in both cats [Stone, 1966; Leceister, 1968; Sanderson and Sherman, 1971; Terao et al., 1982] and monkeys [Bunt et al., 1977] that there is a zone of nasotemporal overlap from which fibers project into both optic tracts. This nasotemporal overlap could, by itself, mediate midline stereopsis. Second, the corpus callosum, which interconnects the two hemispheres, could also play a role in bringing the two eyes' representation together at the single-cell level and thus mediating midline stereopsis.

We have tried to assess the role of callosal projections and of nasotemporal overlap in midline stereopsis by allowing only one of these systems to function at a time. This was done by studying binocular depth responses in cortical neurons of cats in which (1) the visual cortex was removed on one side, eliminating the contribution of the corpus callosum to interhemispheric binocular connectivity; (2) the optic chiasm was sectioned, eliminating the contribution of direct retinal pathways and nasotemporal overlap to cortical binocularity. Assessment of the binocular responses of cortical neurons in these two groups of cat shows that *both* callosal and overlapping retinal pathways contribute to cortical binocular function.

In addition we have embarked on a developmental study of the comparative abilities of callosal versus thalamic inputs to influence the firing patterns of cortical cells. Our findings show that it is possible to produce functional increases or decreases in the efficacy of the callosal pathway by controlling the visual environment early in postnatal life.

METHODS
Surgical Procedures

For visual cortex lesions, cats were anesthetized with intravenous Alfathesin, fixed in a stereotaxic frame and a 3 × 2-cm bone flap, overlying the visual cortex on one side of the brain, was cut through the skull. The dura was incised and retracted and the visual cortex was removed by suction. The lesion included the entire suprasylvian and lateral gyri and the medial bank of the ectosylvian gyrus. The alveus of the hippocampus marked the ventral limit of the lesion with the cingulate gyrus being spared. After suction was complete, Gelfoam was packed loosely in the brain cavity and the bone flap was replaced and reseated with bone wax.

The optic chiasm was sectioned via a transbuccal approach. The animal was anesthetized, fixed upside down in a stereotaxic frame, and after drilling through the roof of the mouth, the optic chiasm was visualized at the base of the brain. It was sectioned under direct vision with a microdissecting knife.

Our methods for recording the responses of cortical neurons were conventional and are described in detail elsewhere [Cynader and Berman, 1972; Cynader and Regan, 1978; Cynader and Mitchell, 1980]. Extracellular recordings were made from single cells located near the border between cortical areas 17 and 18, with receptive fields near the representation of the vertical meridian and 3–10° down from the area centralis. After an initial qualitative characterization of unit responses, including orientation, direction, and binocular properties, we embarked on a quantitative study of neuronal responses to stimuli with varied retinal disparities and directions of depth motion. We studied responses to stimuli moving in the same direction and with the same speed in the two eyes (called in-phase motion) and responses to stimuli moving in opposite directions at the same speeds in the two eyes (called anti-phase motion). Figure 2 shows how motion of an object toward or away from the organism results in opposed motion (anti-phase) on the two retinae. Sideways motion of an object results in the same direction of motion (in-phase) on the two retinae [Beverly and Regan, 1975]. Our procedure involved the measurement of responses to in-phase and anti-phase motion at each of seven different disparities. All stimulus delivery and data collection was performed under computer control.

RESULTS

The effects of unilateral decortication were examined by comparing the responses of cortical neurons in normal and lesioned cats to stimuli presented through each eye. Figure 3 shows two ocular dominance distributions from visual cortical cells found near the area 17-18 border in normal and unilaterally decorticated cats. The ordinate of these distributions represents the percentage of cells encountered, and the abscissa is a seven-point scale of ocular dominance [Hubel and Wiesel, 1962] in which neurons of ocular dominance group 1 are driven only via stimulation of the contralateral eye and neurons in higher ocular dominance groups receive increasingly greater input from the ipsilateral eye. Units in groups 3–5 are highly binocular with equal or near-equal input from the two eyes.

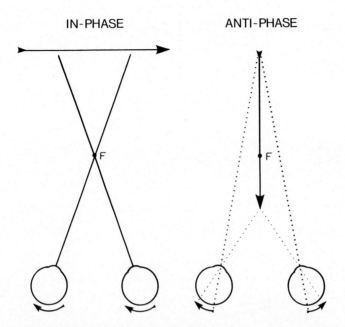

Fig. 2. The perspective of this diagram is from above with the two eyes represented at the bottom of the figure. In these experiments, disparity-specific binocular inter- actions were examined with two types of stimulus movement. Each eye was stimu- lated with an independently controlled optical system. Stimuli moving sideways in the world (in-phase motion) move across the retinae in the same direction (left-hand side). Stimuli presented in anti-phase move across the two retinae in opposite directions (right-hand side), simulating motion toward or away from the animal's nose, or motion-in-depth. In each of the two movement conditions, responses to zero disparity, 3 uncrossed, and 3 crossed disparities were examined. The three crossed disparities represent stimulation in front of the fixation point (F), while stimulation with uncrossed disparities would represent stimulation beyond the fixation plane. For anti-phase motion, illustrated on the right, each trial necessarily involves stimulation over a range of disparities, since by its very nature, motion in depth involves changing disparity. In this case the disparity illustrated represents the *center* of the depth oscillation on a given trial. Responses were also measured through each eye alone.

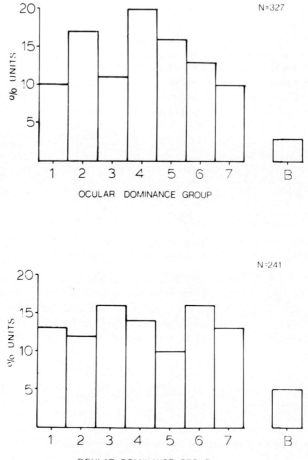

Fig. 3. The distributions of ocular dominance among neurons near the vertical meridian representation of the visual cortex are compared in normal cats and cats with unilateral lesions of the visual cortex. The ordinate represents the incidence of neurons in each ocular dominance group. The abscissa is a seven-point scale of ocular dominance [Hubel and Wiesel, 1962] in which neurons of group 1 are driven exclusively via stimulation of the contralateral eye. Units in higher groups receive a successively greater proportion of their excitatory drive via the ipsilateral eye, with units in group 7 driven exclusively via the ipsilateral eye. Units in groups 3–5 are driven equally or near equally by the two eyes. Units in group B are excited only when the two eyes are stimulated together. In both normal and operated animals many neurons are driven well via stimuli presented through either eye. In the operated animals, there is a small increase in the relative incidence of cells with monocular or near-monocular excitatory drive.

If the corpus callosum were the sole contributor to binocular connectivity of cortical neurons near the vertical meridian, then one would expect that neurons in the operated animals would fall (lower panel of Fig. 3) into ocular dominance groups 1 and 7, representing monocular drive from the contralateral and ipsilateral eyes, respectively. Figure 3 shows that this is not the case. Many neurons in the operated animals are still binocularly activated, and although the ocular dominance distribution of the operated animals is perhaps somewhat more biased toward monocularity than that of normal animals, these data, *in themselves*, do not indicate a major role for callosal projections in midline binocularity. Our findings seem clear, although they are controversial [Dreher and Cottee, 1975; Payne et al., 1980; Blakemore et al., 1983; Payne et al., 1984; Minciacchi and Antonini, 1984; Payne, this volume; Berlucchi, this volume]. Different investigators have obtained varied degrees of increase in the incidence of monocularly driven cells in the cat visual cortex after unilateral decortication or callosal section. It is possible that differences in the survival time after lesion, the layers of cortex examined, and the mode of disruption of callosal function may contribute to the diversity of experimental results.

We can assess cortical binocular connectivity in a more precise way by studying cellular responses to stimuli with different retinal disparities [Barlow et al., 1967; Hubel and Wiesel, 1970b; Cynader et al., 1978; Cynader and Regan, 1978). Figure 4 illustrates the responses of a cortical neuron to stimuli with varied disparities. The figure contains histograms representing responses to 16 repetitions of disparity-specific stimuli and two summary graphs that show how varied disparity conditions affect the neuron's response. We have evaluated binocular responses under two conditions (see Methods), one in which stimuli move in the same direction and at the same speed on the two retinae (in-phase motion) and a second in which stimuli move in opposite directions on the two retinae (anti-phase motion). This corresponds to motion directed toward or away from the observer (see Fig. 2 in Methods). The neuron whose responses are illustrated in Figure 4 showed marked facilitation over the other disparity conditions with in-phase binocular stimulation at the disparity labeled $0°$ in Figure 4. Inhibition was observed with stimulation at the $-2°$ disparity point, representing stimulation beyond the fixation plane. Some facilitation was observed with anti-phase stimulation, but the effects were not nearly so dramatic as those obtained with in-phase stimuli. We have devised a measure, called the "dynamic range," which represents the degree to which binocular stimuli can modulate the firing rate of a given neuron. We define dynamic range as follows:

$$\frac{\text{Maximum number of spikes}}{\text{Minimum number of spikes}}$$

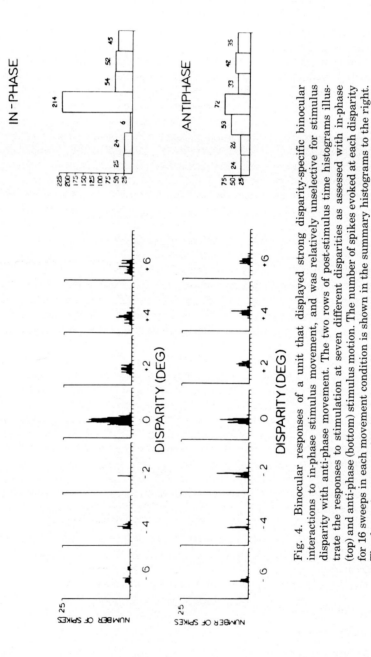

Fig. 4. Binocular responses of a unit that displayed strong disparity-specific binocular interactions to in-phase stimulus movement, and was relatively unselective for stimulus disparity with anti-phase movement. The two rows of post-stimulus time histograms illustrate the responses to stimulation at seven different disparities as assessed with in-phase (top) and anti-phase (bottom) stimulus motion. The number of spikes evoked at each disparity for 16 sweeps in each movement condition is shown in the summary histograms to the right. The dynamic range index for this unit has a value of 214/6 or 35.6.

for all conditions of binocular stimulation. For the neuron illustrated in Figure 4 the dynamic range has a value of 214/6 = 35.6. In a neuron which shows little binocular interactions, i.e., with a relatively flat tuning curve, the dynamic range would be much lower.

We investigated binocular responses in nearly 400 neurons located near the termination zone of the corpus callosum, comparing normal cats with operated animals. The mean value for the dynamic range index for both groups is shown as a function of the depth within the cortex in Figure 5. In normal animals, binocular interactions are strongest in the superficial cortical layers. They then decline to lower values by about 1,000 μm from the surface, corresponding to cortical layer IV, where thalamic input termi-

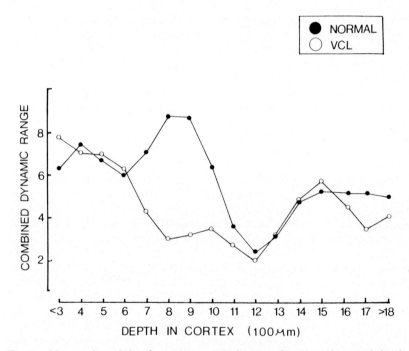

Fig. 5. Mean value of the *dynamic range* index as a function of cortical depth in normal cats and in cats with unilateral lesions of the visual cortex. The dynamic range index has, on average, a high value in the superficial cortical layers, indicating strong binocular interactions, and declines in the middle cortical layers, before rising near the bottom of the cortex. Units affected by decortication were localized within particular cortical layers. Differences between normal and operated cats were largest in a zone around layer III and upper layer IV. Here, decorticate animals showed a substantial drop in the dynamic range index within a region extending from about 700 to 1,100 μm below the cortical surface. The data presented here were smoothed with a three-point Gaussian smoothing function.

nates, and then increase again in strength in the deepest cortical layers. In the operated animals, a similar trend is evident with stronger binocular interactions in the superficial and deep layers than in layer IV, but the operated animals show a substantial difference from normals in the strength of binocular interaction in a zone which ranges from 700 to 1,100 μm below the cortical surface. Here the dynamic range index is consistently higher in normal animals than in unilateral decorticates. These findings allow us to conclude that there is a layer-specific function for callosal connections in cortical depth processing at the vertical meridian. The layer-specific effects that we observe are consistent with anatomical data showing that the superficial layers are zones of heavy callosal terminations [Shatz, 1977; Innocenti, 1980]. These callosal projections appear to make only modest contributions to the ocular dominance distribution of cortical cells, and it remains possible to observe disparity selectivity in some neurons of the operated animals. One function of the callosal projection, however, seems to be that of modulation of binocular responses, especially in the superficial cortical layers, to *enhance* disparity selectivity.

The experiments described above show that the corpus callosum is *necessary* for at least some forms of cortical binocular interactions. We next asked whether the callosal projection was *sufficient* for disparity-specific interactions. To approach this question, we sectioned the optic chiasm in adult cats (see Methods) and allowed the animals 3–4 weeks of recovery before recording single-cell responses from the callosal termination zone at the area 17-18 border. The situation is diagrammed in Figure 9. Sectioning the optic chiasm eliminates retinal pathways crossing to the opposite side of the brain, while leaving uncrossed pathways intact. We would expect, in the absence of any significant callosal projection, to find that all cortical neurons in split chiasm cats were driven only via the ipsilateral eye. Figure 6 shows the ocular dominance distribution actually observed among cortical neurons of the split-chiasm cats. The distribution is heavily skewed in favor of the ipsilateral eye, as would be expected, but nearly 50% of the neurons encountered fall outside ocular dominance groups 6 and 7. This means that they gave clear and vigorous responses to visual stimulation via the contralateral eye. The anatomical evidence (Fig. 9) indicates that these contralateral eye responses must originate from the opposite hemisphere via the corpus callosum, and so the data indicate a robust contribution of callosal input to cortical binocular convergence.

The finding that some cells can be driven by either eye in split-chiasm cats is encouraging, but it does not prove that *disparity-specific* binocular interactions occur in these animals. To test this hypothesis we examined disparity-specific responses of cortical neurons in the split-chiasm cats using the quantitative methods described earlier. Figure 7 illustrates the binocular responses of two neurons encountered near the area 17-18 border in split-chiasm cats. In both cases, the ordinate is the neuron's firing rate and the

CHIASM SECTION

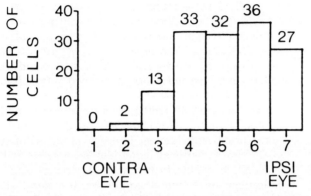

Fig. 6. The distribution of ocular dominance in adult cats in which the optic chiasm has been subjected to mid-sagittal section. Ocular dominance conventions are the same as in Figure 3. The distribution is clearly biased in favor of ipsilateral eye input, but many neurons receive some input via the contralateral eye.

abscissa represents the disparity of the oriented bars. The dotted lines in Figure 7 represent the response to monocular stimulation via the left and right eyes. The two tuning curves illustrated represent responses to in-phase movement (labeled with filled circles) and anti-phase motion (labeled with open squares). For the unit illustrated on the left of Figure 7, responses vary dramatically as a function of the disparity of in-phase stimulation. The unit shows deep inhibition (responses below monocular levels with sideways movement at 0 disparity and marked facilitation at the crossed disparity labeled $+1°$ in Fig. 7. The dynamic range index for this unit has a value of 9.6, a value comparable to that of highly selective neurons in normal cats. The responses to anti-phase stimulation show much less variation with disparity, suggesting that this neuron emphasizes responses to sideways motion rather than motion in depth.

The neuron illustrated on the right-hand side of Figure 7 was encountered on another penetration in a split-chiasm cat. This neuron showed much greater responses for anti-phase motion than would be expected simply by summing the two monocular responses. Responses to in-phase stimuli were weaker, less well tuned to disparity, and approximated the sum of the two monocular responses. These two neurons of Figure 7 thus represent populations of neurons with strong interactions for in-phase and anti-phase stimuli, respectively.

We found that units with disparity-selective responses in the split-chiasm cats tended to be clustered, and individual penetrations, normal to the

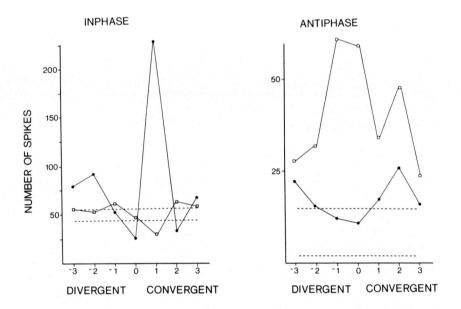

DEPTH SELECTIVITY IN SPLIT CHIASM CATS

Fig. 7. The disparity-specific responses of two neurons encountered near the vertical meridian representation in the cortex of split-chiasm cats. Conventions for this
figure are the same as in Figure 4. The unit whose responses are shown on the left-
hand side of the figure showed marked disparity-specific interactions with in-phase
binocular stimulation (representd by filled circles). Responses could be much greater
than that expected by summing the two monocular responses (two dotted lines in
the figure). The peak of the unit's disparity tuning curve was located at an abscissa
value of 1°, indicating maximum response for convergent disparities in this unit.
Responses to anti-phase stimuli (open squares) were less pronounced and showed
only small variations with disparity. The unit whose responses are illustrated on
the right of Figure 7 showed much stronger responses to anti-phase motion (open
squares) than would be expected from the monocular responses (dotted lines). Responses to in-phase stimulation (filled circles) were weaker and the variation with
stimulus disparity was less pronounced than that for anti-phase responses.

cortical surface, could yield rich or meager harvests of disparity-specific neurons. Moreover, individual penetrations were characterized by neurons that favored either in-phase or anti-phase stimuli. The neuron whose responses are illustrated in left-hand panel of Figure 7 was found on a penetration with several additional neurons, all of which gave vigorous disparity-specific responses to in-phase stimuli, while responses to motion in depth showed less selectivity. The neuron illustrated in the right-hand panel of Figure 7 was clustered with neurons that showed marked binocular interactions associated with motion in depth and relatively weak modulation to sideways motion at different disparities.

Several generalizations emerge from the consideration of disparity-specific responses in split-chiasm cats. First, a subpopulation of neurons in split-chiasm cats shows clear, well-defined, binocular interactions. These interactions can emphasize responses to either sideways motion or to motion in depth, depending on the neuron encountered. The dynamic range index is, on average, lower in the split-chiasm cats than it is in normal cats (Fig. 8), but nearly 50% of the neurons encountered in split chiasm cats achieve a dynamic range of greater than 6 dB, indicating that disparity-specific stimuli can modulate firing by a factor of 4 in these neurons.

Second, the peak of the disparity tuning curve and/or the locus of most-rapid change in response with disparity is generally displaced toward *crossed* disparities, rather than uncrossed or zero disparities in the split-chiasm cats. This indicates that split-chiasm animals emphasize responses to stimuli in front of the fixation plane. Third, when responses of neurons showing strong selectivity for motion in depth are analyzed separately, they show a tendency to prefer motion *toward* the organism rather than *away* from it. No such bias is observed in normal animals [Cynader and Regan, 1978]. Fourth, strong binocular interactions can be observed in neurons that are driven primarily through the ipsilateral eye, falling into ocular dominance groups 6 and 7. This last finding makes it clear that simply studying ocular dominance (Figs. 3, 6) without examining binocular interactions will understate the contribution of the corpus callosum to cortical binocular connectivity.

Development Studies of Callosal Contribution to Cortical Binocularity

In the split-chiasm animals studied above, inputs originating in the two cerebral hemispheres converge onto single cells to allow for disparity-specific responses in cortical neurons. This interhemispheric convergence of input is required for stereoscopic processing just as convergence of inputs from the two eyes is required for stereoscopic processing in unoperated animals. A series of elegant studies [Wiesel and Hubel, 1963, 1965; Hubel and Wiesel, 1965] have shown that the binocular convergence that underlies stereopsis is regulated during development by processes that depend on matching inputs from the two eyes. Failure to achieve congruent inputs to

DYNAMIC RANGE COMBINED

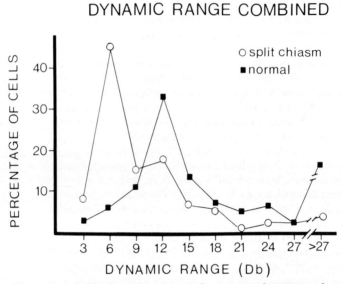

Fig. 8. The value of the dynamic range index among the neuronal population studied in normal and split-chiasm cats. The ordinate represents the incidence of cells whose dynamic range index is given along the abscissa. The dynamic range index is, in general, lower in split-chiasm cats than in normal animals, indicating that binocular stimuli are less effective in modulating units' firing rate in the split-chiasm cats. A population of neurons with large dynamic range values are, however, found in the split-chiasm cats, and nearly 50% of the units encountered display dynamic range value greater than 6 dB.

the two eyes leads to a breakdown of binocularity, and if vision through one eye is impaired relative to the other eye, inputs from the impaired eye become disconnected from the cortex. The functional loss of input is due to a process of binocular competition [Guillery, 1972; Cynader, 1982] which occurs between lateral geniculate axons representing the two eyes [Cynader and Mitchell, 1977].

The split-chiasm preparation offers a unique opportunity to examine the notion of competition as it applies to pathways representing the two cerebral hemispheres, rather than thalamocortical inputs, by arranging for callosal pathways from the two hemispheres to have different utility in vision. The preparation used is shown in Figure 9. Kittens were reared normally from birth until 21 days of age, when they were subjected to surgical section of the optic chiasm and at the same time the left eyelid was sutured shut. The kittens then received visual exposure in a normally lit environment until they were 4 months old. Optic chiasm section restricts visual input from one eye to one hemisphere by severing optic nerve fibers that cross to the

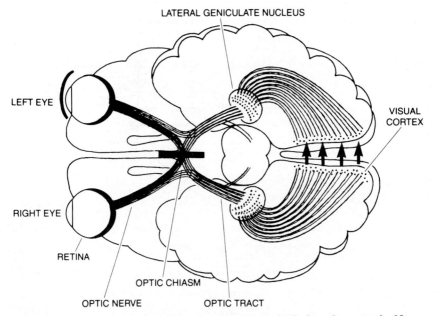

Fig. 9. General organization of the visual system in frontal-eyed mammals. Nerve fibers leave each eye and meet at the optic chiasm where fibers from the nasal hemiretinae cross to the other side of the brain and those from the temporal hemiretinae remain on the same side. Retinal inputs terminate in the LGN whence fibers project to the ipsilateral visual cortex. The corpus callosum interconnects the visual cortices on the two sides of the brain. In the split-chiasm cats whose ocular dominance distribution is shown in Figure 6, the optic chiasm was subjected to mid-sagittal section when the animals were adults. This interrupts retinal input to the opposite side of the brain but leaves ipsilateral input intact. In four additional kittens, the optic chiasm was sectioned 3 weeks after birth, and the left eyelid was sutured shut. For these animals, patterned visual input must take a route from the right eye via the corpus callosum to influence the responses of cells in the left hemisphere. The arrows projecting from the right to the left visual cortex represent the direction of visual information transmission during development.

opposite side of the brain. Suturing the left eyelid prevents visual input from reaching the left visual cortex via the direct ipsilateral pathway through the lateral geniculate nucleus (LGN). The only route by which patterned visual input can reach the left visual cortex in these kittens is a pathway from the right eye through the right LGN and visual cortex, then across the corpus callosum to the left visual cortex. The arrows illustrate the direction that visual input must take across the corpus callosum in order to activate neurons in the left visual cortex.

Figure 10 compares the results of recordings near the 17-18 border in both hemispheres of these specially reared kittens with those of adult split-chiasm cats. A reasonable fraction of neurons encountered in adult split-

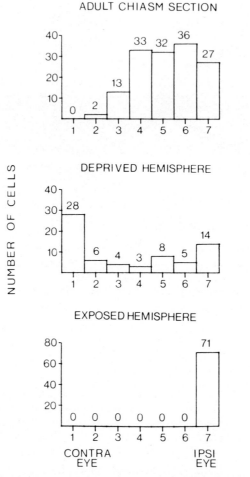

Fig. 10. The distribution of ocular dominance in split-chiasm cats. The top panel contains the same data as Figure 6, showing the distribution of ocular dominance in adult split-chiasm animals. The middle panel, labeled "Deprived Hemisphere," is an ocular dominance distribution from the left hemisphere of the kittens in which the left eyelid was sutured at the same time as the chiasm was sectioned. In this hemisphere most cells received their major input from the eye on the opposite side of the brain despite the chiasm section. In the opposite hemisphere, labeled "Exposed Hemisphere," all cells encountered were influenced only via the exposed eye.

chiasm cats receive inputs from the contralateral eye. (Fig. 10A, see also Fig. 6). Recordings made on the side of the brain ipsilateral to the exposed eye, labeled "Exposed Hemisphere" in Figure 10, show that all units encountered were driven exclusively via stimulation of the exposed eye. No units at all were driven through the eye that had been sutured until the recording session began. This finding indicates a functional loss of inputs originating from the other side of the brain in these animals and mimics the situation in which that hemisphere is inactivated [Berlucchi, 1972; Cynader et al., 1979; Lepore and Guillemot, 1982]. Recording from the side of the brain ipsilateral to the previously deprived eye in these same kittens ("Deprived Hemisphere," Fig. 10), we found that the effectiveness of inputs originating via the contralateral (exposed) eye was greatly enhanced relative to that found in adult split-chiasm cats. Inputs from this eye were clearly more effective than inputs from the deprived eye in driving most cortical cells. This indicates a substantial increase in the effectiveness of inputs originating on the side of the brain receiving visual stimulation during development relative to those from the deprived eye.

These results show that the functional effectiveness of callosal connections can be markedly enhanced or diminished on different sides of the same brain. In effect, the corpus callosum has been transformed from a bidirectional pathway into a one-way route. Information originating in the "exposed" hemisphere flows to the "deprived" hemisphere but not in the reverse direction. These physiological findings are supported by the results of anatomical studies that show that the terminal field of the corpus callosum is markedly expanded in the "deprived" hemisphere relative to the "exposed" hemisphere [Cynader et al., 1981b]. This induced functional asymmetry shows that the postnatal exposure history of the animal can modify the effectiveness of cortical output pathways in a similar manner to that by which it alters the effectiveness of inputs to the cortex [Wiesel and Hubel, 1963, 1965; Cynader and Mitchell, 1977].

Figure 11 is taken from Sperry [1974] and reminds us that many aspects of human performance are marked by asymmetries between the functional capabilities of the two hemispheres. In some cases, the basis of these asymmetries is already present at birth, [e.g., Geshwind, 1977], but in other cases, asymmetries may be established by selective exposure in postnatal life. It may be possible to at least partially overcome preexisting genetically determined functional asymmetries between the two hemispheres using techniques similar to the ones that we have employed here to modify interhemispheric connectivity or, alternatively, to create new asymmetries experimentally. If one considers the situation in which left-handed children are trained to use the right hand for writing, or in which baseball players are trained to hit from both sides of the plate, one can see formal similarities with the processes that we have described here in the visual cortex. It is possible that callosal connections are being modified in these situations, just as they are in our kittens.

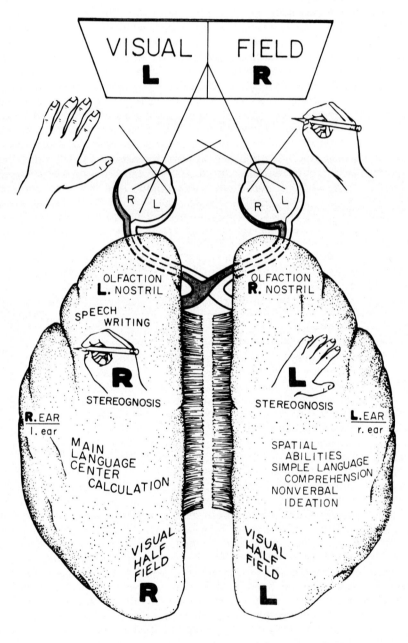

Fig. 11

A striking feature of the modifiability of thalamocortical binocular connectivity is that it occurs only during a well-defined critical period [Hubel and Wiesel, 1970a; Olson and Freeman, 1980; Cynader et al., 1980] during the first few months of a kitten's life. We still have little information on the nature or duration of a critical period for modification of *interhemispheric* binocular connectivity. In preliminary experiments, using cats subjected to chiasm section and monocular suture at different ages, we have obtained evidence that interhemispheric binocular connections can be modified in much older subjects than can thalamocortical connections. This suggests that interhemispheric processing functions may retain plasticity well into adulthood in humans as well.

SUMMARY AND CONCLUSIONS

Our findings show that callosal connections are both necessary and sufficient for stereoscopic binocular interactions in some neurons encountered at the cortical representation of the vertical midline. Cortical binocular interactions are reduced when interhemispheric communication is prevented by unilateral decortication and can still be observed in split-chiasm cats. The binocular interactions mediated by the corpus callosum can be altered by controlling the visual exposure conditions of the developing organism. We have used controlled visual exposure early in life to induce an asymmetry in the callosal projection, changing it from a bidirectional to a functionally unidirectional pathway.

REFERENCES

Barlow HB, Blakemore C, Pettigrew JD (1967): The neural mechanism of binocular depth discrimination. J Physiol (Lond) 193:327–342.

Berlucchi G (1972): Anatomical and physiological aspects of visual functions of the corpus callosum. Brain Res 37:371–392.

Berlucchi G (1980): Recent advances in the analysis of the neural substrates of interhemispheric communication. Satellite Symposium of the International Brain Research Organization, Pisa, Italy.

Beverly KI, Regan DM (1975): The relationship between discrimination and sensitivity in the perception of motion in depth. J Physiol 249:387–398.

Blakemore C, Diao Y, Pu M, Wang Y, Xiao Y (1983): Possible functions of the interhemispheric connexions between visual cortical areas in the cat. J Physiol (Lond) 337:331–349.

Bunt AH, Minkler DS (1977): Foveal sparing, new anatomical evidence for bilateral representation of the central retina. Arch Ophthalm 95:1445–7.

Fig. 11. Segregation of different functional properties in the two hemispheres in humans. Each hemisphere is specialized for certain tasks and these functional asymmetries may result from preexisting genetic predispositions [Geshwind, 1977]. The exposure history of the organism may also play a role in setting up (or reversing) hemispheric asymmetries.

Cynader M (1982): Competitive neuronal interactions underlying amblyopia. Hum Neurobiol 1:35–39.

Cynader M, Berman N (1972): Receptive-field organization of monkey superior colliculus. J Neurophysiol 35:187–201.

Cynader M, Dobbins A, Gardner JC, Lepore F, Guillemot JP (1979): Binocular interactions across the corpus callosum. Soc Neurosci Abstr 5:781.

Cynader M, Gardner J, Douglas RM (1978): Neural mechanisms of stereoscopic depth perception in cat visual cortex. In Cool S, Smith EL, III (eds): "Frontiers of Visual Science." Berlin, Heidelberg, New York: Springer, pp 373–390.

Cynader M, Lepore F, Guillemot JP (1981a): Interhemispheric compeition during postnatal development. Nature 290:139–140.

Cynader M, Lepore F, Guillemot JP, Feran M (1981b): Competition Interhemispherique au cours du developpement Post-Natal. Rev Can Biol 40:47–51.

Cynader M, Mitchell DE (1977): Monocular astigmatism effects on kitten visual cortex development. Nature 270:177–178.

Cynader M, Mitchell DE (1980): Prolonged sensitivity to monocular deprivation in dark-reared cats. J Neurophysiol 43:1026–1040.

Cynader M, Regan DM (1978): Neurons in cat parastriate cortex sensitive to direction of motion in three-dimensional space. J Physiol (Lond) 274:549–569.

Cynader M, Timney BN, Mitchell DE (1980): Period of susceptibility of kitten visual cortex to the effects of monocular deprivation extends beyond six months of age. Brain Res 91:545–550.

Dreher B, Cottee LJ (1975): Visual receptive-field properties of cells in area 18 of cat's cerebral cortex before and after acute lesions in area 17. J Neurophysiol 38:735–750.

Geshwind N (1977): Anatomical asymmetry as the basis for cerebral dominance. Fed Proc 37:226–236.

Grusser OJ, Grusser-Cornehls U (1978): Physiology of vision. In: Schmidt RF (ed) "Fundamentals of Sensory Physiology." New York, Heidelberg, Berlin: Springer-Verlag, chapter 4.

Guillery RW (1972): Binocular competition in the control of geniculate cell growth. J Comp Neurol 144:117–127.

Hubel DH, Wiesel TN (1962): Receptive fields, binocular interaction and functional architecture in the cat's visual cortex. J Physiol (Lond) 160:105–154.

Hubel DH, Wiesel TH (1965): Binocular interaction in striate cortex of kittens reared with artificial squint. J Neurophysiol 288:1041–1059.

Hubel DH, Wiesel TN (1970a): The period of susceptibility to the physiological effects of unilateral eye closure in kittens. J Physiol (Lond) 206:419–436.

Hubel DH, Wiesel TN (1970b): Cells sensitive to binocular depth in area 18 of macaque monkey cortex. Nature 225:41–42.

Innocenti GM (1980): The primary visual pathway through the corpus callosum: Morphological and functional aspects in the cat. Arch Ital Biol 118:124–188.

Leicester J (1968): Projection of the visual vertical meridian to cerebral cortex of the cat. J Neurophysiol 31:371–382.

Lepore F, Guillemot JP (1982): Visual receptive field properties of cells innervated through the corpus callosum in the cat. Exp Brain Res 46:413–424.

Minciacchi O, Antonini A (1984): Binocularity in the visual cortex of the adult cat does not depend on the integrity of the corpus callosum. Behav Brain Res 13:183–192.

Mitchell DE, Blakemore C (1970): Binocular depth perception and the corpus callosum. Vis Res 10:49–54.

Myers RE (1962): Transmission of visual information within and between the hemispheres. A behavioral study. In Mountcastle VB (ed): "Interhemispheric Relations and Cerebral Dominance." Baltimore: Johns Hopkins Press, pp 51–73.

Olson CR, Freeman RD (1980): Profile of the sensitive period for monocular deprivation in kittens. Exp Brain Res 39:17–21.

Payne BR, Elberger AJ, Berman N, Murphy H (1980): Binocularity in the cat visual cortex is reduced by sectioning the corpus callosum. Science 207:1097–1098.

Payne BR, Pearson HE, Berman N (1984): Role of corpus callosum in functional organisation of cat striate cortex. J Neurophysiol 52:570–594.

Sanderson K, Sherman M (1971): Nasotemporal overlap in visual field projected to lateral geniculate nucleus in the cat. J Neurophysiol 34:453–466.

Shatz CJ (1977): Anatomy of interhemispheric connections in the visual system of Boston Siamese and ordinary cats. J Comp Neurol 173:497–518.

Sperry RW (1961): Cerebral organization and behavior. Science 133:1749–1757.

Sperry RW (1974): Lateral specialization in the surgically separated hemispheres. In Schmitt FO, Worden FG (eds): "The Neurosciences: Third Study Program." Cambridge, MA: MIT Press, pp 5–19.

Stone J (1966): The naso-temporal division of the cat's retina. J Comp Neurol 126:585–599.

Terao N, Akihiro I, Maeda T (1982): Anatomical evidence for the overlapped distribution of ipsilaterally and contralaterally projecting neurons to the lateral geniculate nucleus in the cat retina: A morphologic study with fluorescent tracers. Invest Ophthalm 23:796–798.

Wiesel TN, Hubel DH (1963): Single cell responses in the striate cortex of kittens deprived of vision in one eye. J Neurophysiol 26:1003–1017.

Wiesel TN, Hubel DH (1965): Comparison of the effects of unilateral and bilateral eye closure on cortical unit responses in kittens. J Neurophysiol 28:1029–1040.

Two Hemispheres—One Brain:
Functions of the Corpus Callosum, pages 211–229
© 1986 Alan R. Liss, Inc.

The Role of the Corpus Callosum in Midline Fusion

FRANCO LEPORÉ, MAURICE PTITO, AND JEAN-PAUL GUILLEMOT
*Département de Psychologie, (F.L.), Centre de Recherches en Sciences
Neurologiques (F.L., M.P.), Université de Montréal, Québec H3C 3J7; Groupe de
Recherches en Neuropsychologie, Université du Québec à Trois-Rivières G9A
5H7 (M.P.); Département de Kinanthropologie, Université du Québec à Montréal
(J.-P.G.) H3C 3P8, Canada*

The two hemispheres of the brain are each capable of functioning independently of the other, and for the most higher-order sensory and motor activities, each controls principally the opposite side of the body or, for distance receptors, the contralateral hemifield. In normal organisms, each side is made aware of, and participates in, the activities of the other side through a series of interconnecting commissures. The most important of these, at least in terms of the number of its component axons, is the corpus callosum (CC). Despite its anatomical proeminence, however, it is only during the last three decades that its more obvious functions have started to be described [see Colonnier, this volume].

There is general agreement that the pioneering work of Roger Sperry and his numerous students and collaborators constitutes the cornerstone of the present body of knowledge concerning commissural, and especially callosal, function. In the first series of experiments with Ronald Myers it was demonstrated that CC is involved in the interhemispheric transfer of monocularly learned visual pattern discriminations in cats [Myers, 1956; Myers and Sperry, 1958]. These studies were extended to the somatosensory system [Stamm and Sperry, 1957] and, with Gazzaniga and Hamilton, among others, to primates and humans [Gazzaniga, 1966; Gazzaniga et al., 1962; Hamilton and Gazzaniga, 1964; Hamilton et al, 1968].

Studies of the pattern of anatomical projections of callosal neurons has suggested a major role for CC, namely, that of uniting the hemibodies or, for distance receptors, the hemifields. The elegant studies of Jones and collaborators [Jones and Powell, 1968; Jones et al., 1979, this volume; Heath and Jones, 1971], Kaas and collaborators [this volume] and Innocenti and his group [Innocenti, 1980,1981, this volume], among others [Zeki, 1970; Sanides, 1978a,b; Seagraves and Rosenquist, 1982a,b; Van Essen et al., 1982; Pandya and Seltzer, this volume] have shown that neurons that either send their axons through the callosum or receive callosal afferents from the contralateral hemisphere are situated in areas of cortex in which the mid-line of the visual or somatosensory fields are located.

Electrophysiological studies, carried out mainly in the cat, have tended to support this "midline fusion hypothesis" of callosal function [Hubel and Wiesel, 1967; Berlucchi, 1972, 1981; Lepore and Guillemot, 1982; Tassinari et al. 1985]. The experiments to be described below addressed this question in a systematic manner using various electrophysiological approaches to study the visual and somatosensory callosal systems.

VISUAL CALLOSAL ORGANIZATION: RECORDING FROM CORTICAL VISUAL AREAS

The major thalamic recipient zones in the cat cortex are areas 17 and 18. These areas have been shown by anatomy to be connected interhemispheri-cally, areas 17 projecting to contralateral areas 17 and 18, while the latter projects to its homologue in the other hemisphere. To study electrophysiolog-ically the receptive field (RF) properties of callosal neurons, a number of approaches are possible. One could, for example, record in that part of cortex that has been shown anatomically to be callosally connected. This corre-sponds to a small strip of cortex representing the vertical midline situated in the transition zones between 17 and 18. The problem with this approach is that one does not know, unless this approach is complemented with electrical stimulation of the opposite hemisphere, whether a particular unit under investigation is in fact callosally activated. A more direct approach, introduced by Berlucchi and collaborators [Berlucchi and Rizzolatti, 1968] and presented in Figure 1 is particularly useful for studying callosally activated neurons. Essentially this uses a split-chiasm preparation, which limits each eye's input to a single hemisphere. Any binocularly driven cortical cell recorded in the visual cortex must in all probability be receiving an ipsilateral geniculocortical input and a contralateral callosal input.

Results obtained in our laboratory using this preparation have been presented in extenso elsewhere [Lepore and Guillemot, 1982]. In general, we found that about one-third of the units situated in the border region of areas 17 and 18 were binocularly driven in the split-chiasm preparation. This proportion is similar to that reported by others [Berlucchi and Rizzo-latti, 1968; Cynader et al., 1981], although no callosal responses using this preparation have also been observed [Yinon et al., 1982, 1984; Milleret and Buser, 1984]. It may be of interest with respect to this point to mention that in a more recent experiment using the same preparation [Lepore and Sam-son, unpublished], we stimulated simultaneously, but independently, the two eyes when a contralateral receptive field could not be detected by the usual means. Under these conditions, more than two-thirds of all cells, including those that would normally have been classed as monocular, were clearly affected by the contralateral eye stimulation. These interaction effects, therefore, illustrate that the callosum has a much greater influence

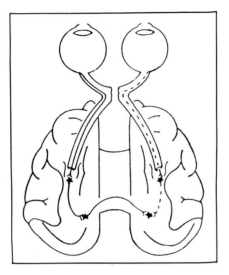

Fig. 1. Split-chiasm preparation used to record callosal recipient neurons. Binocular cells are activated ipsilaterally via thalamocortical inputs and contralaterally via callosal inputs.

on postsynaptic neurons than the binocular results derived from RF studies would suggest.

The RF properties of binocular units in the split-chiasm cats were in general quite similar for each eye with respect to most parameters: orientation and directional specificity, preferred velocity, size and elevation in visual space. The major differences were that the callosal response was generally weaker than the ipsilateral thalamocortical response and that the two RF's were situated in separate hemifields. What was, however, particularly interesting for the present discussion was that the two medial borders of the RF's either approached or straddled the vertical meridian (VM). This is precisely what would be predicted by the midline fusion hypothesis.

To quantify this preferential relationship between the medial border of the RF's and VM, the transformation indicated in the inset of Figure 2 was carried out on all units recorded in the chiasmatomized cats [Lepore and Guillemot, 1982]. The results thereby obtained for callosally activated cells (the binocular units) are presented in Figure 2a and those found for the monocular units are shown in Figure 2b. It must be noted that these two types of units were often recorded during the same penetration and do not represent sampling biases across the cortical surface. The results are quite clear: nearly all binocular units have RF's whose medial borders for each eye either touch or straddle the VM, whereas many monocular units, which

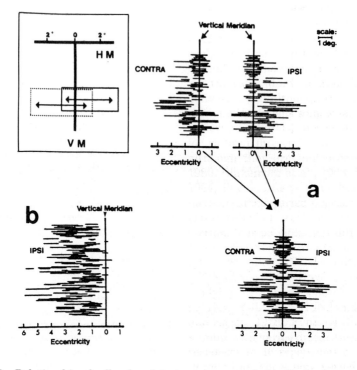

Fig. 2. Relationship of callosal recipient neurons recorded in the border regions of areas 17 and 18 with the vertical meridian. The inset on the upper left-hand corner illustrates the receptive field transformations expressed by a line joining the medial to the lateral border of each field. This transformation is applied to each receptive field. a. The figures on the upper right-hand corner represent the monocular fields of the binocular units, whose combined receptive fields are shown in the figure on the bottom right-hand corner; b. Receptive field representations of the monocular units.

presumably have no direct relation with CC, have RF's whose medial borders do not touch the VM.

The midline fusion hypothesis seems, therefore, to be confirmed for the primary visual cortex. This comes as little surprise since most anatomical and physiological studies have demonstrated, as indicated above, that callosal efferent and recepient zones are situated in parts of the cortex wherein the center of the visual field is represented. This, however, is not the case for "higher-order" visual areas, such as lateral suprasylvian visual area, where callosal projecting neurons have been found throughout most of the area, at least as far out as 40° eccentricity [Seagraves and Rosenquist, 1982a,b]. This may be taken as indicating that the midline fusion hypothesis only applies to primary visual areas. However, a close examination of the RF properties of neurons recorded in lateral suprasylvian visual areas in split-chiasm cats confirms even more strikingly the midline fusion hypothesis for this area. These units were recorded in Professor Berlucchi's laboratory with Dr. Antonella Antonini [Antonini et al., 1983]. Applying the same transformation as in Figure 2 for lateral suprasylvian area neurons, the results shown in Figure 3 were obtained. They indicate that although many units have large RF's, some being larger than the screen on which the stimuli were projected, the medial border of the RF's for each eye either touched or straddled the VM. In mapping studies, where isocontours are drawn using the center of a RF, many of these units would be considered quite eccentric with respect to the VM. The monocular units, unrelated to callosal function, have similar RF's in terms of sizes and visual field location, but the medial borders of only a limited number of units approach or straddle VM.

RECORDING FROM VISUAL CC IN CATS

In the previous series of experiments, the activity of callosal recipient cells was recorded in split-chiasm cats. The spatial organization of their RF's both in the primary and "higher-order" visual cortex was consistent with the midline fusion hypothesis of callosal function. The neurons from which these responses were obtained, however, were not in fact callosal neurons. Their activity was postsynaptic to the callosal axon and represented the integration of this and of a thalamocortical input. This first-order transformation of the callosal input might actually mask activity unrelated to VM in the sense that this type of information might in fact be transmitted through the callosum but is reorganized in some hierarchical fashion in the postsynaptic neuron such that the resultant RF is related to VM. This would apply particularly well to the units with large RF's found in lateral suprasylvian cortex.

To determine more precisely the nature of the information going through CC, axonal activity was recorded directly from the posterior portion of CC. This region has been shown by anatomy, physiology, and behavior [Myers, 1962; Berlucchi et al., 1967; Hubel and Wiesel, 1967; Seagraves and Rosenquist, 1981a,b; Ptito and Lepore, 1983] to be related to visual function. Representative results obtained during one penetration are presented in Figure 4, which also shows a schematic representation of the recording site. Most units were binocularly driven and the ocular dominance distribution of some 60 axons that were recorded resembled the typical distribution obtained from the primary visual cortex or from the lateral suprasylvian area. All RF sizes were found, although there was a tendency for axons to have RF properties more like neurons of the lateral syprasylvian area than area 17. However, about one-quarter had simple type RF's, suggesting that they might have originated in the latter area. Since no simple type RF's

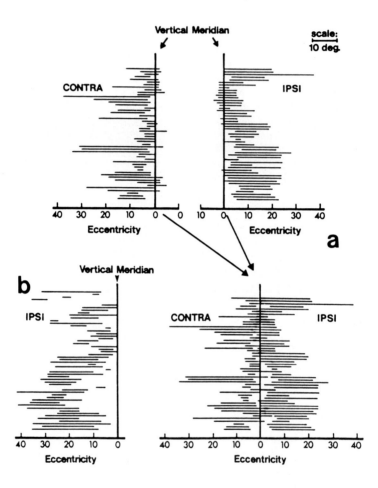

Fig. 3. Relationship of callosal recipient neurons recorded in the lateral suprasylvian area with the vertical meridian. (See description of transformations in Fig. 2). a. The two top figures represent the monocular fields of the binocular units, whose combined receptive fields are shown in the figure on the bottom right-hand corner; b. Receptive field representations of monocular units.

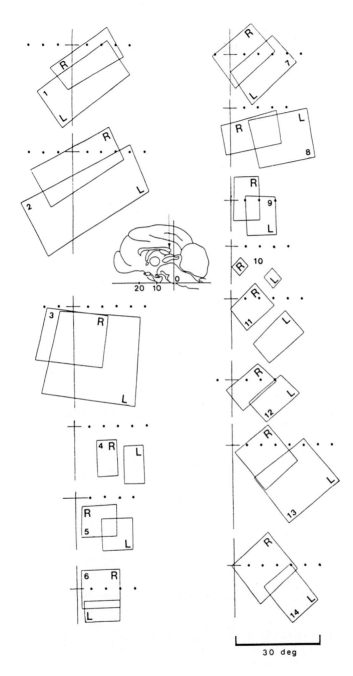

Fig. 4. Visual receptive fields of callosal axons. Inset: approximate anteroposterior location of recording site.

were found in the split-chiasm cats, this confirms to some degree the hypothesis formulated above, namely, that some transformation takes place in the postsynaptic cell partially innervated through the callosum.

The principal difference in RF organization, which was in fact completely predictable, between these axons and the neurons recorded in the split-chiasm preparation was that in the former the two RF's of binocular units were situated in the same hemifield. The midline fusion hypothesis, however, was clearly supported by these data. If one considers the border of the most medial of the two RF's, its close relationship with the VM is evident.

Minor exceptions to this rule were, however, found in this preparation. One example is cell 10 from the penetration presented in Figure 4. In all, four such units were found. It is not clear what the function of these units is, nor what happens to them once they contact the postsynaptic neuron, since similar units were never found in the split-chiasm cat. It is possible that these units connect with units having large, composite RF's, which then reach the VM.

In conclusion, therefore, the RF properties of cells, particularly their position in visual field with regards to VM, recorded in both the primary visual cortex and in the lateral suprasylvian visual area, support the hypothesis that one of the principal functions of the corpus callosum is to unite the two visual hemifields to insure continuity across the midline. This hypothesis was also confirmed by direct callosal axonal recording, since most of the RF's obtained overlapped or were situated near the VM.

RECORDING FROM SOMATOSENSORY CALLOSAL AXONS IN THE CAT

Recording callosal recipient or projecting neurons in the visual system would suggest that nearly all these cells are concerned with midline fusion. However, close inspection of the data indicates that most RF's were not only close to the VM but also to the horizontal meridian, with a preponderance of units having RF's in lower visual field. This clustering around the point of intersection of the two meridians, which corresponds to the area centralis in the cat, supports a second major function of the callosum, mainly demonstrated through neurobehavioral studies, namely, that of assuring the interhemispheric transfer of learned discriminations. Since visual discrimination learning requires the area centralis, it is possible that many of the callosal axons or the neurons present in the callosal recipient zone were not involved in midline fusion but were there to assure that discriminated material became accessible to the two hemispheres. In this case, the position of these neurons near the vertical meridian would be coincidental with the fact that the area centralis is coextensive with VM. We therefore looked for a system where the structures involved in fine discrimination and midline fusion would be widely separated in terms of their RF positions. The somatosensory system was deemed to be ideal for such studies since the structures involved in midline fusion, that is, the axial and para-axial body regions and those responsible for fine discrimination, namely, the forepaws, are widely separated from each other. Morevoer, the organization of head somesthesia is much like that of vision, in the sense that the head is a highly sensitive region, with fine and varied somatosensory RF's, yet most of the crucial structures are situated close to the midline.

We recorded directly from somatosensory callosal axons in the anterior portion of the callosum (A 16 ± 2 mm). Representative examples of RF's are presented in Figures 5 and 7. Figure 5 illustrates the RF's of axial and para-axial, as well as distal, portions of the body. In all, 73 units were found, and these responded to one or another of a series of stimuli: air puffs, light pinches, squeezes, stroking, etc. Moreover, most were rapidly adapting (75%), although some slowly adapting axons were also found. The units mainly responded to unilateral stimulation and the RF's were generally quite large, occupying in some cases a large portion of the hemibody. In others, the RF's were clearly bilateral. Pertinent to the present discussion, nearly all RF's touched or straddled the body midline. This is convincingly demonstrated by transforming the RF data along the lines of the transformations to which

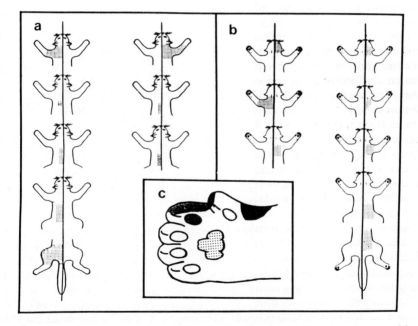

Fig. 5. Somatosensory receptive fields of callosal axons in the cat, represented by darkened or stippled surfaces. a. Dorsal view; b. Ventral view; c. Forepaw.

visual RF's were submitted in Figure 2. In this case, each somatosensory RF is represented by a line passing through its anteroposterior center and extending to the two lateral borders (see inset to Fig. 6). The summary results of this transformation for all RF's recorded on the trunk are presented in Figure 6 (a, ventral view; b, dorsal view). It is evident from these results that all axial somatosensory RF's have a preferred relationship with the body midline. This furnishes added proof that one of the principal functions of the callosum is, for the somatosensory system, to unite the two hemibodies, as it was, for the visual system, to join the two visual hemifields.

The results obtained on the trigeminal system of the head appear to be somewhat more complicated. These are presented in Figure 7. It is clear from Figure 7a that many RF's resemble those obtained for the trunk; i.e., they are fairly large, are mainly unilateral, and more adapt rapidly to repeated stimulation then adapt slowly. Those representing the mouth, tongue, and nose regions on the other hand, are rather small. However, in agreement with the midline fusion hypothesis, most RF areas extend to the midline.

This, however, is not the case with the few specialized RF's represented in Figure 7b; simple tooth, whiskers, perioral, or bilateral corneal RF's. These do not fit the fusion hypothesis or, for them to do so, one must postulate, as we did for the few visual callosal axons that also did not fit the hypothesis, that these units input to cells having large, composite RF's that do in fact include the midline.

Fig. 5c illustrates another series of units that do not appear to fit the midline fusion hypothesis. Nearly 5% of these axons were recorded in the callosum. Given their rather small size and extended distance from the midline, they appear to be involved more with intermanual transfer than midline fusion. The conclusion one is tempted to draw from these units and from those having specialized RF's obtained for the trigeminal system (Fig. 7) is that the corpus callosum is not only involved with midline fusion (visual and somatosensory) but also with the fine discrimination that is at the basis of interhemispheric transfer.

RECORDING FROM SOMATOSENSORY CORPUS CALLOSUM OF THE MONKEY

The results presented above indicate that some callosal neurons are probably not involved in midline fusion since they have RF's restricted to the extremities and thus are far removed from the body midline. These data can, however, be reconciled with the midline fusion hypothesis if one assumes a functional midline instead of purely an anatomical one. As far as the trunk is concerned, these are coextensive. The extremities, on the other hand, although widely separated in body space, come together whenever an animal manipulates a small object with its forepaws and forearms. The corpus callosum would in this case help to control intermanual coordination to assure smooth flow of information from one hand to the other. This is precisely what is happening when information goes from one hemifield or axial hemibody to the other.

If this hypothesis is correct, namely, that forepaw and forearm RF's are the physiological substrates of a functional midline, one would expect that a more "manipulative" animal would have proportionately more callosal units representing the extremities. We thus recorded somatosensory RF's of callosal neurons in rhesus monkeys, first, to confirm the generality of the midline fusion hypothesis for the axial body regions and, second, to determine whether this animal, which uses much more frequently and efficiently than the cat its arms and hands in coordinated manipulative activities, has proportionately more callosal axons transmitting information about these body regions.

Results obtained in two monkeys support quite strongly the midline fusion hypothesis for axial body regions. Some representative results are presented in Figure 8. As was the case for the cat, somatosensory RF's that could be mapped with one or more of a series of mechanical stimuli were found on most body regions. Rapidly adapting axons were most frequent than slowly adapting ones, as were unilateral RF's compared to bilateral. Most of the RF's concerned the trunk or the face and were either large in the former case or relatively small in the latter. In agreement with the midline fusion hypothesis, most axial and para-axial RF's, including those of the head, either touched or straddled the body midline. The second hypothesis, postulating that because the monkey is a more "manipulative" animal and shows more bimanual activity than the cat it should have proportionately more callosal axons concerned with the hands and forearms, was not confirmed. If anything, fewer axons responded to stimulation of the extremities in relation to the trunk and head region than in the cat.

DISCUSSION AND CONCLUSION

In the series of electrophysiological experiments presented above, we have attempted to confirm the hypothesis that one of the principal functions of CC is to assure continuity across the spatial or body midlines. This "midline fusion hypothesis" was shown to apply to different visual structures, namely, primary visual areas 17 and 18, and as has recently been shown, area 19 [Tassinari et al., 1985] and "higher-order" areas such as the lateral suprasylvian, which had been shown anatomically [Seagraves and Rosenquist, 1982a,b] to contain callosal neurons throughout most of its extent. The apparent eccentric position of these callosal neurons, however, is reconciled with the midline fusion hypothesis by the fact that they have large RF's whose medial borders extend to the VM. We have also shown that not only callosal recipient but also projecting neurons are involved in midline fusion of the visual hemifields.

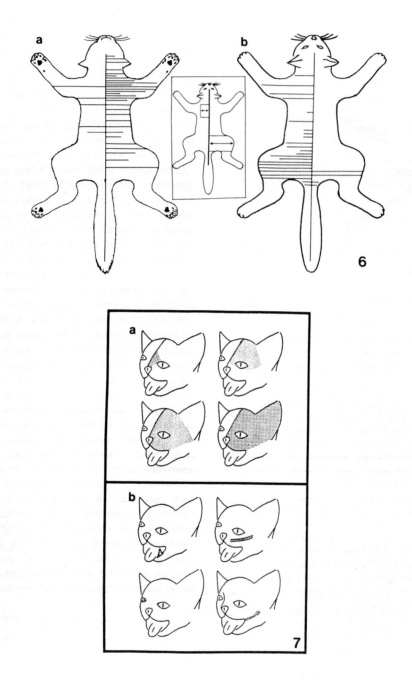

The fusion hypothesis was not only confirmed across visual structures, but also across sensory modalities. In the somatosensory system, as indicated previously, most cells were involved with the body midline.

A particularly convincing example of this is shown in Figure 9. In this figure are represented the RF's of two out of three polymodal fibers recorded in the rostral part of the splenium. Based on Pandya and Seltzer's [this volume] anatomical demonstrations in monkeys, this region of the CC probably transmits information from parietal cortex. The figure illustrates the results for one of the two fibers having bilateral RF's (Fig. 9a) and for

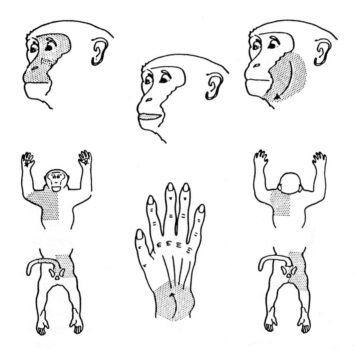

Fig. 8. Somatosensory receptive fields of callosal axons for the monkey. Each field is represented by a stippled surface. The arrows indicate that the unit responded only to movement of the joint.

Fig. 6. Relationship of trunk somatosensory receptive fields with body midline. Each receptive field is represented by a line traversing the anteroposterior center of each field (see inset). a. Ventral view b. Dorsal view.

Fig. 7. Somatosensory receptive fields of callosal axons for the trigeminal system in the cat. Each field is represented by a stippled surface. a. Receptive fields extending to midline; b. Receptive fields that did not extend to midline.

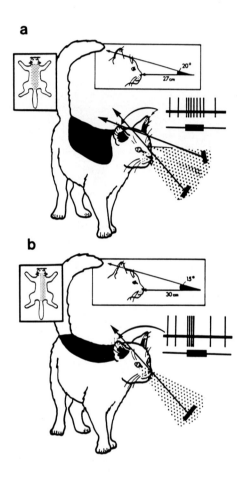

Fig. 9. Tri-modal receptive fields recorded in posterior callosal axons. Insets in upper left-hand corners represent the somatosensory fields. Insets in upper right represent the angle and direction at which the visual stimulus had to be displaced to evoke the best response. Auditory responses are schematically illustrated by the spike pictorial. a. Bilateral receptive fields, b. Unilateral receptive fields.

the axon having unilateral RF's (Fig. 9b). These units responded to visual, somatosensory, and auditory stimulation. In the case shown in Figure 9a, the axon discharged to a dark visual stimulus approximately 10×20 cm in size, moving toward the head of the animal at an angle of $20°$ from the horizontal and just missing the head. The somatosensory RF is shown schematically in the inset, the best stimulus being soft, moving strokes applied to the appropriate skin region. The auditory stimulus was a low screeching sound presented anywhere in the field in front of the animal. About the same type of stimuli were needed to excite the neuron represented in Figure 9b. However, in this case, the unit only responded when the stimuli were presented unilaterally. Precise mapping with visual or somatosensory stimulation revealed that the medial borders of the RF's extended to the midline.

We have not yet systematically examined the auditory cortex. However, a number of electrophysiological studies suggest that the hypothesis generally might hold for this modality. Many units in the primary auditory cortex are sensitive to binaural stimulation [Hall and Goldstein, 1968; Brugge et al., 1969; Eisman, 1974; Sovijärvi and Hyvärinen, 1974; Imig and Adrian, 1977; Imig and Brugge, 1978; Middlebrooks et al., 1980]. The nature of the interaction can be variable, producing either facilitation (also termed summation [Imig and Adrian, 1977; Imig, et al., this volume] or excitatory-excitatory [E-E] [Middelbrooks and Pettigrew, 1981] or inhibition (suppression or excitatory-inhibitory [E-I]) in the sense that a unit that is excited by stimulation of the contralateral ear either increases or decrease its response level, respectively, when the ipsilateral ear is also stimulated. Callosal neurons appear to belong mainly to the E-E category. A recent study [Middlebrooks and Pettigrew, 1981] looking at the spatial organization of the RF's of primary auditory cortex neurons described three types of units: omnidirectional units, which could be driven by stimuli presented anywhere in front of the cat; and hemifield and axial units, which responded mainly to contralateral ear stimulation. Since omnidirectional units appear to be mainly of the E-E type, as seems to be the case for callosal neurons [Imig and Adrian; Imig et al, this volume], it is possible that many are in fact the same neurons and that their sensitivity to stimulation across auditory space reflects their participation to midline fusion for this sensory modality.

An important question concerns the process by which the activity of callosal neurons becomes restricted to the midline. It appears that both genetic and experiential factors contribute to this restriction of the zone of influence of these neurons. At birth, callosal neurons are distributed throughout most of the primary visual, auditory, and somatosensory cortices [Innocenti and Frost, 1979; Innocenti and Caminiti, 1980; Innocenti, 1981; Feng and Brugge, 1983]. After the first postnatal month, this "exuberant" projection [Innocenti et al., 1977] becomes restricted to a narrow cortical strip representing the immediate surroundings of the VM. However, already at birth, at least for the visual system, Innocenti [this volume] demonstrated that only callosal axons projecting to this region extend into the gray matter, whereas those projecting beyond this zone terminate in underlying white matter. If the animal is subjected to normal visual experience, the transitory callosal projections disappear and only those axons concerned with the midline maintain their synaptic connectivity. If, on the other hand, visual experience is abnormal, as for example, in the case of monocularly sutured animals or those raised with natural or artificial strabismus [Shatz, 1977a,b; Lund, et al., 1978; Lund and Mitchell, 1979a,b; Innocenti and Frost, 1979, 1980], a different pattern of representation may develop. Which connexions disappear and which are maintained can probably best the explained by Berlucchi's [1981] neuronal "competition" hypothesis: if callosal and thalamocortical inputs to a cell have coextensive RF's and have similar properties, they will synchronously activate the cell and thereby survive. If, on the other hand, they have different properties, or have RF's that are discontinous at the midline, the weaker of the two inputs, generally the callosal input, will disappear and the cell will only be activated by the stronger thalamocortical input. Of course, this clustering of RF's about the midline need not only assure perceptual continuity of stimuli that straddle the two hemifields but can also be responsible for a number of other functions carried out near midline, namely, that of permitting the development of eye alignment and visual acuity [Elberger, 1979,1982, this volume], nonspecific facilitation [Payne, this volume], and stereoperception [Elberger, 1980; Ptito et al., this volume].

ACKNOWLEDGMENTS

The experiments were made possible in part by grants from NSERC and FCAC to each author. Thanks are also extended to Ms. Louise Prevost, Christiane Provençal, Dominique Petit, and Marie-Claude Paradis and to Mr. Louis Richer for their help in the experimentation.

REFERENCES

Antonini A, Berlucchi G, Lepore F (1983): Physiological organization of callosal connections of a visual lateral suprasylvian cortical area in the cat. J Neurophysiol 49:902–921.

Berlucchi G (1972): Anatomical and physiological aspects of visual functions of corpus callosum. Brain Res 37:371–392.

Berlucchi G (1981): Recent advances in the analysis of the neural substrate of interhemispheric communication. In Pompeiano O, Ajmone-Marsan C, (eds): "Brain Mechanisms of Perceptual Awareness and Purposeful Behavior." New York: Raven Press, pp 133–152.

Berlucchi G, Rizzolatti G (1968): Binocularly driven neurons in visual cortex of split-chiasm cats. Science 159:308–310.

Berlucchi G, Gazzaniga MS, Rizzolatti G (1967): Microelectrode analysis of transfer of visual information by the corpus callosum. Arch Ital Biol 105:583–596.

Brugge JF, Dubrovsky NA, Aitkin LM, Anderson DJ (1969): Sensitivity of single neurons in the auditory cortex of cat to binaural stimulation: Effects of varying interaural time and intensity. J Neurophysiol 52:1005–1024.

Cynader MS, Lepore F, Guillemot JP (1981): Inter-hemispheric competition during postnatal development. Nature 290:139–140.

Eisman JM (1974): Neural encoding of sound location: An electrophysiological study in auditory cortex (AI) of the cat using free field stimulation. Brain Res 75:203–214.

Elberger AJ (1979): The role of the corpus callosum in the development of interocular eye alignment and the organization of the visual field in the cat. Exp Brain Res 36:71–85.

Elberger AJ (1980): The effect of neonatal section of the corpus callosum on the development of depth perception in young cats. Vision Res 20:177–187.

Elberger AJ (1982): The corpus callosum is a critical factor for developing maximun visual acuity. Dev Brain Res 5:350–353.

Feng JZ, Brugge JF (1983): Postnatal development of auditory callosal connections in the kitten. J Comp Neurol 214:416–426.

Gazzaniga MJ (1966): Interhemispheric communication of visual learning. Neuropsychologia 4:183–189.

Gazzaniga MJ, Bogen JE, Sperry RW (1962): Some functional effects of sectioning the cerebral commissures in man. Proc Natl Acad Sci 48:1765–1769.

Hall JL, Goldstein MH (1968): Representation of binaural stimuli by single units in primary auditory cortex of unanesthetized cats. J Acoust Soc Am 43:456–461.

Hamilton CR, Gazzaniga MS (1964): Lateralization of learning of color and brightness discriminations following brain bisection. Nature (Lond.) 201:220.

Hamilton CR, Hillyard SA, Sperry RW (1968): Interhemispheric comparison of color in split brain monkeys. Exp Neurol 21:486–494.

Heath CJ, Jones EG (1971): The anatomical organization of the suprasylvian gyrus of the cat. Ergebn Anat Entw Gesch 45:1–64.

Hubel DH, Wiesel TN (1967): Cortical and callosal connections concerned with the vertical meridian of visual fields in the cat. J Neurophysiol 30:1561–1573.

Imig TJ, Adrian HO (1977): Binaural columns in the primary field (AI) of cat auditory cortex. Brain Res 138:211–257.

Imig TJ, Brugge JF (1978): Sources and terminations of callosal axons related to binaural and frequency maps in primary auditory cortex of the cat. J Comp Neurol 182:637–660.

Innocenti GM (1980): The primary visual pathway through the corpus callosum: Morphological and functional aspects in the cat. Arc Ital Biol 118:124–188.

Innocenti GM (1981): Growth and reshaping of axons in the establishment of visual callosal connections. Science 212:824–827.

Innocenti GM, Caminiti R (1980): Postnatal shaping of callosal connections from sensory areas. Exp Brain Res 38:381–394.

Innocenti GM, Frost DO (1979): Effects of visual experience on the maturation of the efferent system to the corpus callosum. Nature 28:231–234.

Innocenti GM, Frost DO (1980): The postnatal development of visual callosal connections in the absence of visual experience or of the eyes. Exp Brain Res 39:365–375.

Innocenti GM, Fiore L, Caminiti R (1977): Exuberant projection into the corpus callosum from the visual cortex of newborn cats. Neurosci Lett 4:237–242.

Jones EG, Powell TPS (1968): The commissural connections of the somatic sensory cortex in the cat. J Anat 103:433–455.

Jones EG, Coulter JD, Wise SP (1979): Commissural columns in the sensory-motor cortex of monkeys. J Comp Neurol 188:113–134.

Lepore F, Guillemot JP (1982): Visual receptive field properties of cells innervated through the corpus callosum in the cat. Exp Brain Res 46:413–424.

Lund RD, Mitchell DE (1979a): The effects of dark-rearing on visual callosal connections of cats. Brain Res 167:172–175.

Lund RD, Mitchell DE (1979b): Asymmetry in the visual callosal connections of strabismic cats. Brain Res 167:176–179.

Lund RD, Mitchell DE, Henry GH (1978): Squint-induced modifications of callosal connections in cats. Brain Res 144:169–172.

Middlebrooks JC, Pettigrew JD (1981): Functional classes of neurons in primary auditory cortex of the cat distinguished by sensitivity to sound location. J Neurosci 1:107–120.

Middlebrooks JC, Dykes RW, Merzenich MM (1980): Binaural response specific bands in primary auditory cortex (AI) of the cat: Topographical organization orthogonal to isofrequency contours. Brain Res 181:31–48.

Milleret C, Buser P (1984): Receptive field sizes and responsiveness to light in area 18 of the adult cat after chiasmotomy. Postoperative evolution; role of visual experience. Exp Brain Res 57:73–81.

Myers RE (1956): Function of corpus callosum in interocular transfer. Brain 79:358–363.

Myers RE (1962): Transmission of visual information within and between the hemispheres: a behavioral study. In Mountcastle VB (ed): "Interhemispheric Relations and Cerebral Dominance." Baltimore: John Hopkins Press, pp 52–73.

Myers RE, Sperry RW (1958): Interhemispheric communication through the corpus callosum: mnemonic carry over between the hemispheres. Arch Neurol Psychiatr 80:298–303.

Ptito M, Lepore F (1983): Interhemispheric transfer in cats with early callosal transection. Nature 301:513–515.

Sanides D (1978a): The retinotopic distribution of visual callosal projections in the suprasylvian visual areas compared to the classical visual areas (17, 18, 19) in the cat. Exp Brain Res 33:435–444.

Sanides D (1978b): The visuotopic distribution of the callosal projection in the cat. Neurosci Lett 1:S 382.

Seagraves MA, Rosenquist AC (1982a): The distribution of the cells of origin of callosal projections in cat visual cortex. J Neurosci 2:1079–1089.

Seagraves MA, Rosenquist AC (1982b): The afferent and efferent callosal connections of retinotopically defined areas in cat cortex. J Neurosci 2:1090–1107.

Shatz CJ (1977a): Anatomy of interhemispheric connections in the visual system of Boston Siamese and ordinary cats. J Comp Neurol 173:497–518.

Shatz CJ (1977b): Abnormal interhemispheric connections in the visual system of Boston Siamese cats: A physiological study. J Comp Neurol 171:229–245.

Sovijärvi ARA, Hyvärinen J (1974): Auditory cortical neurons in the cat sensitive to the direction of sound source movement. Brain Res 73:455–471.

Sperry RW (1961): Cerebral organization and behavior. Science 133:1749–1757.

Stamm SJ, Sperry RW (1957): Function of corpus callosum in contralateral transfer of somesthetic discrimination in cats. J Comp Physiol Psychol 50:138–143.

Tassinari G, Di Stefano M, Minciacchi D, Antonini A (1985): Interhemispheric influences on area 19 of the cat. Exp Brain Res (in press).

Van Essen DC, Newsome WT, Bixby JL (1982): The pattern of interhemispheric connections and its relationship to extrastriate visual areas in the macaque monkey. J Neurosci 2:265–283.

Yinon U, Hammer A, Podell M (1982): The hemispheric dominance of cortical cells in the absence of direct visual pathways. Brain Res 232:187–190.

Yinon U, Podell M, Goshen S Deafferentation of the visual cortex (1984): The effects on cortical cells in normal and in early monocularly deprived cats. Exp Neurol 83:486–494.

Zeki SM (1970): Interhemispheric connections of prestriate cortex in monkey. Brain Res 19:63–75.

Two Hemispheres—One Brain:
Functions of the Corpus Callosum, pages 231–254
© 1986 Alan R. Liss, Inc.

Role of Callosal Cells in the Functional Organization of Cat Striate Cortex

BERTRAM R. PAYNE

Department of Anatomy, Medical College of Pennsylvania, Philadelphia, Pennsylvania 19129

INTRODUCTION

The contribution of interhemispheric connections to cerebral cortical function has been studied primarily in patients who have undergone surgical transection of the corpus callosum [see Sperry, 1966, 1970, 1974; Gazzaniga, 1970; Gazzaniga and LeDoux, 1978, for reviews]. These studies have examined the role of the corpus callosum in integrating the actions of association areas in temporal, parietal, and frontal lobes of the two hemispheres. In these patients it has not been possible to examine the role played by callosal connections in integrating information processing in primary sensory areas in the two hemispheres. In an effort to understand the role played by callosal connections in such areas it is necessary to turn to animal models. For these studies area 17 of the cat's occipital lobe was chosen for the following reasons: (1) It is a primary sensory area that sends fibers to, and receives fibers from, the contralateral hemisphere via the corpus callosum. (2) Area 17 can be subdivided into three stereotyped zones according to the origin and termination of callosal fibers and also contains a point-to-point map of the contralateral half of visual space. Each callosal zone contains a representation of a different portion of the visual field, and it is therefore possible to specify in which callosal zone a cell is located by the position of its receptive field in visual space. (3) The receptive field properties of neurons in area 17 are relatively well understood, and any changes in their properties after surgical section of the callosal pathway are more likely to be detected than in other cortical regions where the properties of neurons are less well understood.

I will describe some anatomical and electrophysiological experiments that my colleagues and I have carried out to define some of the underlying principles of the organization and function of neurons whose fibers contribute to the corpus callosum.

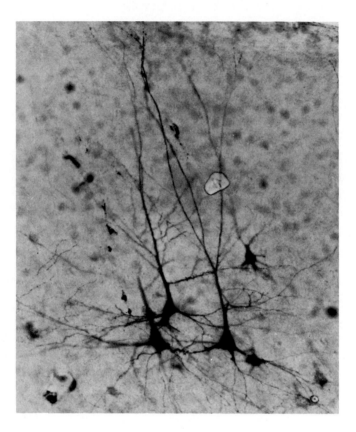

Fig. 1. Photomicrograph of callosal cells in the border region between areas 17 and 18 filled with horseradish peroxidase reaction product.

Fig. 2. Drawing of five neurons shown in Figure 1. All of these neurons are contained within *one* 70-μm-thick section. Oxidized diaminobenzidine reaction product appears to fill the cells and their processes completely, since large numbers of dendrites and spines can be seen. The three neurons on the left are pyramidal cells with prominent apical dendrites that can extend up to 400 μm into layer 1. Note also profuse network of basal dendrites, extending laterally up to 300 μm from the cell somata. Many of the dendrites, both apical and basal, bear large numbers of spines. The two neurons on the right are stellate cells, their dendrites appear less well directed than the dendrites on the pyramidal cells. The dendrites of stellate

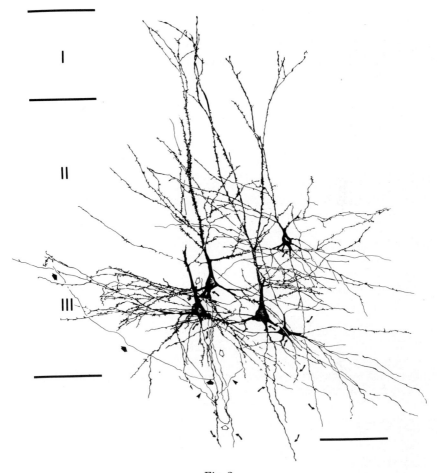

Fig. 2

cells rarely reach layer 1. In addition, the distribution of the spines on these dendrites is relatively sparse. Axons are indicated by arrows. Descending axons to the white matter of all five neurons are marked by curved arrows. The axon collaterals of the left-hand pyramidal cell are indicated by filled and open, broad and narrow arrowheads. All these collaterals ascend toward the pial surface. One collateral is arciform (open, broad arrowhead); as it ascends it passes almost parallel to the descending portion of the axon. The remaining collaterals ascend somewhat obliquely through the cortex. Scale bar at bottom right = 100 μm. Plano-Apo ×100 oil-immersion objective, N.A. 1.35. Achromat-Aplanat Condensor, N.A. 1.35.

Based on studies of the topography of callosal connections and on the effects of callosal transection, it is suggested that callosal cells modulate activity related to specific regions of visual space in both ipsilateral and contralateral hemispheres.

ORGANIZATION OF CALLOSAL CONNECTIONS IN AREA 17

Cells that project axons through the corpus callosum have characteristic morphologies and laminar distributions, and they project to well-defined locations in the contralateral hemisphere. On the basis of the origin and termination of callosal projections, we have divided area 17 into three zones: a callosal terminal zone, a callosal cell zone, and an acallosal zone [Payne et al., 1986]. Area 17 contains a well-ordered, point-to-point map of the contralateral half of visual space [Tusa et al., 1978], and neurons in each of the three callosal zones respond to stimuli in different portions of the visual field. The zone of origin of callosal projections was defined using retrograde transport of horseradish peroxidase from terminal sites in the contralateral hemisphere. This procedure also provided the opportunity to observe and describe the morphology and laminar distribution of callosal cells. The zones of termination and laminar distribution of callosal projections were defined either by anterograde transport of tracers such as tritiated amino acids or by stains for degenerating fibers after lesions to the callosal pathway.

Laminar Distribution and Morphology of Callosal Cells

In area 17, callosal cells are a somewhat heterogeneous population distributed over a number of cortical layers. The majority of callosal cells are pyramids located in the supragranular layers; they bear large numbers of dendritic spines and have a number of locally arborizing axon collaterals (Figs. 1,2) [Naporn et al., 1984a,b]. Other morphological types, including stellate and intermediate forms, are also shown in the summary diagram (Fig. 3). More callosal cells are concentrated in the supragranular than infragranular layers, and no callosal cells have been observed in layer 5. In addition to their long-ranging axon collaterals, callosal cells also have local axon collaterals that project most commonly to the supra- and infra-granular layers and rarely to layer 4. Therefore, while many callosal cells have a similar morphology and laminar location, many are not easily classified. This heterogeneity of cell morphology and laminar distribution suggests that the different types of callosal cells may have different roles in information processing in area 17.

Laminar Distribution of Callosal Terminals

Autoradiographic procedures after transport of tritiated amino acids from a large number of visual areas in one hemisphere to the contralateral hemisphere reveal a differential laminar distribution in area 17. The label

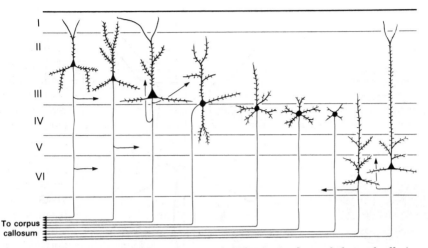

Fig. 3. Summary diagram of the laminar distribution and morphology of cells in the region of the border between areas 17 and 18 that project to the contralateral hemisphere via the corpus callosum. Also shown is the laminar distribution of local axon collaterals (arrowheads). Callosal cells may have a pyramidal, stellate, or intermediate morphology and can be found in all layers except layer 5. There are five times more pyramidal cells in the superficial layers than cells in other layers or with other morphologies.

is densest in layers 1, 3, 5, and 6 (Fig. 4, right column). Injections restricted to only one or two areas in the contralateral hemisphere show that projections from homotopic locations terminate in different layers than projections from heterotopic locations. Projections from areas 17 and 18 in one hemisphere to homotopic sites in the contralateral hemisphere are densest in layers 1 and 3 and relatively light in layers 5 and 6. Projections from heterotopic locations, such as lateral suprasylvian areas or area 19 in the contralateral 3 [Payne et al., 1986]. It is interesting that the layers that contain high-density label are the same layers into which ipsilateral local collaterals of callosal cells project. Local and distant axon collaterals of callosal cells may therefore show some selective affinity during development and form contacts with cells in particular layers regardless of whether the target cells are located in the ipsilateral or contralateral hemisphere. This similarity in the laminar projections of local and long-ranging collaterals of callosal cells suggests that the local collaterals in the same hemisphere and long-ranging collaterals in the contralateral hemisphere play a similar role in information processing.

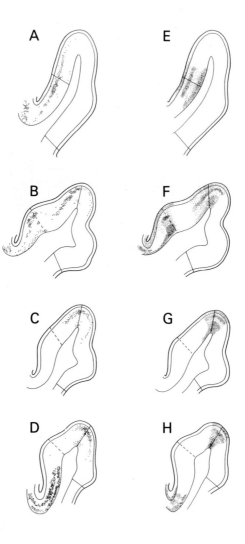

Fig. 4. Demonstration of the extent of the callosal cell zone (A–D) and callosal terminal zone (E–H) in areas 17 and 18 after 40 injections of a mixture of horseradish peroxidase and tritiated proline were made into all visual areas in the contralateral

Regional Distribution of Callosal Cells and Terminals

Callosal cells and terminals in area 17, besides having a characteristic laminar position, also have a characteristic regional distribution. This regional distribution divides area 17 into three callosal zones (Fig. 4). Within area 17 the cortical territory containing either callosal cells or callosal terminals is similar at all rostrocaudal levels. (1) Callosal cells extend 3.5–4 mm from the border with area 18 and occupy the lateral half of area 17, the medial half being devoid of labeled callosal cells. (2) In contrast, all callosal terminals in area 17 are located within 1 mm of the border with area 18. While the callosal cell zone partially overlaps the terminal zone, the cell zone also includes more medial regions of cortex. (3) The third zone, referred to as acallosal, occupies the remainder of area 17 and contains neither callosal cells nor terminals.

REPRESENTATION OF THE VISUAL FIELD IN CALLOSAL CELL AND TERMINAL ZONES

The organization of these callosal zones has implications for the types of information relayed to, and received from, the contralateral hemisphere. In terms of visual field coordinates, the origin and termination of some of the callosal projections will be matched topologically, while others will not. While area 17 contains a point-to-point representation of visual space, the representation of these different points is not equal [Tusa et al., 1978]. In the center of the visual field, $(1 \text{ mm})^2$ of cortex views approximately $(1°)^2$ of visual space. In the fields 20° from the center, the same amount of cortex views approximately $(5°)^2$ of visual space. Since the callosal cell zone occupies a larger region of cortex than the terminal zone, we can therefore predict that the cell zone will contain a representation of more of the visual field than the terminal zone and that not all interhemispheric connections will be matched visuotopically. Specifically, the greater region of visual

---

hemisphere. Horseradish-peroxidase -containing cells and silver grains are denoted by dots. Tetramethylbenzidine was the chromogen used to visualize the horseradish peroxidase. Pairs of sections (A+E, B+F, etc.) are adjacent sections and are taken from four representative levels in the brain. These levels are at Horsley-Clarke P4, APO, A4, and A9 and represent elevations of approximately 0°, −5°, −10°, and −20° to −25° in the map of the visual field, respectively. Note that while the width of the callosal cell and terminal zones at the area 17/18 border varies at different rostrocaudal levels, the variability is all in area 18. The width of the callosal cell and terminal zones in area 17 is constant at all rostrocaudal levels. Note relatively low density of silver grains in layers 2 and 4. Solid lines crossing cortical layers represent borders of area 17. Interrupted line represents the border between area 18 and area 19. Medial is to the right.

space represented in the callosal cell zone must converge on a smaller representation of visual space in the callosal terminal zone. To determine which regions of visual space are represented in the cell and terminal zones, experiments combining either anterograde or retrograde pathway tracing techniques and electrophysiological mapping techniques were carried out [Payne et al., 1986].

Callosal Terminal Zone

Experiments to determine the representation of visual space in the callosal terminal zone show that more of inferior space than central space is represented in this zone. The locations of the receptive fields of neurons located within the callosal terminal zone are shown for two different rostrocaudal levels of area 17 in Figures 5 and 6. Figure 5 shows that caudal in area 17, close to the representation of the area centralis, virtually all cells within the terminal zone have receptive fields within 1° of the vertical midline. At a more rostral location in area 17, and a more inferior location in the visual field, cells have receptive fields up to 3° or 4° from the midline of the visual field (Fig. 6).

Reconstructions of electrode tracks made at other rostrocaudal levels in the same animal and comparisons with our own and published maps of area 17 [Tusa et al., 1978] allow us to define the region of visual space repre-

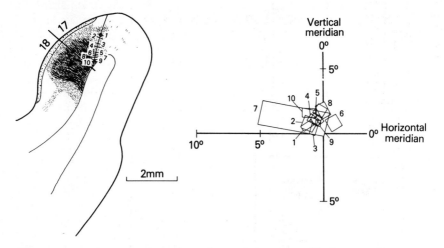

Fig. 5. Reconstruction of an electrode track into area 17 of a cat after corpus callosum transection and after staining the section for degenerating fibers. Left: Electrode track reconstruction of the sites of ten neurons recorded within the zone of degeneration. Right: Size and location of the receptive fields of the neurons relative to the principal meridians of the visual field. All units had receptive fields clustered within 1° or so of the 0° vertical meridian.

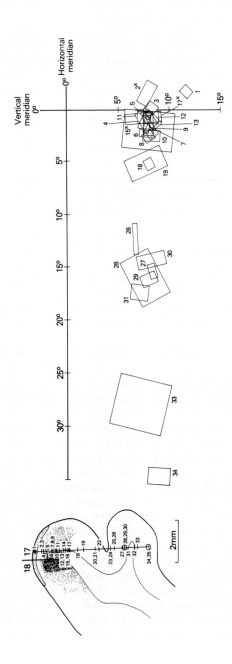

Fig. 6. Reconstruction of an electrode track into area 17 of the same cat after corpus callosum transection. Left: Electrode track reconstruction of the sites of 35 recorded units of which 17 were located in the zone of degeneration. Degeneration occupies approximately one-tenth of the width of area 17 at this rostrocaudal level. Right: Size and location of the receptive fields relative to horizontal and vertical meridians. All units in the zone of degeneration have receptive fields confined to within 3° to 4° of the vertical meridian.

sented in the callosal terminal zone. This reconstruction shows that more of inferior visual space than of central space is represented in the terminal zone (Fig. 7, right-hand side). Neurons in the terminal zone at the representation of central visual space view the 1° of visual space adjacent to the vertical midline. Neurons in the terminal zone in the representation of fields distant to central visual space view up to 5° adjacent to the midline.

The region of visual space represented in the callosal terminal zone is similar to that viewed by cells in the nasotemporal division of the retina [Illing and Wässle, 1981]. The nasotemporal division is a zone that separates populations of ganglion cells in nasal retina that project exclusively to the contralateral side of the brain from those in temporal retina that project exclusively to the ipsilateral side of the brain. This zone contains a population of cells, some of which project contralaterally and others that project

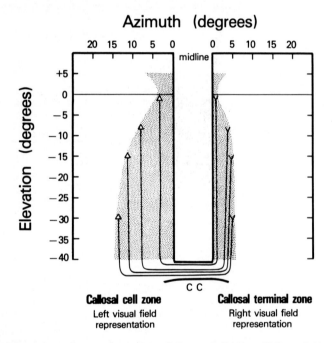

Fig. 7. Diagrammatic representation of the organization of the origin and termination of callosal projections to and from area 17 *in terms of visual field coordinates*. Left: Neurons in the callosal cell zone with receptive fields in one hemifield. These neurons (triangles) view a limited region of visual space and send information about that spatial location along axons in the corpus callosum to neurons in the contralateral hemisphere. Neurons in the contralateral hemisphere are located in the callosal terminal zone and view locations on the midline or in a limited region of the contralateral hemifield.

ipsilaterally. Illing and Wässle [1981] have shown that the nasotemporal division is much narrower in the center of the retina than at more peripheral locations. However, like the constancy in width of the callosal terminal zone at different rostrocaudal levels, there is constancy of width in the nasotemporal division in terms of the number of intercell spacings between the purely contralaterally projecting population and the purely ipsilaterally projecting population. The similarity between the region of visual space represented in the callosal terminal zone and that viewed by ganglion cells in the nasotemporal division suggests a causal relationship between the organization of these two regions and that a fixed number of ganglion cells provide the direct afferent input, via the retino-thalamo-cortical path, to the callosal terminal zone at all rostrocaudal locations in area 17.

One possible explanation for the similarity between the nasotemporal division and the callosal terminal zone may lie in the fact that in the nasotemporal division adjacent ganglion cells can project to different hemispheres. Consequently, there are likely to be deficiencies such as an incomplete map and decreased acuity in the representation of visual information in both hemispheres. The simplest role for projections of some callosal cells into the terminal zone may be to redress these natural deficiencies in visual system wiring caused by such an imprecise decussation zone in the retina. To examine this possibility, we have determined which regions of visual space are represented in the callosal cell zone of area 17 to see if callosal input could redress these deficiencies.

Callosal Cell Zone

Experiments to determine the representation of visual space in the callosal cell zone show that, like the terminal zone, less of central visual space than of inferior visual space is represented. However, at any given level in area 17, more space is represented in the cell zone than in the terminal zone. The locations of the receptive fields of neurons located within the callosal cell zone are shown for three different rostrocaudal levels of area 17 in Figure 8. Caudal in area 17, close to the representation of the area centralis, neurons in the callosal cell zone have receptive fields within 4° of the 0° vertical meridian. At more rostral locations in area 17, and inferior in the map of visual space, neurons in the cell zone have receptive fields up to 8° from the midline. At the most rostral level examined, at the representation of elevations −15° to −25°, neurons in the cell zone have receptive fields up to 14° from the midline. The larger representation of the visual field in the callosal cell zone compared with the callosal terminal zone means that some callosal cells can redress the deficiencies caused by an imprecise zone of decussation in the retina.

Integration of Visual Field Information in Callosal Cell and Terminal Zones

The organization of the termination and origin of the callosal projections in area 17 are summarized in terms of visual field coordinates in Figure 7.

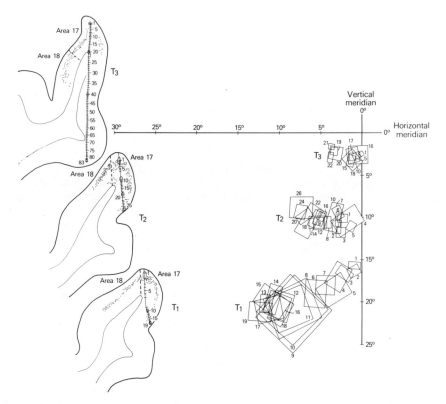

Fig. 8. Reconstruction of electrode tracks into area 17 after multiple injections into the contralateral hemisphere of wheat germ agglutinin conjugated to horseradish peroxidase. Each dot represents one labeled cell. Left: Distribution of labeled cells and reconstructed electrode tracks. Top section is caudal and bottom section is rostral in area 17. Right: Size and location of the receptive field of cells recorded in the callosal cell zone relative to horizontal and vertical meridians. (For the sake of clarity, not all receptive fields have been reproduced.)

This summary shows that some regions connected by callosal axons are relatively well-matched topologically while others are not. Callosal neurons relay information about specific regions of the visual field on one side of the midline to neurons in the terminal zone in the contralateral hemisphere with receptive fields close to or on the other side of the midline. In the representation of central visual space, callosal cells view up to 4° lateral to the midline and project to cells in the contralateral hemisphere with receptive fields up to only 1° on the other side of the midline. At representations of inferior visual space callosal cells may have receptive fields up to 15° from the midline and project to neurons in the terminal zone in the contralateral hemisphere with receptive fields up to 5° into the other hemifield. There will also be some callosal neurons with receptive fields close to the midline that project to neurons in the contralateral hemisphere with receptive fields also close to the midline.

The connections between callosal cells viewing regions adjacent to the midline and neurons in the contralateral hemisphere with receptive fields also close to the midline will be relatively well-matched topologically. These connections can serve to redress deficiencies in visual system wiring. Other callosal connections from cells nearer to the edge of the callosal cell zone, viewing up to 15° into one hemifield, and projecting to cells in the callosal terminal zone of the contralateral hemisphere, with receptive fields up to 5° on the other side of the midline, will be mismatched topologically by up to 20°. These non-topologically matched callosal connections presumably subserve different functions. One possible role for them is that they may be similar to the normal, long-distance, intracortical connections found in area 17. These connections are not matched topologically and may have a modulatory or facilitatory role in cortical function [Payne et al., 1984b].

Callosal projections to and from area 17 may act either as modulators of neuronal activity or act as a relay of specific visual information. The studies of others have shown that intracortical axons in cat area 17 may project several millimeters within area 17 [Gilbert and Wiesel, 1979]. The origin and termination of these long projections cannot be matched topologically. In many cases, these cells presumably contribute to receptive field properties without providing an excitatory drive to their target neurons, since a lack of congruence of binocular receptive fields of more than a few degrees, or neurons with receptive fields at more than one location in the visual field, have not been detected in area 17. These non-topologically matched projections presumably modulate the responses of neurons to activation of other afferent pathways, such as those coming from other cortical areas or from the thalamus. For example, it is known that stimuli presented in regions of visual space outside of the classically defined receptive field can influence the response properties of individual cortical neurons [Nelson and Frost, 1978]. The long, intrinsic connections of cortical neurons may form a morphological substrate for this effect. Cells located in the body of area 17 have many options as to the targets of their intrinsic projections, since they are able to project their axons in any direction. However, for cells located close to the border between areas 17 and 18, the possible targets within the same area are more limited. Cells located close to the border have more options medially than laterally, and the number of options for intrinsic connections decreases with increasing proximity to the 17/18 border. Therefore, cells located close to the area 17/18 border may have to project to the contralateral hemisphere in order to reach appropriate target neurons within area 17 (Fig. 9). In accord with this suggestion of the relative numbers of options available medially and laterally, it has been shown that callosal cells are densest at the lateral border of area 17 and less dense at more medial locations (see Fig. 4A–D). Such interhemispheric projections may then act to facilitate the responses of cells to stimuli presented in the hemifield represented in the contralateral area 17. These callosal cells are then similar to other neurons that form long, intracortical connections except their target neurons are located in the contralateral hemisphere and have receptive fields on the opposite side of the midline.

The anatomical and electrophysiological mapping experiments described above suggest that many callosal cells may be involved in processing of visual information at a rather subtle level since the experiments have revealed the lack of topological congruence in some of the callosal connections. Neurons with multiple receptive fields are rarely, if ever, recorded in area 17 of normal, intact cats. In addition, neurons with receptive fields beyond 1° into the ipsilateral hemifield, let alone 15° into that hemifield, have not been recorded in area 17. It is therefore unlikely that many of the callosal inputs are of sufficient strength to drive a significant number of cells. However, intracellular recording experiments have revealed that afferent input from callosal fibers is excitatory and that a great many cells are influenced by stimulation of the callosal pathway [Toyama et al., 1974; Singer et al., 1975]. Therefore, inputs from callosal cells may serve to raise excitability levels and summate with excitatory inputs from other sources to drive neurons in the callosal zones of area 17. This is presumably also the case for the local, ipsilateral and, long-ranging, axonal contralateral projections of callosal cells. Other investigators using different techniques have come to similar conclusions [Clare et al., 1961; Landau et al., 1961; Lassonde, this volume].

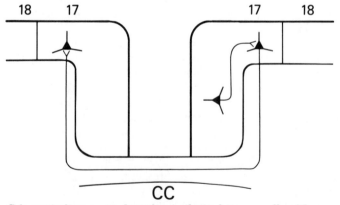

Fig. 9. Schematic diagram to show the similarity between cells with axon collaterals confined to the area in which the parent cell is located and cells whose principal axon passes through the corpus callosum to the contralateral hemisphere.

Other intracortical connections over short distances will be relatively well matched topologically and may be like callosal connections concerned directly with the midline of the visual field. These callosal connections may encode for small disparities about the midline of the visual field, while the local intracortical connections may provide the anatomical substrate for detection of small disparities at locations somewhat lateral to the midline.

Support for such an idea that some callosal cells are involved in disparity detection about the midline comes from the study of Mitchell and Blakemore [1970], who showed that in a human subject disparity detection and depth perception close to the midline is abolished by surgical section of the corpus callosum. However, no impairment in depth perception was found for locations more lateral in the visual field. Such a result is apparent when one considers that cells in each hemisphere that view regions close to the midline will be deafferented of disparate information arising in the contralateral hemisphere by the section, whereas those cells that view locations lateral to the midline will be unaffected by the surgery.

ROLE OF CORPUS CALLOSUM IN THE BINOCULARITY OF NEURONS IN AREA 17 OF CAT STRIATE CORTEX

To test these ideas about the role of callosal connections in the function of neurons in area 17, the corpus callosum was sectioned in adult cats and the responses of neurons in area 17 were compared with those recorded in area 17 of anesthetized, intact cats. This experimental paradigm partially deafferents cells in the 1 mm of cortex in the callosal terminal zone and axotomizes a population of neurons in the 3.5–4-mm-wide strip of the callosal cell zone. In the cell zone, callosal cells may undergo retrograde changes after axotomy that decrease the excitability of these cells, as has been described for ventral horn cells (see Payne et al., [1984a] for a more detailed discussion). This reduced excitability of axotomized callosal neurons will result in less activity in all axon collaterals, and this will reduce the effectiveness of the input that neighboring cortical cells normally receive via the local collaterals of the callosal cells. In other words, these neighboring cells are functionally partially deafferented. Callosum transection should have no effect on the zone, which contains neither callosal cells nor terminals.

We have made electrophysiological recordings from neurons in the three callosal zones in the rostral part of area 17, both in normal cats and in cats with various survival times after surgical transection of the corpus callosum [Payne et al., 1984a]. Receptive fields of neurons were plotted and the data analyzed with reference to accurate localization of the principal meridians of the visual field and to the callosal zones [Payne et al., 1981]. In intact cats, there is a gradient in the proportion of neurons that can be activated by both eyes (Fig. 10). The gradient extends from the midline, where 75–80% of recorded neurons are binocular, to the representation of far temporal visual space where neurons can only be driven by one eye [Berman et al., 1982]. The region containing the highest proportion of binocular neurons is coincident with the callosal cell zone [Payne et al., 1986]. After transection of the corpus callosum, there is a significant reduction in the proportion of neurons that can be driven by both eyes (Fig. 10). Other receptive field properties, including orientation and direction selectivity and their columnar organization, appear to be unaffected [Payne et al., 1984b].

The decrease in binocularity is confined to the callosal zones, but the extent of the callosal zones affected varies with the duration of the postoperative period. In the first few weeks, there is a decrease in the proportion of neurons that could be activated by both eyes. This decrease in binocularity is confined to neurons within the callosal cell zone. At more lateral locations, the neurons are just as likely to be binocular as in normal cats. Furthermore, within the cell zone binocularity is reduced the most in the

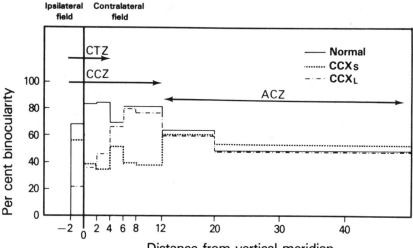

Fig. 10. Percent binocularity of neurons in normal cats (solid line) and in short-term (up to 7 weeks postoperative—dotted line) and long-term (up to 42 weeks postoperative—interrupted line) cats according to distance of their receptive fields from the vertical meridian. In short-term animals binocularity of neurons is reduced up to 12° from the vertical meridian. This reduction in binocularity occurs only in the callosal cell zone (CCZ), which also encompasses the callosal terminal zone (CTZ). In the long-term animals binocularity of neurons is reduced only up to 4° from the vertical meridian. This reduction in binocularity occurs only in the callosal terminal zone. In the long-term animals, neurons in the callosal cell zone outside of the terminal zone show recovery of binocularity. In both groups of animals, binocularity of neurons in the acallosal zone (ACZ) is unaffected by section of the corpus callosum.

supragranular layers, somewhat less in the infragranular layers, and is unchanged in layer 4 [Payne et al., 1984b]. The layers in which binocularity is reduced are precisely the ones that receive local and long-distance axon collaterals from callosal cells.

Since there is a reasonable amount of residual binocularity in the cell zone after transection, the result suggests that while the binocularity of some neurons in area 17 is reinforced by inputs from cells with axons projecting through the corpus callosum, for other neurons, binocularity is not dependent on callosal input. As expected, normal numbers of binocular neurons are recorded in the acallosal region of area 17 after callosum transection. Similar results showing a reduction in binocularity in the primary visual cortex of cats after interruption of the callosal pathway have been obtained by Dreher and Cottee [1975], Elberger [1981], and Blakemore et al. [1983]. Results by other investigators suggest little or no change in binocularity after interruption of the callosal pathway; however, the location of the recorded neurons relative to the callosal zones is unclear or recordings were taken from unanesthetized animals [see chapters in this volume by Berlucchi, by Cynader, and by Elberger for more details].

To investigate whether callosal cells can recover from the effects of axotomy, we examined cats 8–10 months after transection of the corpus callosum. The results show that there is a differential recovery of neurons following corpus callosum transection. The decrease in binocularity observed in the terminal zone is permanent, whereas the decrease in the part of the cell zone outside the terminal zone is only temporary. Eight to ten months after transection of the corpus callosum, the proportion of neurons that could be activated by both eyes was reduced relative to normal. However, the reduction was confined to those neurons in the callosal terminal zone (Fig. 10). These results are in contrast to those obtained from cats recorded within a few weeks of transection, where the decrease in binocularity extended beyond the terminal zone to include neurons in the rest of the cell zone.

The changes in binocularity in the callosal terminal zone are permanent, presumably because the region is partially deafferented and because neurons with processes confined to the central nervous system cannot regenerate lost portions of their axons and reinnervate deafferented targets. The temporary changes in the callosal cell zone may be due to changes in levels of excitability of callosal neurons after axotomy. Reversible changes in excitability have been demonstrated in a number of other systems in which axons have been damaged. These changes are associated with a number of other morphological, biochemical, and physiological changes; and they have been characterized most fully in axotomized motor neurons (see Payne et al., [1984a] for a more detailed discussion). Examples of the time course of some of these changes after axotomy are compared with the time course of changes in binocularity in the callosal cell zone of area 17 after section of the corpus callosum in Figure 11.

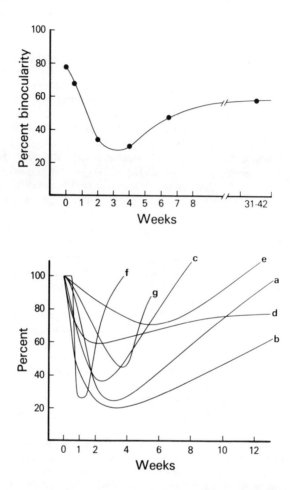

Fig. 11. Top: Binocularity of neurons in the callosal cell zone of area 17 as a function of time after corpus callosum transection. The initial point represents control data obtained from normal animals. The data at 2 and 4 weeks approximate the maximum decrease in binocularity as a result of corpus callosum transection. Data pooled from weeks 31–42 demonstrate some recovery of binocularity. The recovery is confined to the region of cortex containing callosal cells but outside the callosal terminal zone (see Fig. 10). There is no recovery in the callosal terminal zone, and as a result, overall values do not return to normal levels. Curve fitted by eye. Bottom: Time course of the retrograde effects of axotomy alone (curves a–f) or in conjunction with deafferentation (curve g). Data have been redrawn from a number

The curves show the time course of alterations in neuronal excitability and related alterations in morphology and biochemistry. For example, the time course of synaptic stripping and reattachment following axotomy are shown for hypoglossal neurons in curves a and b and for alpha-motor neurons in curve d. It is interesting to note that the time course of the reduction in binocularity after section of the callosum is similar to the time course of many of these retrograde changes after axotomy.

These data show that after corpus callosum transection some cells are partially deafferented of callosal input and can only be activated by one eye. Since callosal neurons are unable to regenerate their long-ranging axon collaterals, these effects are permanent. The data also suggest that after callosum transection callosal neurons undergo retrograde changes that may cause depression in their activity. This depression in activity functionally partially deafferents neighboring neurons of input from modulatory and facilitatory influences. Together, these data suggest that callosal cells appear to provide an essential but nondriving input to cells in the ipsilateral hemisphere. This ipsilateral input allows neighboring cortical neurons to respond to stimuli presented to both eyes (Fig. 12).

SUMMARY AND CONCLUSIONS

The organization of the callosal pathway and the differential responses of neurons to corpus callosum transection allow us to suggest two ways by which callosal cells may be operating in the normal functioning of the cortex. Some callosal connections are topologically organized, while others are not, suggesting that some callosal connections provide a direct drive to their target neurons, while others provide only a facilitatory input. These actions of callosal cells and their long-ranging axon collaterals may be similar, in many respects, to the actions of local, intracortical axon collaterals of callosal or other cells. It is possible to consider the neurons with topologically matched afferent connections operating as part of a logic "or" gate (Fig. 13). For example, in the case of a binocular neuron in area 17, afferents relaying information from one eye may have their origin in the thalamus, while afferents relaying information from the other eye may have their origin in the contralateral hemisphere. Activity along either pathway may be able to drive the cell. In contrast, neurons may have

---

of published studies (see below). In each study the normal data has been set at 100% and the experimental data show the percent change relative to normal as a function of time since axon damage. In all studies the effects of axon damage take at least 1 week and up to 5 weeks to show their maximal change. Curve a from Sumner [1975], Figure 6; b from Sumner [1975], Figure 4; c from Sumner and Sutherland [1973], Figure 7; d from Chen [1978], Table 1; e from Sumner and Watson [1971], Figure 2; f from Baker et al. [1981], Figure 6; and g from Echlin [1975], Figure 1. Curves have been fitted by eye (figure reproduced with permission from Payne et al. [1984a]).

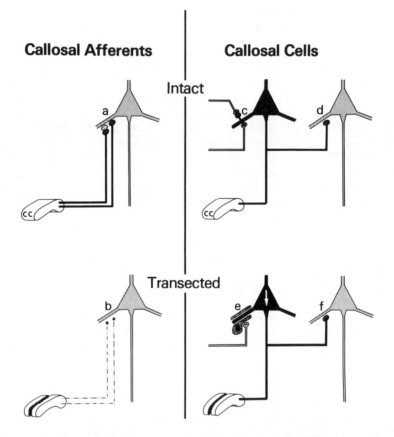

Fig. 12. Diagram outlining the events that we propose result from transection of the corpus callosum and that may explain the reduction in binocularity in the callosal terminal and cell zones. In normal animals the role of distant and local axon collateral terminals is to provide excitatory driving or essential facilitatory inputs to postsynaptic cells. These inputs allow the postsynaptic cell to respond to inputs arising from both eyes. Upper left: In intact cats, cells in the callosal terminal zone receive inputs onto dendritic shafts or their spines from long-ranging axons that pass through the corpus callosum (cc) from cells located in the contralateral hemisphere (a). Lower left: Following corpus callosum transection, axon segments

topologically matched afferents relaying information from both eyes via the thalamus. However, if the thalamic input from one eye is located on more distal parts of the dendrites, it may be insufficient to depolarize the cell body beyond threshold. If callosal terminals are located at strategic positions closer to the cell body, this callosal input may, in conjunction with excitation of the afferents at more distal dendritic locations, depolarize the cell membrane sufficiently to activate the cell. In this case the callosal input is operating as part of a logic "and" gate.

Callosum transection causes degeneration of the long-ranging axons, resulting in permanent, partial deafferentation and permanent removal of modulating afferents. Callosum transection may also cause temporary retrograde changes in callosal cells that reduce the efficacy of the local collateral modulation of neighboring cells.

Taken together, these results suggest a means by which callosal cells modulate the activity of other cortical neurons in both the contralateral and ipsilateral hemispheres [see also Lassonde, this volume]. Inputs from callosal neurons allow cells to respond to input arriving from the eyes via the thalamus—nondriving callosal cells of intact cats operate as part of a logic "and" gate, while driving callosal neurons operate as part of a logic "or" gate.

It is likely that many callosal cells influence the responses of neurons not only in the contralateral hemisphere but also in the same hemisphere. This is shown especially in the experiments where surgical section of the

---

separated from their cell bodies degenerate, and inputs to cells in the callosal terminal zone are removed (b). Excitability decreases and the neuron can then only respond to stimuli presented to one eye. Since central axons do not regenerate, the reduction in responsivity and the decrease in binocularity in this region is permanent. Upper right: In intact cats, callosal cells (black) receive afferent input onto dendrites and their spines from neighboring or distant cells (c). Callosal cells not only have axons passing through the corpus callosum to cells in the contralateral hemisphere but also have local axon collaterals that terminate on dendrites of neighboring cells (d). Lower right: Following corpus callosum transection, callosal cells down-regulate production of receptors (arrow), thus decreasing the ability of afferent fibers to influence these cells. Synaptic stripping may occur in which synaptic terminals are removed from the callosal cells and synaptic clefts are invaded by glial cell processes (e). As a result of these changes, the callosal cells themselves become more difficult to activate, and in turn their ability to influence neighboring cortical cells via local axon collaterals is reduced (f). This decreased transmission of afferent information reduces the facilitory input to neighboring cells, and these neighboring cells are thus less likely to be driven by both eyes. These changes may be reversible and lead to a recovery in binocularity. With time, there may be an up-regulation of receptor synthesis and possibly a reformation of synapses onto callosal cells. Callosal cells are then able to raise their excitability level and facilitate the responses of neighboring cells; thus both eyes become effective in driving these neighboring cells once again.

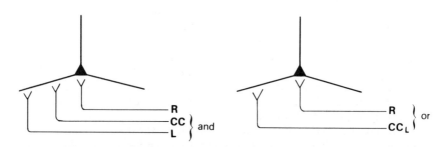

Fig. 13. Schematic diagram outlining the ways callosal cells may operate as part of a logic "and" gate (left) or logic "or" gate (right). Left ("and" gate): A neuron receives afferent input from both the left (L) and right (R) eyes via the thalamocortical pathway. These inputs terminate on dendrites close to or distant from the cell body. Callosal input terminates at strategic locations closer to the cell body than the distal inputs onto the dendrite. The differential distribution of afferents from the two eyes onto the dendrites means that activity in the right eye, in this case, is more likely than activity in the left eye to activate the postsynaptic neuron. However, simultaneous activity in callosal axons (CC) will increase the probability that activity in the left eye will depolarize the cell body sufficiently for activation of the cell. Activation of the cell by the left eye requires the thalamocortical pathway "and" callosal cells to be active at similar times. Right ("or" gate): In this case the neuron receives afferent driving inputs from the right eye along the thalamocortical pathway (R) and from the left eye via callosal cells (CC_L). Therefore, the cell can respond to input from either the thalamocortical pathway or callosal cells.

corpus callosum can lead to significant physiological changes. Some of these physiological changes may be permanent, while others may show recovery of normal function. The results from these studies show that the effects of lesions of the central nervous system, including the corpus callosum, are not simple to interpret since retrograde changes, as a result of axotomy, may be occurring in addition to anterograde changes as a result of deafferentation. Knowledge of the relative contribution of anterograde and retrograde changes to the loss of function is crucial to understanding the basis of recovery of function after lesions in the central nervous system.

ACKNOWLEDGMENTS

I would like to thank Andrea Elberger, Douglas Labar, Hazel Murphy, Atania Naporn, and Helen Pearson for their participation in various experiments described here, and Nancy Berman, in whose laboratory much of this work was carried out. I would also like to thank Timothy Cunningham and Michael Goldberger for their valuable discussions, and Ann Repka and Mary Wilkes for providing valuable technical support. The preparation of this manuscript was supported by a grant from the National Institutes of Mental Health (MH 38399).

REFERENCES

Baker R, Delgado-Garcia J, McCrea R (1981): Morphological and physiological effects on cat abducens motorneurons. In Flohr M, Precht W (eds): "Lesion Induced Neuronal Plasticity in Sensorimotor Systems." Berlin: Springer Verlag, pp 51–63.

Berman N, Payne BR, Labar D, Murphy EH (1982): Functional organization of neurons in cat striate cortex: Variations in ocular dominance and receptive field type with cortical laminae and location in the visual field. J Neurophysiol 48:1362–1377.

Blakemore C, Diao Y-C, Pu M-L, Wang Y-K, Xiao Y-M (1983): Possible functions of the interhemispheric connections between cortical areas in the cat. J Physiol Lond 337:331–350.

Chen DH (1978): Qualitative and quantitative study of synaptic displacement in chromatolyzed spinal neurons of the cat. J Comp Neurol 177:635–664.

Clare MH, Landau WM, Bishop GH (1961): The cortical response to direct stimulation of the corpus callosum in the cat. Electroencephalogr Clin Neurophysiol 13:21–33.

Dreher B, Cottee LJ (1975): Visual receptive-field properties of cells in area 18 of cat's cerebral cortex before and after acute lesions in area 17. J Neurophysiol 38:735–750.

Echlin F (1975): Time course of development of supersensitivity to topical acetylcholine in partially isolated cortex. Electroencephalogr Clin Neurophysiol 38:225–233.

Elberger AJ (1981): Ocular dominance in striate cortex is altered by neonatal section of the posterior corpus callosum in the cat. Exp Brain Res 41:280–291.

Gazzaniga MS (1970): "The Bisected Brain." New York: Appleton Century Crofts.

Gazzaniga MS, LeDoux JE (1978): "The Integrated Mind." New York: Plenum Press.

Gilbert CD, Wiesel TN (1979): Morphology and intracortical projections of functionally characterised neurons in the cat visual cortex. Nature 280:120–125.

Illing R-B, Wässle H (1981): The retinal projection to the thalamus in the cat: A quantitative investigation and a comparison with the retinotectal pathway. J Comp Neurol 202:265–286.

Landau WM, Bishop GH, Clare MH (1961): The interactions of several varieties of evoked response in visual and association cortex of the cat. Electroencephalogr Clin Neurophysiol 13:43–53.

Mitchell DE, Blakemore C (1970): Binocular depth perception and the corpus callosum. Vision Res 10:49–54.

Naporn A, Berman N, Payne BR (1984a): Morphology of callosal cells in areas 17 and 18 of cat visual cortex. Invest Ophthalmol (Suppl) 25:211.

Naporn A, Berman N, Payne, BR (1984b): Morphology of callosal cells in area 19 and lateral suprasylvian visual areas in cat visual cortex. Neurosci Abstr 10:932.

Nelson JI, Frost B (1978): Orientation-selective inhibition from beyond the classic visual receptive field. Brain Res 139:359–365.

Payne BR, Berman N, Naporn A (1986): The structural and functional organization of the callosal projections in area 17 of cat cerebral cortex. (In preparation.)

Payne BR, Berman N, Murphy EH (1981): A quantitative assessment of eye alignment in cats after corpus callosum transection. Exp Brain Res 43:371–376.

Payne BR, Pearson HE, Berman N (1984a): Deafferentation and axotomy of neurons in cat striate cortex: Time course of changes following corpus callosum transection. Brain Res 307:201–215.

Payne BR, Pearson HE, Berman N (1984b): Role of the corpus callosum in the functional organization of cat striate cortex. J Neurophysiol 52:570–594.

Singer W, Tretter F, Cynader M (1975): Organization of cat striate cortex: A correlation of receptive field properties with afferent and efferent connections. J Neurophysiol 38:1080–1098.

Sperry RW (1966): Brain bisection and consciousness. In Eccles JC (ed): "Brain and Conscious Experience." New York: Springer-Verlag, pp 298–313.

Sperry RW (1970): Cerebral dominance in perception. In Young FA, Lindsley DB (eds): "Early Experience and Visual Information Processing in Perceptual and Reading Disorders." New York: New York Academy of Sciences.

Sperry RW (1974): Lateral specialization in the surgically separated hemispheres. In Schmitt FO, Worden FG (eds): "The Neurosciences, Third Study Program." Cambridge, Massachusetts: MIT Press, pp 5–20.

Sumner BEH (1975): A quantitative analysis of boutons with different types of synapses in normal and injured hypoglossal nuclei. Exp Neurol 49:406–417.

Sumner BEH, Sutherland FI (1973): Quantitative electron microscopy on the injured hypoglossal nucleus in the rat. J Neurocytol 2:315–328.

Sumner BEH, Watson WE (1971): Retraction and expansion of the dendritic trees of motorneurons of adults induced in vivo. Nature 233:273–275.

Toyama K, Matsunami K, Ohno T, Tokashiki S (1974): An intracellular study of neuronal organization in the visual cortex. Exp Brain Res 21:45–66.

Tusa RJ, Palmer LA, Rosenquist AC (1978): The retinotopic organization of area 17 (striate cortex) in the cat. J Comp Neurol 185:657–678.

Two Hemispheres—One Brain:
Functions of the Corpus Callosum, pages 255–266
© 1986 Alan R. Liss, Inc.

Effects of Sensory Experience on the Development of Visual Callosal Connections

DOUGLAS O. FROST AND GIORGIO M. INNOCENTI

Section of Neuroanatomy, Yale University School of Medicine, New Haven, Connecticut 06510 (D.O.F.); Institut d'Anatomie, Faculté de Médecine, Université de Lausanne, Lausanne, Switzerland (G.M.I.)

INTRODUCTION

In normal adult cats, the first and second visual areas (V_1 and V_2) in the two cerebral hemispheres are interconnected through the corpus callosum (CC) by neurons (callosal neurons) that have a characteristic bilaminar depth distribution and are restricted to the region of the boundary between cytoarchitectonic areas 17 (V_1) and 18 (V_2) [Innocenti and Fiore, 1976; Shatz, '77b; Sanides and Donate-Oliver, 1978; Innocenti, 1980]. In newborn kittens the callosal neurons have already acquired a bilaminar radial distribution, but they are distributed across the entire tangential extent of areas 17 and 18 (and other visual cortical areas); the adult distribution is acquired gradually over the first three postnatal months by the elimination of the callosal projections from most of area 17 and part of area 18 [Innocenti et al., 1977; Innocenti and Caminiti, 1980]. In this process, some area 17 and 18 neurons eliminate their callosal axon and presumably make connections in the hemisphere in which they are located [Innocenti, 1981a; Koppel and Innocenti, 1983]. A similar reshaping of an "exuberant" juvenile distribution of callosal neurons occurs in the auditory cortex of cats [Feng and Brugge, 1983] and in the somatosensory areas of cats [Innocenti and Caminiti, 1980] and rats [Ivy and Killacky, 1981; O'Leary et al., 1981]. In recent years it has become clear that the overproduction and elimination of neural connections is a pervasive phenomenon in the development of the central and peripheral nervous systems [reviewed in Innocenti, 1981b]. There are even examples of transient juvenile projections between functional systems that are not connected in mature brains [Stanfield et al., 1982; Frost, 1984; Innocenti and Clarke, 1984; Innocenti, this volume].

Here we review a series of experiments designed to investigate the role of early postnatal visual experience in the development of visual callosal connections. Our three principal questions were the following: (i) Is normal visual experience necessary for the normal maturation of callosal connections? (ii) How is the developmental process influenced by particular aspects of abnormal visual experience? (iii) How are the effects of vision dependent upon the developmental stage at which it is experienced?

In all of our cats, we filled areas 17 and 18 with horseradish peroxidase (HRP) by making multiple, 0.5 µl injections of 30–40% HRP into the lateral and posterolateral gyri. The injections also spread into other visual areas. After a 2-day survival time, the cats were perfused and serial sections of their brains were processed using standard procedures for HRP histochemistry [see Innocenti and Frost, 1979, 1980; Innocenti et al., 1984 for details]. The distributions of retrogradely labeled callosal neurons were charted for individual sections using a computer microscope [Glaser and Van der Loos, 1965]. Serial section reconstructions of the distributions of callosal neurons in areas 17 and 18 as well as statistical analyses of the numbers of callosal neurons in different groups of cats were also made using a computer.

In all of these experiments, we focused our attention on area 17. The distribution of callosal neurons in normal cats is subject to individual variability. In area 17 this variability is limited, thus facilitating the comparison of normal and experimentally reared cats. There is a greater variability in the distribution of callosal neurons in other areas; this is presumably related to greater variation in the visual field representation and/or larger single-unit receptive fields in those areas [Innocenti, 1980; Berlucchi, 1981]. The effects of the various experimental rearing paradigms are less clear for subzone c than for subzone a and are not presented here.

VISUAL CALLOSAL CONNECTIONS IN NORMAL CATS

In normal adult cats, the cortical volume containing callosal neurons (callosal efferent zone, CZ) consists of two radially separated laminae, located in layers III/IV and VI (subzones a and c, respectively; see Fig. 1A). Subzone a is wider and richer in callosal neurons. Most neurons in subzone a lie in the lateral part of area 17, and in medial area 18, although particularly rostrally, scattered callosal neurons are sometimes found as far medially in area 17 as the suprasplenial sulcus (Figs. 1A, 2A). The lateral boundary of subzone a, which lies in area 18, is irregular and susceptible to individual variation. Callosal neurons are generally found along the medial banks and sometimes down to the fundi, of the lateral and postlateral sulci (Figs. 1A, 2A).

At the ages at which experimental rearing was started, callosal neurons are found throughout areas 17 and 18 and are more densely packed than in adults [Innocenti and Caminiti, 1980]. The tangential distribution of callosal neurons appears to be mature by 3 months postnatally. The radial distribution of callosal neurons in newborn kittens is bilaminar, as in adults [Innocenti and Caminiti, 1980]. The tangential distribution of callosal neurons appears to be mature by 3 months postnatally. The radial distribution

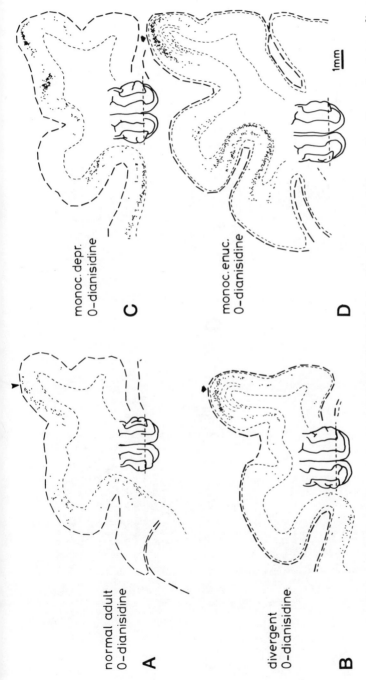

normal adult
0-dianisidine

A

monoc. depr.
0-dianisidine

C

divergent
0-dianisidine

B

monoc. enuc.
0-dianisidine

D

1mm

Fig. 1. Computer-microscope charts of the distribution of HRP-labeled callosal neurons in coronal sections at corresponding rostrocaudal levels of the postlateral gyri of (A) a normal adult cat (B) a 288-day-old cat reared from eye opening (day 9) with divergent strabismus, (C) a 146-day-old cat reared from eye opening (day 8) with monocular eyelid suture, and (D) a 124-day-old cat subjected to monocular enucleation on postnatal day 1. The eyelid-sutured and enucleated cats were injected contralateral to the open or remaining eye, respectively. All sections were reacted with ortho-dianisidine. Each HRP-labeled neuron is represented by one dot. Thick broken lines represent the cortical surface, while thinner lines represent the lower boundaries of layers I and IV–VI; filled arrowheads point to the cytoarchitectonic boundary between areas 17 and 18.

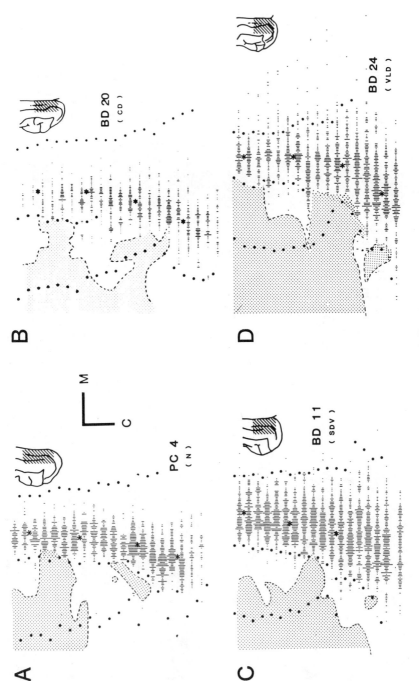

Fig. 2

of callosal neurons in newborn kittens is bilaminar, as in adults [Innocenti and Caminiti, 1980].

CALLOSAL CONNECTIONS IN CATS REARED WITH VISUAL DEPRIVATION BY EYELID SUTURE OR ENUCLEATION

In order to determine whether visual experience is necessary for the normal maturation of the CZ, we deprived kittens of pattern vision by suturing both eyelids shut on postnatal days 6–7 (before the time of normal eye opening about day 8) or by bilateral enucleation on postnatal days 1–4. Both groups of cats were raised to at least 3 months of age.

In cats reared with binocular deprivation by eyelid suture (BD cats), callosal neurons appear to have normal morphologies and are found within the normal radial boundaries of subzones a and c (Fig. 3). However, there are only about half as many callosal neurons in subzone a of BD cats as there are in normal cats [Innocenti et al., 1984]. The bulk of these neurons is concentrated in a restricted zone straddling the area 17-18 border, between the crown of the gyri and the fundi of the lateral and postlateral sulci (Figs. 2B, 3). In some BD cats the CZ appears somewhat narrower than in normal cats.

In cats subjected to neonatal binocular enucleation (BEE cats) the radial distribution and morphology of callosal neurons appear normal. In areas 17 and 18 callosal neurons are more numerous than in BD cats but less numerous than in normal cats [Innocenti and Frost, 1980]. The majority of callosal neurons is found, as in normal cats, between the fundus of the

---

Fig. 2. Computer reconstructions of subzone a in (A) a normal adult cat (PC 4; N), (B) a cat that was deprived by binocular eyelid suture until sacrifice at 175 days (BD 20; CD), (C) a cat that was deprived of vision by bilateral eyelid suture until day 37 (BD 11; SDV) and then normally reared until day 147, and (D) a cat that had 10 days of normal vision, followed by 99 days of binocular deprivation by eyelid suture (BD 24; VLD). At the end of the rearing period BD 11 had developed a large degree of divergent strabismus. The reconstructions are flattened views of the lateral and postlateral gyri (hatched areas in corresponding insets of dorsal views of brains traced from photographs). Dotted lines represent from lateral to medial, the fundi of the lateral, postlateral, and suprasplenial sulci. The asterisks mark the boundary between areas 17 (medially) and 18 (laterally). The neurons in subzone a of each section were projected onto a line running parallel to the pial surface and 400 μm deep; the line was divided into bins of 100 μm, and the number of neurons in each bin was represented by a line segment whose length is proportional to the number of neurons in the bin (shortest segments = 1 neuron). Each row of line segments represents one section. Stippling indicates regions of areas 18 and 19 that are continuous with the reconstructed parts of the callosal zone, and within which there is a very high density of labeled callosal neurons. All sections were reacted with the tetramethylbenzidine technique. Scale lines represent 2 mm. M = medial; C = caudal.

PX 22 dab   BD 1 dab   BEE 13 dab

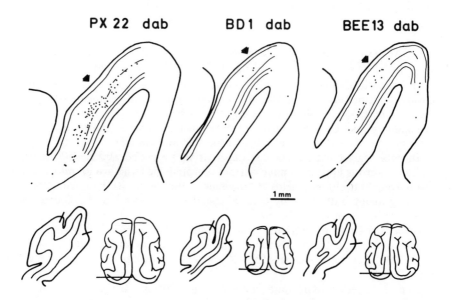

Fig. 3. Computer-microscope charts of the distribution of HRP-labeled callosal neurons in coronal sections at corresponding rostrocaudal levels of the postlateral gyri of a normal adult cat (PX 22), a cat (BD 1) raised with bilaterally sutured eyelids, and a cat (BEE 13) that had been bilaterally enucleated on postnatal day 2. All sections were reacted with the diaminobenzidine technique. Each HRP-labeled neuron is represented by one dot. The drawings at the top are enlargements of the region denoted in the corresponding low-power drawings. The rostrocadual levels are indicated on drawings made from dorsal-view photographs of the corresponding brains. In each section thinner lines mark the lower boundaries of layers I and III–V; a filled arrow points to the cytoarchitectonic boundary between areas 17 and 18.

postlateral (or entolateral) sulcus and the crowns of the lateral and postlateral gyri. However, additional callosal neurons in subzone a are frequently found in area 17 medial to the crowns of the lateral and postlateral gyri, extending as far as the fundus of the suprasplenial sulcus and occasionally farther (Fig. 3). In the rostral half of the CZ, neurons in the medial part of the area 17 become about as numerous as in the lateral part of the CZ. Thus, although BEE cats have less callosal neurons in subzone a than normal cats, the CZ extends further into the periphery of area 17 than in normal cats.

These results suggested the following conclusions:

1. Binocular visual deprivation by eyelid suture or enucleation accentuates the normally occurring loss of juvenile callosal axons. Therefore, normal vision has a stabilizing influence on juvenile callosal connections.

However, since some callosal axons are stabilized even in BD and BEE cats, other stabilizing influences, including nonvisual ones, must exist.

2. Binocular enucleation eliminates both normal visual experience and signals emanating from the retina independent of vision. Since in BEE cats, callosal neurons are both more numerous and more widespread than in BD cats, it appears that signals from the retina destabilize juvenile callosal connections, either directly or by inhibiting nonvisual influences that stabilize juvenile callosal connections [see Innocenti and Frost, 1980 for details]. The influence of the retina may be underestimated in our experiments owing to the formation of functional retinogeniculate projections several weeks before birth [Shatz 1983; Shatz and Kirkwood, 1984; Stretavan and Shatz, 1984].

3. It is clear that the postnatal development of callosal connections is under the control of multiple, interacting influences that differ in the magnitude or quality of their effects. In BEE cats, callosal neurons are abnormally widespread across the cortical surface despite the fact that they are less numerous than normal. This apparently paradoxical result could be explained if the multiple influences on callosal development are weighted in different ways in determining different characteristics of the callosal system.

CALLOSAL CONNECTIONS IN CATS REARED WITH MONOCULAR VISION OR SYMMETRIC STRABISMUS

We next consider whether the development of the corpus callosum responds specifically to particular aspects of visual experience.

In normal adult cats, the midline of the binocular visual field (vertical meridian) is projected onto the retinal line of decussation, and both are represented in area 17 at the area 17-18 border. In normal cats, callosal neurons become restricted to the region of the area 17-18 border. Since two of the putative functions of the corpus callosum are unification of the two visual hemifields and the synthesis of binocular disparity information for stereopsis in the region of the vertical meridan [Berlucchi, 1972, 1981; Doty and Negrao, 1973, Blakemore et al., 1983], we asked whether the callosal zone would remain in the region of the area 17-18 border when the representation of the vertical meridan is shifted into the periphery of area 17 by symmetric convergent or divergent strabismus.

We found that in adult cats raised with symmetric strabismus produced by bilateral section of the medial or lateral recti muscles on postnatal days 6–9, callosal neurons remain concentrated in the region of the area 17-18 border, although subzone a extends further medially in area 17 than in normal cats (compare Figs. 1A and 1B) [see also Innocenti and Frost, 1979]. Callosal neurons reach the fundus of the suprasplenial sulcus along almost all of its rostrocaudal extent, and some callosal neurons are found between the fundi of the suprasplenial and splenial sulci. Thus, convergent or divergent strabismus during the period that exuberant callosal connections are normally eliminated leads to the stabilization of some callosal axons that would have been lost, although it does not produce a displacement of the CZ into the periphery of area 17 where the vertical meridian is represented.

We next asked whether the expansion of the CZ in strabismic cats was due to some direct effect of strabismus such as the projection of the vertical meridian onto the retinal periphery, and hence the periphery of area 17, or the generation of abnormal afferent signals from the extraocular muscles. Alternatively, this expansion might have been related to the loss of binocular convergence onto cortical neurons, which is another consequence of strabismus [Hubel and Wiesel, 1965].

To examine this issue, we raised cats that were monocularly enucleated at 1 day of age (MEE cats) or that had one eye sutured shut on days 6–8, just before normal eye opening (MD cats). Both groups of cats were raised to 3 or more months of age. Monocular eyelid suture [Wiesel and Hubel, 1965] and monocular enucleation both eliminate binocularity in cortical neurons, while the vertical meridian is still projected onto the retinal line of decussation and hence onto the area 17-18 border, as in normal cats.

In both MD and MEE cats, as in strabismic cats, callosal neurons are distributed much further into the periphery of area 17 than in normal cats (Fig. 1: compare C and D, respectively, to A) [see also Innocenti and Frost, 1979]. This result suggests that there is a relationship between the loss of binocularity by cortical neurons and the increase in the size of the CZ. Those types of visual experience that abolish cortical binocularity also appear to stabilize some juvenile callosal connections that would normally be eliminated.

The effects of strabismus, monocular enucleation, and monocular eyelid suture on the number of callosal neurons are currently under study. However, it is clear that none of these manipulations stabilizes all of the callosal connections present in newborn kittens. This finding further supports the inference made from observations in BD and BEE cats that factors independent of visual experience influence the stabilization or elimination of juvenile callosal axons.

TIME DEPENDENCE OF VISUAL INFLUENCES ON CALLOSAL DEVELOPMENT

In an additional series of experiments [Innocenti et al., 1984], we investigated the role of temporal factors in the influence of visual experience on callosal development.

We first determined that the effects of rearing from birth with binocular eyelid suture are fully and irreversibly expressed by 3 months of age: the number and distribution of callosal neurons do not change significantly in BD cats raised beyond 3 months of age; 2 months of normal visual experience following rearing to 3 months with binocular eyelid suture does not restore the normal number or distribution of callosal neurons.

We raised two cats for 1 month with binocular eyelid suture followed by 3½ months' exposure to a normal visual environment. These cats developed a divergent strabismus during the period when their eyes were open. They had significantly more callosal neurons than normal cats. They also resembled one BD cat sacrificed at 1 month of age, one normal 1-month-old cat, and all our adult cats raised from eye opening with strabismus, in that their CZs extended further into the periphery of area 17 than in normal cats (Fig. 2: compare C and A). These preliminary results suggest that the effects of binocular lid suture are not yet expressed at 1 month of age. They also suggest that the effects of strabismus, even from the time of eye opening, may not be expressed until after 1 month of age, and that the callosal axons from the periphery of area 17 that are stabilized by strabismus are those that would have been lost during the second and third postnatal months.

Finally, some kittens were allowed to open their eyes normally on day 8 and to have 10–21 days of normal vision before both eyes were sutured shut for 2½–8½ months. Surprisingly, these cats had slightly more callosal neurons than normal cats, although the difference was not statistically significant. In addition, as in MD cats, MEE cats, cats reared from eye opening with strabismus and cats reared with 1 month of binocular eyelid suture followed by vision, the CZ in these cats was wider than normal (Fig. 2: compare D and A). Thus, the loss of callosal connections induced by binocular eyelid suture during the second and third postnatal months can be prevented by brief periods of normal visual experience during the first postnatal month. The results obtained in kittens reared with vision followed by binocular eyelid suture also indicate that normal vision can have both stabilizing and destabilizing effects on juvenile callosal axons: visual experience during the first postnatal month has a quick and potentially long-lasting stabilizing influence on a fraction of the juvenile projections. However, this stabilization is apparently reversible over the following 1 or 2 months, since if visual experience continues normally, it will provoke the elimination of some of the previously stabilized connections, namely, those from the more peripheral parts of area 17.

DISCUSSION

The preceding results are consistent with the notion that multiple visual and nonvisual factors influence the development of the corpus callosum. Since changes in the number and distribution of callosal neurons are not always correlated, the multiple influences on callosal development are weighted in different ways in determining the various characteristics of the callosal system.

Normal visual experience is necessary to the normal maturation of the CZ: although some callosal connections are stabilized in BD and BEE cats, the normally occurring loss of callosal projections is exaggerated in these cats. Normal vision has both stabilizing and destabilizing effects on juvenile callosal connections according to the developmental stage at which it is experienced. Signals from the retina seem to have a destabilizing effect independent of vision.

The results of these experiments suggest how at least one particular aspect of visual experience affects the development of callosal connections. Rearing conditions known to disrupt the binocularity of cortical neurons all result in the stabilization of callosal projections from the periphery of area 17, which would normally have been eliminated.[1] Presumably, the loss of binocularity is due to a modification in the maturation of the geniculocortical pathway; thus the development of thalamocortical and callosal connections may be interrelated.

It is likely that the effects of visual experience and of the integrity of the retina on the development of other (intrinsic and extrinsic) cortical connections are similar to those on the corpus callosum. Callosal connections probably reproduce for limited portions of the representation of the sensory periphery, anatomical features, and functions otherwise typical of intracortical and/or ipsilateral association connections. Operations that in each hemisphere take place within and among cortical columns may take place between the two hemispheres via groups of neurons connected by the corpus callosum in such a way as to reconstitute columnar units and intercolumnar interactions [Hubel and Wiesel, 1967; Innocenti, 1980]. Thus, the disruptive consequence of abnormal rearing on callosal connections may be paradigmatic for similar effects of abnormal rearing on other cortical connections.

Our results also demonstrate that a normally transient, neocortical population of projection neurons can provide a substrate for altered neuronal connectivity in that some of these neurons can be stabilized as a consequence of abnormal sensory experience early in life ("efferent plasticity"— Innocenti [1979]). Thus, it seems likely that the abnormal callosal projections of Siamese cats [Shatz, 1977a,b], which resemble those of our strabismic cats, are related to the squint-induced loss of binocularity in Siamese cats [Hubel and Wiesel, 1971] rather than to a direct action of the mutant gene on callosal connections. Normally transient projection neurons can also be stabilized following surgical manipulations of the structures in which they terminate [Hollyday and Hamburger, 1976; Caminiti and Innocenti, 1981].

Finally, we note that the modifiability of callosal and other cortical connections by neonatal sensory experience is probably extremely important during normal development. Since interocular distance and ocular alignment change in early postnatal life [Olson and Freeman, 1978] devel-

---

[1]Cats given 10–21 days of normal visual experience followed by 2½–8½ months of binocular eyelid suture have a similarly expanded CZ. The status of cortical binocularity is not known for these cats.

opmental mechanisms must be sensitive to changing visual input in order to assure that the final pattern of cortical connectivity will be appropriately matched to the definitive position and alignment of the eyes. It is attractive to view the modifications we observed in MEE, MD, and strabismic cats as partial compensation for the disturbance of the binocular visual field, although the adaptiveness of the changes remains to be demonstrated.

REFERENCES

Berlucchi G (1972): Anatomical and physiological aspects of visual functions of corpus callosum. Brain Res 37:371–392.

Berlucchi G (1981): Recent advances in the analysis of the neural substrates of interhemispheric communication. In Pompeiano O, Ajmone-Marsan C (eds): "Brain Mechanisms and Perceptual Awareness." New York: pp 133–152.

Blakemore C, Diao Y, Pu M, Wang Y, Kiao Y (1983): Possible functions of the interhemispheric connections between visual cortical areas in the cat. J Physiol 337:331–349.

Caminiti R, Innocenti GM (1981): The postnatal development of somatosensory callosal connections after partial lesions of somatosensory areas. Exp Brain Res 42:53–62.

Doty RW, and Negrao N (1973): Forebrain commissures and vision. In Jung R (ed): "Handbook of Sensory Physiology." Berlin: Springer, Vol VII/3, Part B, pp 543–582.

Feng JZ, Brugge JF (1983): Postnatal development of auditory callosal connections in the kitten. J Comp Neurol 214:416–426.

Frost DO (1984): Axonal growth and target selection during development: retinal projections to the ventrobasal nucleus and other "nonvisual" structures in neonatal syrian hamsters. J Comp Neurol 230:576–592.

Glaser EM, Van der Loos H (1965): A semi-automatic computer microscope for the analysis of neuronal morphology. IEEE Trans Bio-Med Eng 12:22–31.

Hollyday M, Hamburger V (1976): Reduction of the naturally occurring motor neuron loss by enlargement of the periphery. J Comp Neurol 170:311–320.

Hubel DH, Wiesel TN (1965): Binocular interaction in striate cortex of kittens reared with artificial squint. J Neurophysiol 28:1041–1059.

Hubel DH, Wiesel TN (1967): Cortical and callosal connections concerned with the vertical meridian of visual fields in the cat. J Neurophysiol 30:1561–1573.

Hubel DH, Wiesel TN (1971): Aberrant visual projections in the siamese cat. J Physiol 218:33–62.

Innocenti GM (1980): The primary visual pathway through the corpus callosum: Morphological and functional aspects in the cat. Arch Ital Biol 118:124–188.

Innocenti GM (1981a): Growth and reshaping of axons in the establishment of visual callosal connections. Science 212:824–827.

Innocenti GM (1981b): Transitory structures as substrates for developmental plasticity of the brain. In Van Hof MW, Mohn G (eds): "Functional Recovery from Brain Damage." Dev Neurosci 13:305–333.

Innocenti GM, Caminiti R (1980): Postnatal shaping of callosal connections from sensory areas. Exp Brain Res 38:381–394.

Innocenti GM, Clarke S (1984): Bilateral transitory projection to visual areas from auditory cortex in kittens. Dev Brain Res 41:27–32.

Innocenti GM, Fiore L (1976): Morphological correlates of visual field transformation in the corpus callosum. Neurosci Lett 2:245–252.

Innocenti GM, Fiore L, Caminiti R (1977): Exuberant projection into the corpus callosum from the visual cortex of newborn cats. Neurosci Lett 4:237–242.

Innocenti GM, Frost DO (1979): Effects of visual experience on the maturation of the efferent system to the corpus callosum. Nature 28:231–234.

Innocenti GM, Frost DO (1980): The postnatal development of visual callosal connections in the absence of visual experience or of the eyes. Exp Brain Res 39:365–375.

Innocenti GM, Frost DO, Illes J (1985): Maturation of visual callosal connections in visually deprived kittens: A challenging critical period. J Neurosci 5:255–267.

Ivy GO, Killackey HP (1981): The ontogeny of the distribution of callosal projection neurons in the rat parietal cortex. J Comp Neurol 195:367–389.

Koppel H, Innocenti GM (1983): Is there a genuine exuberancy of callosal projections in development? A quantitative electron microscopic study in the cat. Neurosci Lett 41:33–40.

O'Leary DDM, Stanfield BB, Cowan WM (1981): Evidence that the early postnatal restriction of the cells of origin of the callosal projections is due to the elimination of axonal collaterals rather than to the death of neurons. Dev Brain Res 1:607–617.

Olson GR, Freeman RD (1978): Eye alignment in kittens. J Neurophysiol 41:848–859.

Sanides D, Donate-Oliver F (1978): Identification and localization of some relay cells in the cat visual cortex. In Brazier MAB, Petsche H (eds): "Architectonics of the Cerebral Cortex." New York: Raven Press, pp 227–234.

Shatz C (1977a): Abnormal interhemispheric connections in the visual system of Boston Siamese cats: A physiologic study. J Comp Neurol 171:229–246.

Shatz CJ (1977b): Anatomy of interhemispheric connections in the visual system of Boston Siamese and ordinary cats. J Comp Neurol 173:497–518.

Shatz CJ (1983): The prenatal development of the cat's retinogeniculate pathway. J Neurosci 3:482–499.

Shatz CJ, Kirkwood PA (1984): Prenatal development of functional connections in the cat's retinogeniculate pathway. J Neurosci 4:1378–1397.

Sretavan D, Shatz CJ (1984): Prenatal development of individual retinogeniculate axons during the period of gestation. Nature 308:845–848.

Stanfield BB, O'Leary DDM, Fricks C (1982): Selective collateral elimination in early postnatal development restricts cortical distribution of rat pyramidal tract neurones. Nature 298:371–373.

Wiesel TN, Hubel DH (1965): Comparison of the effects of unilateral and bilateral eye closure on cortical unit responses in kittens. J Neurophysiol 28:1029–1040.

SECTION IV
ANIMAL BEHAVIOR

Two Hemispheres—One Brain:
Functions of the Corpus Callosum, pages 269–279
© 1986 Alan R. Liss, Inc.

Interhemispheric Mnemonic Transfer in Macaques

ROBERT W. DOTY, JAMES L. RINGO, AND JEFFREY D. LEWINE

Center for Brain Research, University of Rochester, Rochester, New York 14642

INTRODUCTION

The real challenge is not "two hemispheres, one brain," but rather "two brains, one mind." Most human beings, at least, will testify to a unity of conscious experience. However, the ingenious analysis of Sperry and his colleagues shows that when the surgeon's knife healingly severs the forebrain commissures, the price of the therapy is a peculiarly divided consciousness. The right brain no longer knows what transpires in the left, yet each can be induced to report its own experiences and memories, and each displays appreciations that are unequivocally human [e.g., Sperry et al., 1979]. Thus, it must be presumed that in normal life it is the forebrain commissures that somehow imperceptibly knit the neural events of each hemisphere into an experiential unity. While this may be no more miraculous than the unity prevailing between events in frontal versus occipital areas of the same hemisphere, or for that matter the effortless creation of a spatially and temporally continuous visual world from the manifold digital events transmitted from the retina, the fascination of the unity forged from interhemispheric transactions is the paradox that the initial, and essential, neural pathway can now be precisely specified, but the fundamental character of the interchange required for conscious unity cannot even be guessed at.

Of course, arguments are sometimes advanced that only the left, speaking hemisphere is the seat of truly human consciousness and, if so, then no hemispheric "interchange" is required for "unification." However, this position has the obvious flaw of denying humanity to those individuals in whom the left hemisphere has been removed surgically. One of the most fascinating and best studied of such cases is that reported by Schepelmann et al. [1976]. Although this patient had evidence of a left hemisphere lesion (massive angioma) present by at least the age of 5, left hemispherectomy was not performed until he was 35 years old. Preoperative assessment showed a subnormal intellectual level and problems with language (sensory aphasia, dyslexia, trouble finding the proper word). Since these problems were essentially the same postoperatively, it must be presumed that the left, pathological hemisphere was nonfunctional, probably for most of the patient's life. Yet this does not indicate that the right hemisphere had, therefore, become the "dominant" hemisphere in the sense in which that term is usually employed for the "speaking hemisphere," since the linguistic deficiency displayed by the right hemisphere postoperatively is congruent with that for individuals who possessed a truly "dominant, speaking" left hemisphere prior to its surgical removal [e.g., Smith, 1966; Gott, 1973].

The patient of Schepelmann et al., most clearly reveals the usual and well-known deficiency of the right hemisphere for the production of speech. The patient had an IQ of roughly 80; could, unassisted, use railway or air transportation from home to hospital for follow-up visits; appreciated jokes or a play on words; understood speech very well even when conversation was passing among as many as five people. His own speech production, however, was painfully limited: 78% of his "utterances" were limited to 1–5 words (up to 10 words making up 94%), and a vocabulary of 20 words constituted 82% of his usage in a total spoken vocabulary of about 150 words. Almost none of these spoken words were nouns or verbs, and except for the second person plural (in German) all uses of verbs were in the present tense. In other words, there was a clear dichotomy between general intellectual level and the ability to formulate thoughts into speech (or writing). A particularly dramatic example of this is given by Gott [1973], in which her subject, with only the right hemisphere remaining, could count objects correctly if done seriatim, and could then write the correct number; but could not correctly read the number she had written, although she could indicate it by counting on her fingers! Further exploration of limitations in the right hemisphere's ability to translate between visual and auditory linguistic spheres can be found in the work of Zaidel and Peters [1981] and Zaidel [this volume].

Again, it might be argued that, although the right hemisphere is capable of an independent if somewhat different mental life, in the intact individual it is so submerged by the "dominance" of the left that its contribution to conscious experience is essentially nil. If so, then there is no role for the forebrain commissures in producing anything but a unified sensorium, e.g., the "seamless" visual field. The inaccuracy of such a concept, however, is indicated by the "expert testimony" of the noted neuroanatomist, Alf Brodal [1973], reporting the consequences of his own loss of a rather limited portion of his right hemisphere. There were subtle, but profound, disturbances even of his linguistic abilities, the whole man clearly having been diminished by this localized, unilateral loss. While Brodal tends to explain the deficiencies in terms of corticopontine and corticospinal pathways, i.e., as loss of motor control, it seems to us that a more likely explanation is von Monakow's "diaschisis," the massive loss of commissural input to the left hemisphere pursuant to the lesion on the right. Even with Tomasch's figure [1954] of

200,000,000 fibers for the human corpus callosum with light microscopy, and taking account of the uneven distribution of callosal fibers, the input to certain cortical areas might be reduced by the order of 10% following such a lesion; and there is reason to believe that the true figure may perhaps be larger by a factor of four, as per the findings of Koppel and Innocenti [1983], were callosal fiber counts made with the electron microscope.

From such considerations it is thus evident that the "nondominant" hemisphere alone can sustain a human mentality, and that disruption of activity in this "nondominant" hemisphere alters mental life despite presence of the "dominant" hemisphere. It is, therefore, logical to conclude that the forebrain commissures, known to be necessary for interhemispheric communication, are indeed continuously active in achieving normal mental unity from the potentially separable mental products of the two hemispheres. The experiments to be summarized here test, for the first time in animals, the operation of these commissures in achieving the interhemispheric communication necessary for such unification. Extensive previous work [see Doty and Negrão, 1973; Butler, 1979, for reviews] has demonstrated that at least one of the forebrain commissures must be intact for the interhemispheric transfer of discrimination habits, i.e., the learning of "rules"; but the interhemispheric communication of visual memories, i.e., memory for "events" [Squire, 1982], has received only passing attention [Hamilton et al., 1968]. It is shown herein that either the anterior commissure (AC) or the splenium of the corpus callosum (CC) are capable of highly efficient interhemispheric transfer of pictorial memory, an achievement that a priori would seem essential to formation of a unified experience from two hemispheres.

METHODS

The experiments have been performed on juvenile, male *Macaca nemestrina*. The novel features of the procedure are, first, that the optic chiasm is transected via the transphenoidal approach, following Downer [1959], and, second, that the animal is required to perform a delayed-matching-to-sample (DMS) task, using trial-unique photographic slides [Overman and Doty, 1979], with one eye and hemisphere viewing the "sample" and the other responding for the "match." Thus, without the chiasm, what the animal views with, say, the left eye goes directly only to the left hemisphere; the question is then, can the right eye and hemisphere subsequently recognize what the left has seen; and, if so, what commissure(s) are necessary to achieve this mnemonic comparison, and what are the parameters of the phenomenon. In addition to allowing such a test for interhemispheric transfer, the paradigm also readily permits testing whether one hemisphere is equivalent to the other, and for different types of visual material, when the mnemonic comparison is made intrahemispherically, i.e., when the same eye is used for both the "sample" and the "match"; or whether one hemisphere may be more proficient than the other in the roles of "sending" versus "receiving" the information, i.e., whether the mnemonic transfer goes better in one direction, e.g., right to left, than in the other.

The animal is drawn daily into a chair [Glassman et al., 1969] and placed before three vertically stacked panels on which the images are rear-projected. The vertical orientation of these panels makes allowance for the restricted visual field following transection of the optic chiasm. The monkey is provided with a mask bearing solenoid-operated shutters so that vision can be restricted to either selected eye. The "sample" image is projected onto the middle panel, and the monkey responds by pressing it, for which it receives a small quantity of fruit juice or water (depending upon its preference). The image on the panel is then extinguished and a delay of 0–15 seconds ensues. Two images are then projected upon the upper and lower panels, one of which is identical with the "sample." If the monkey presses this panel, which matches the sample, it receives a substantial allotment of fluid, whereas if the other image is selected, it receives a puff of air to the face, and the start of the next trial is delayed. Fifty or more "sample" images are utilized for each daily run, and each image is unique for the session.

A second, potentially more difficult procedure is used to achieve longer time delays between presentation of the "sample" and the test for its recognition. This is the running "list" procedure developed by Gaffan [e.g., 1977]. In this situation there are only two panels in the vertical stack. Images are presented seriatim on the upper panel at 10-second intervals. If it is the first time that the image has been viewed in that session, the monkey presses the panel on which it appears and receives a small quantity of fluid. However, if the image has appeared previously in that session, the monkey must indicate its recognition by pressing the lower, blank panel, for which it receives a much larger reward. Striking the upper panel in such a circumstance merely results in the air puff and a loud auditory signal. Of course, in this situation the animal makes a certain number of "false-positive" responses, i.e., it strikes the lower panel on the first presentation of the image, so that this rate of irrelevant responding must be deducted from its correct identifications to obtain the true level of recognition achieved. Again, the arrangement is such that the eye viewing either the initial or repeated presentation is controlled via shutters. The animals view 100–280 images per session; and the inventory of photographic slides is sufficiently large that about 2 weeks elapses before reuse of a particular image is required.

RESULTS
Delayed Matching to Sample

Perhaps the most important, certainly the most fundamental, result is that following transection of the optic chiasm interocular comparisons in the DMS task are equally as good as comparisons made with the same eye (and hemisphere). In other words, the forebrain commissures are as efficient in the interhemispheric transfer of visual information as are the decussating fibers of the optic nerves. If both the AC and CC are completely transected in addition to the chiasm, then such interocular comparisons are no better than chance.

The next question to be examined was whether the AC might differ from the CC in either the efficiency of such mnemonic evaluations, or in the type of visual material that could be compared. Two animals were thus prepared, both with optic chiasm transected. In one the AC and all of the CC except the posterior 5 mm of the splenium was also cut; and in the other all of the CC was cut but the AC was left intact. Both animals were able to recognize with one eye and hemisphere a wide variety of images perceived 2–10 seconds earlier by the other eye and hemisphere [Doty et al., 1982, 1985; Doty, 1985]. The accuracy of performance depended upon the nature of the material presented, but in any event the level of interhemispheric matching was in each case equivalent to that achieved intrahemispherically. For images of complex, colored objects, accuracy with a 10-second delay in a well-trained animal was often perfect for a run of 50 trials (e.g., 8 errors in 1,500 trials!).

With some rather minor exceptions, it made no difference which hemisphere viewed the image first; nor for intrahemispheric comparisons was one hemisphere any different from the other regardless of which hand was in use. The types of material included complex objects in full color (e.g., fruits, flowers, tools, electronic components, packages, toys); the same objects presented as projected colorless photographs; pure, diffuse color; human faces; alphanumeric symbols; and matching of the *number* of identical objects. The latter was a particularly difficult task, especially since the animals had long experience with choosing on the basis of difference in objects. Another task proved even more difficult, choosing between Japanese kanji (up to six strokes), which were employed in the hope that they would serve as definable geometric patterns. Even after training for more than 2,000 trials, some of the monkeys still lingered at chance levels of performance for intrahemispheric comparison or with both eyes open, whereas human observers, literate in Western languages but unschooled in Chinese or Japanese, could make the proper selections at a 10-second delay with 100% accuracy and without difficulty.

The only difference of possible significance noted between transections of the AC versus CC was on another animal (with only partial section of the chiasm) 60 days after the transection of the CC. When called upon for the first time to make an interhemispheric mnemonic comparison in this condition, it displayed a noticeable uncertainty and hesitation, although it achieved a level of 97% correct for the 37 choices it did make from the 50 presentations. In subsequent sessions no such hesitancy appeared; and the animal with only the splenium displayed not the slightest hesitation in its comparable first session. The animal with only the AC remaining (and chiasm totally transected) was examined only 31 days after complete division of the CC. While it displayed no evident hesitation when first called upon to make interhemispherically guided choices, its accuracy here was, at first, markedly poorer than when performing with intrahemispheric comparisons. Over the ensuing weeks, the interhemispheric performance gradually improved, until it was indistinguishable from that intrahemispherically.

Several months of observations on these animals, plus another with only the optic chiasm transected, demonstrated a remarkable similarity in the performance of the two hemispheres in a given animal. Using several hundred different images of different types over a period of months, each hemisphere was tested several times intrahemispherically with each of the items. This yielded a highly significant correlation between the errors made by each hemisphere, and this in turn was indistinguishable from the correlation between repeat errors made by each hemisphere itself. Since there was much less correlation between the errors made by the three animals, the high level of correlation between hemispheres in the same animal must arise more from some underlying individual strategy, rather than simply being inherent in the material. To date an adequate examination of this phenomenon has not been made on the same animal before and after full transection of the forebrain commissures.

The List Paradigm

With the list procedure there was also no evidence of a difference in the capability of the AC versus the splenium. There is, however, a surprising difference in the accuracy of interhemispheric transfer in this task compared to the DMS procedure.

If there are many items intervening between initial presentation and ultimate test of recognition, the running list procedure becomes much more difficult than the DMS. Unlike the latter, where no further memory is required once the "match" has been made, in the list situation, with increasing numbers of presentations intervening before the test of recognition ensues, a substantial inventory of previously seen images must be stored and available upon demand at any time within the series. Furthermore, when the image is presented for the second time, it appears alone, whereas with the DMS situation a second cue is available, the "non-match" image. Despite this difficulty of the running list, after considerable training a macaque is able to perform this mnemonic task with consistent proficiency; our best animal to date being able to maintain performance above chance levels for inter- or intrahemispheric comparisons after 12 minutes in which 46 intervening images were seen.

Yet, unlike the DMS procedure, the performance here for intrahemispheric recognition is always better than when an interhemispheric operation is required. Under the conditions where the intrahemispheric recognition is 95% accurate, the comparable interhemispheric level is about 70% [Lewine and Doty, 1983]. It was reasoned that some of this difference might lie in the fact that each eye gets a slightly different view of the image [e.g., Hamilton and Tieman, 1973]. Thus, an optical arrangement was introduced that doubled each image so that each eye might then have essentially the same view of it. For some 200 trials this effected a complete elimination of the difference between inter- versus intrahemispheric performance by one monkey; but ultimately with this and other monkeys the intrahemispheric accuracy remains significantly better than interhemispherical accuracy despite this use of doubled images. Since with the DMS procedure, the inter- versus intrahemispheric performance is the same, we are inclined to conclude that the interhemispheric mnemonic processing in the list situation is complicated by some factor of interference, perhaps conflicting appraisals by the two hemispheres (see Discussion).

In one macaque, with at least 92% of the optic chiasm transected, after some 20,000 trials with the list procedure, the posterior 10 mm of the CC was also divided, thus leaving the AC, the genu, and part of the body of the CC for effective interhemispheric communication in the test situation. This loss of the splenium at first reduced interhemispheric performance to chance levels, while reducing intrahemispheric performance by only 8%. Over the next several months of training, however, the interhemispheric performance improved to the point where accuracy was only about 10% less than it had been before the splenial transection. The remainder of the CC was then transected, and interhemispheric performance again fell to chance; but with intensive training it has come to a point where statistically significant identification can be made at slightly above chance levels interhemispherically at intervals of 6–50 seconds with 0–4 intervening items.

DISCUSSION

These experiments demonstrate unequivocally in macaques that the immediate past experience of one hemisphere is readily available to the other, so long as one of the forebrain commissures is intact. There is certainly no a priori reason to believe that the same is not true in man, and that the forebrain commissures thus unify one's perception of the past, despite differing hemispheric aptitudes.

There are still a number of puzzles, however. Perhaps most obvious is the difference between man and macaque in the efficiency with which the AC seems to transfer visual information. Although there may still be some uncertainty as to whether the AC is entirely comparable to the CC in this regard in macaques [see Butler, 1979], no sustained difference could be found in the present exploration. It might be argued that the AC is much smaller than the splenium and therefore that the latter should be able to convey a greater amount of information; but this neglects the probability that a great variety of signals irrelevant to the present task may traverse the splenium, so that in actuality the relevant interhemispheric transfer could easily be equivalent in the two structures despite a large difference in total number of fibers.

This line of reasoning is to some degree less convincing for the human case, since the difference in size of splenium versus the AC is perhaps an order of magnitude greater than in macaques. Nevertheless, in some human individuals the AC is apparently able to effect transfer of mnemonic visual information with a reliability entirely equal to that reported above for macaques [Risse et al., 1978]; but in most individuals examined this ability has been rudimentary or absent [McKeever et al., 1981; Sidtis et al., 1981; Gazzaniga, 1983; Holtzman, 1984]. Holtzman [1984] remarks that one patient with the CC cut and the AC remaining could describe (with his left hemisphere) the visual perception of his left visual field only as a "shadowy blob," and could not tell whether two pictures presented simultaneously to right and left visual fields were the same or different. Of course, there are two very significant differences in most of these human studies compared with our procedures with macaques: (a) all material is presented tachistoscopically (and we have not tried this with our animals), and (b) in most instances the left hemisphere is called upon to verbalize information presented to the right hemisphere. The right hemisphere is unlikely to be adept at generating such verbal translation, and it may also be that the AC lacks adequate interconnection with linguistic areas.

Two other factors may be mentioned in this connection. First, is the large degree of variation in size of the human AC, a feature readily discerned by casual observation, and quantified by Tomasch [1957], who found a wide range in number of fibers (2.5–4 million). Second, is our incidental recognition that some period of learning may be required by the monkeys when first called upon to use their AC to make interhemispheric mnemonic comparisons. While not a strong effect, it nevertheless suggests that the restriction of normal pathways makes some noticeable initial difference in the animal's response to a familiar task, and it is possible that in man the great difference in the characteristics of operation of the two hemispheres and differences in mental "set" magnify the situation seen in macaques to the point where some special "trick" or training might be required to achieve efficient use of the AC.

The striking correlation in our experiments between errors committed by each hemisphere upon intrahemispheric testing is not entirely unexpected. Sperry et al. [1956] found that each hemisphere in cats with the chiasm and CC transected, but the AC intact, displayed remarkably similar characteristics in the progresssive learning of a visual discrimination. It seems likely that in both cat and macaque these hemispheric similarities arise from the inherent genetic and experiential backgrounds of the hemispheres rather than from a unifying effect of the remaining commissure; but this important point is yet to be proven. Were the correlation between the hemispheres actually attributable to the commissures, however, it would make even more puzzling the ability to detect hemispheric specialization in human subjects by lateralizing the input.

The fact that DMS performance is the same for the intra- versus interhemispheric mode, while with the list paradigm intrahemispheric recognition is consistently better than interhemispheric recognition, may reflect subtle changes in behavioral strategy demanded by the two tasks. In the DMS situation the hemisphere called upon to respond has, in essence, two unequivocal cues in its field of view: the image that the other hemisphere perceived, and the image that it did not. In the list situation, on the other hand, the responding hemisphere has before it an image that it has not previously seen, i.e., a veridical image, and must contrast this with the memory, presented at least initially by the other hemisphere. It must then extract from that paler mnemonic store whether or not the veridical image is part of that store. In other words, it must contrast a present image, which it definitely has not seen, with a nonpresent image provided via the other hemisphere. There is thus some opportunity for conflict in the appraisals of the two hemispheres, and it seems possible that this could well account for the much poorer inter- as compared with intrahemispheric performance in the list procedure, where the two are essentially identical in the DMS task.

SUMMARY

In macaques with transbuccal division of the optic chiasm the ability of each of the forebrain commissures, the corpus callosum and the anterior commissure, independently to support interhemispheric mnemonic comparisons of visual images was assayed in different animals. Two behavioral tasks were used: delayed-match-to-sample (DMS), in which on each trial a choice is made between two images, one of which has been seen via the other hemisphere; and a list procedure, in which a running series of images is presented and the task is to recognize previously viewed images regardless of the hemisphere used for initial viewing. In both instances, in contrast to certain human data, the AC was found to be equally as proficient as the CC and, depending upon the complexity of the material or the task, very high levels of accuracy were achieved. With the DMS task interhemispheric performance was equal to that intrahemispherically (initial viewing and subsequent choice made by the same hemisphere), whereas in the list situation interhemispheric performance was distinctly less accurate than with the intrahemispheric condition. It is reasoned that this result is peculiar to the list procedure, since here with a repeated image the two hemispheres have conflicting appraisals as to whether the image has or has not been seen before. In any event, the experiments in sum firmly support the view that the forebrain commissures provide a continuously available mechanism for unifying the past experiences of the two hemispheres.

ACKNOWLEDGMENTS
This work was supported by grant BNS-8208583 from the National Science Foundation.

REFERENCES

Brodal A (1973): Self-observations and neuro-anatomical considerations after a stroke. Brain 96:675–694.

Butler SR (1979): Interhemispheric transfer of visual information via the corpus callosum and anterior commissure in the monkey. In Steele Russell I, van Hof MW, Berlucchi G (eds): "Structure and Function of Cerebral Commissures." London: Macmillan, pp 343–357.

Doty RW (1984): Some thoughts, and some experiments, on memory. In Butters N, Squire L (eds): "The Neuropsychology of Memory." New York: Guilford Press, pp 330–339.

Doty RW, Gallant JA, Lewine JD (1982): Interhemispheric mnemonic transfer in *Macaca nemestrina*. Abstr Soc Neurosci 8:628.

Doty RW, Lewine JD, Ringo JL (1985): Mnemonic interaction between and within cerebral hemispheres in macaques. In Alkon DL, Woody CD (eds): "Neural Mechanisms of Conditioning." New York: Plenum (in press).

Doty RW, Negrão N (1973): Forebrain commissures and vision. In Jung R (ed): "Handbook of Sensory Physiology. Vol VII/3B: Central Processing of Visual Information, Part B." Berlin: Springer Verlag, pp 543–582.

Downer JL de C (1959): Changes in visually guided behaviour following midsagittal division of optic chiasm and corpus callosum in monkey (*Macaca mulatta*). Brain 82:251–259.

Gaffan D (1977): Monkeys' recognition memory for complex pictures and the effect of fornix transection. Q J Exp Psychol 29:505–514.

Gazzaniga MS (1983): Right hemisphere language following brain bisection, a 20-year perspective. Am Psychol 38:525–537.

Glassman RB, Negrão N, Doty RW (1969): A safe and reliable method for temporary restraint of monkeys. Physiol Behav 4:431–434.

Gott PS (1973): Language after dominant hemispherectomy. J Neurol Neurosurg Psychiatry 36:1082–1088.

Hamilton CR, Hillyard SA, Sperry RW (1968): Interhemispheric comparison of color in split-brain monkeys. Exp Neurol 21:486–494.

Hamilton CR, Tieman SB (1973): Interocular transfer of mirror image discrimination by chiasm-sectioned monkeys. Brain Res 64:241–255.

Holtzman JD (1984): Interactions between cortical and subcortical visual areas: evidence from human commissurotomy patients. Vision Res 24:801–813.

Koppel H, Innocenti GM (1983): Is there a genuine exuberancy of callosal projections in development? A quantitative electron microscopic study in the cat. Neurosci Lett 41:33–40.

Lewine JD, Doty RW (1983): Transcallosal mnemonic processing is inferior to intrahemispheric processing in *Macaca nemestrina*. Abstracts Soc Neurosci 9:651.

McKeever WF, Sullivan KF, Ferguson SM, Rayport M (1981): Typical cerebral hemisphere disconnection deficits following corpus callosum section despite sparing of anterior commissure. Neuropsychologia 19:745–755.

Overman WH Jr, Doty RW (1979): Disturbance of delayed match-to-sample in macaques by tetanization of anterior commissure versus limbic system or basal ganglia. Exp Brain Res 37:511–524.

Risse GL, LeDoux J, Springer SP, Wilson DH, Gazzaniga MS (1978): The anterior commissure in man: Functional variation in a multisensory system. Neuropsychologia 16:23–31.

Schepelmann F, Prüll G, Fellmann A, Becker W, Rössing H (1976): Klinisches Bild, Verhalten der motorischen Aktivität, elektroenzephalographische, neuropsychologische und linguistische Befunde bei einem Fall von linkseitiger Hemisphärektomie. Fortschr Neurol Psychiatr 44:381–432.

Sidtis JJ, Volpe BT, Wilson DH, Rayport M, Gazzaniga MS (1981): Variability in right hemisphere language function after callosal section: evidence for a continuum of generative capacity. J Neurosci 1:323–331.

Smith A (1966): Speech and other functions after left (dominant) hemispherectomy. J Neurol Neurosurg Psychiatry 29:467–471.

Sperry RW, Stamm JS, Miner N (1956): Relearning tests for interocular transfer following division of optic chiasma and corpus callosum in cats. J Comp Physiol Psychol 49:529–533.

Sperry RW, Zaidel E, Zaidel D (1979): Self recognition and social awareness in the deconnected minor hemisphere. Neuropsychologia 17:153–166.

Squire LR (1982): The neuropsychology of human memory. Ann Rev Neurosci 5:241–273.

Tomasch J (1954): Size, distribution and number of fibers in the human corpus callosum. Anat Rec 119:119–135.

Tomasch J (1957): A quantitative analysis of the human anterior commissure. Acta Anat (Basel) 30:902–906.

Zaidel E, Peters AM (1981): Phonological encoding and ideographic reading by the disconnected right hemisphere: Two case studies. Brain Lang 14:205–234.

Two Hemispheres—One Brain:
Functions of the Corpus Callosum, pages 281–297
© 1986 Alan R. Liss, Inc.

The Role of the Corpus Callosum in Visual Development

ANDREA J. ELBERGER

Department of Neurobiology and Anatomy, The University of Texas Medical School at Houston, Texas 77030

For a long time, investigations of the functions of the cerebral commissures were conducted using adults of different species because it was assumed that commissures such as the corpus callosum performed a single, major function of uniting the overlapping or duplicated information processed in each cerebral hemisphere for each separate modality. In terms of the sensory modalities this meant that the callosum provided the mechanism for joining the two halves of the body or of space. For the visual system, support for this concept came from anatomical studies demonstrating that the corpus callosum interconnected regions of the visual cortex representing the vertical meridian [reviewed in Berlucchi, 1972]. This idea was also supported by physiological studies showing that the visual receptive fields of cortical cells whose axons form the corpus callosum (callosal neurons) overlapped or abutted the vertical meridian in almost every case [Berlucchi et al., 1967; Hubel and Wiesel, 1967; Shatz, 1977]. However, more recent studies have shown that this traditional view does not hold for callosal connections between all visual cortical regions, nor does it hold for all the callosal connections of regions where this probably is the case [e.g., Segraves and Rosenquist, 1982a,b]. Evidence will be presented from recent studies using behavioral, physiological, and anatomical techniques [Elberger, 1979, 1981, 1982a,b, 1984a–c; Elberger and Smith, 1983, 1984; Elberger et al., 1983a,b] to show that the corpus callosum plays multiple roles in the functions of the visual system. To this end, three major points will be emphasized:

1. There is a heterogeneity of functions of callosal neurons; some functions will be considered direct, or primary, in that callosal input at a given point in development is required for that visual function to be maximally

Andrea J. Elberger's current address is Department of Anatomy, The University of Tennesee Center for the Health Sciences, Memphis, TN 38163 developed; some functions will be considered indirect, or secondary, in that callosal input at a given point in development enables the visual system functions to develop more efficiently, but the callosal input is not necessary for development of that visual function; callosal neurons may not play any role in some visual system functions.

2. There is a critical period for the role of the corpus callosum in the development of the visual system, and that critical period is completed by the end of the first postnatal month.

3. The alterations of visual functions resulting from neonatal corpus callosum section are due to the interruption of callosal inputs during the callosal critical period, and are not due to secondary changes resulting from the callosal surgery.

Finally, speculations as to how the corpus callosum develops in order to perform these multiple roles will be discussed briefly.

The research presented emphasizes corpus callosum connections related to the visual system in cats of different ages. One approach that has been utilized to assess the functions of the corpus callosum has been to sever the callosal fibers and measure any changes in the visual system that result. This method has successfully been used for cats at all stages of development. Extensive modifications of the surgical method developed for adult cats [Myers, 1956] have been made so that the surgery can be performed on kittens as young as the day of birth with minimal or no cortical lesions resulting; these modifications have been detailed elsewhere [Elberger, 1980, 1982b, 1984c].

ROLE OF THE CORPUS CALLOSUM IN BASIC VISUAL FUNCTIONS
Visuomotor Behaviors

Paw placing was studied in terms of the age of onset in control (9 normal and 2 sham-operated) and corpus callosum (CC)-sectioned (16, surgery 12–19 postnatal days) cats. Beginning at 20 days of age, each cat was held by the investigator and slowly lowered over an 18-in distance to a visually patterned surface. A positive response, when the cat could see the surface below, was indicated by extension of the front paws as if to jump to the surface; a negative response was indicated by failure to extend the paws. The positive response quickly increased from chance to a significant 70% frequency over a 2-day period. The CC-sectioned cats did not show a significant positive response (mean = 31.56; SD = 2.39) until 4 days after this appeared for the controls (mean = 27.91; SD = 1.90) [Elberger, 1982b] (Fig. 1). This difference is statistically significant (Mann-Whitney U-test, P = .002), indicating that neonatal CC section delays the normal development of paw placing but does not prevent its occurrence.

Object avoidance was studied in terms of the age of onset in control (2 normal, 2 sham-operated) and CC-sectioned (11, surgery 12–19 postnatal days) cats. Each cat was allowed to locomote around ten randomly placed

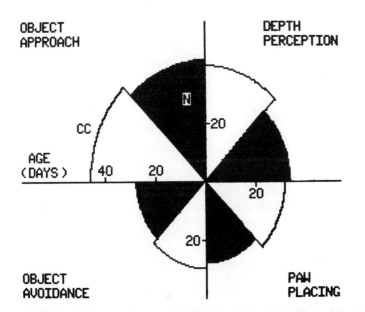

Fig. 1. Role of the corpus callosum in four visual functions. The solid sections represent the data from normal controls, the open sections represent the data from the neonatal CC-sectioned cats. The length of the radius indicates the mean age in days at which each group correctly performed the visual task on every trial. Within each marked quadrant, the mean difference between the performance of the two groups of cats on that task is shown by the difference between the radius of the open versus filled sections. Neonatal section of the corpus callosum causes delays ranging from 3 to 6 days in the acquisition of these four functions, but since each function eventually does develop, the corpus callosum role is indirect, or secondary.

multifaceted objects on a visually nontextured surface beginning at 20 days of age. A negative score was given every time a cat bumped into an object during a 2-minute period; successful object avoidance was declared when 70% or more of the trials had no negative scores. The CC sectioned cats met this criterion (mean = 30.18; SD = 2.79) 3 days after the controls did (mean = 27.67; SD = 3.06) [Elberger, 1982b] (Fig. 1). This difference was statistically significant (U-test, P < .002), indicating that neonatal CC section also delays the normal development of object avoidance without preventing its occurrence.

Object approach detection was studied in terms of the age of onset in control (2 normal, 2 sham-operated) and CC-sectioned (11, surgery 12–19 postnatal days) cats. Beginning at 20 days of age each cat was held by the investigator while an irregularly shaped object was moved slowly over a distance of 25 in toward the cat at its eye level. A positive response was scored if the cat used its paw to touch the object as if to ward off its approach.

The CC-sectioned cats met a 70% positive criterion (mean = 46.09; SD = 4.06) 4 days after the controls did (mean = 42.33; SD = 2.52) [Elberger, 1982b] (Fig. 1). This difference is statistically significant (U-test, P < .002), indicating that neonatal CC section delays the normal development of this behavior without preventing its occurrence.

These three representative tests of visuomotor behaviors that develop at a relatively early age illustrate functions of the corpus callosum that may be considered secondary, or indirect, because the normal visual function eventually develops without callosal input to the visual cortex. In addition to neonatal corpus callosum section, significant alterations in the quantity or quality of early visual experience have a secondary effect on the development of these functions. This can be demonstrated following dark-rearing or surgically produced divergent strabismus [see discussion in Elberger, 1982b]. However, lesioning a significant component of the visual pathway can eliminate the ability to perform these tasks or prevent them from developing in the first place, depending on the age at which the lesion was made. This primary effect can be demonstrated following bilateral ablation of 17, 18, 19, and lateral suprasylvian (LS) cortical areas in adult cats [see discussion in Elberger, 1982b]. Since surgical section of the corpus callosum results in a very specific bilateral cortical lesion (only the cortical cells giving rise to callosal fibers are involved), these results indicate that the callosal neurons are not a source of critical processing for visuomotor information, even in the neonate. Evidently, the non-callosal neurons of areas 17, 18, 19, and LS are responsible for this processing. Without callosal interconnections there is a reorganization of the processing of visual information for visuomotor coordination that takes place during a period of 3–4 days (Fig. 1), thus the callosal role is secondary.

Depth Perception and Stereopsis

Development of depth perception was investigated in terms of the age at which a visual cliff was reliably perceived. Each cat was required to choose between descending to a checkerboard surface that appeared close by or one that appeared far away, the "visual cliff"; in fact, the two surfaces were equidistant. Control (four normal) and CC-sectioned (five, surgery 15–19 and 29 postnatal days) cats were tested beginning at 20 days of age. All CC-sectioned cats did not completely avoid the visual cliff (at 39 days) until 6 days after all controls did (at 33 days) [Elberger, 1980] (Fig. 1). The difference in visual behavior is statistically significant (F = 25.95; df = 1, 20; P < .001), indicating that neonatal corpus callosum section delays the development of depth perception but does not prevent its occurrence. Thus the callosal role in this visual function is secondary. The ability to avoid a visual cliff can be eliminated (a primary role) in the adult cat only if 90% or more of the neocortical projection of the dorsal lateral geniculate nucleus (LGNd) is ablated [Cornwell et al., 1976]. These cortical regions also have callosal interconnections, so it must be the non-callosal neurons in these areas that are responsible for the visual cliff response. Since many visual cues, either monocular or binocular, can be used to perform this discrimination, this suggests that the callosal input to the visual cortex allows one set of visual cues to be utilized in the discrimination. However, a different set of visual cues may be utilized successfully in the absence of callosal input, but the reorganization of visual processing requires a period of approximately 6 days (Fig. 1).

The callosal role in stereopsis was investigated in terms of performance on a stereoacuity task after interruption of callosal input. This task measured the difference between monocular and binocular depth perception abilities and thereby provided an assessment of the animal's capacity for fine stereopsis. Control (one normal, one sham-operated) and CC-sectioned (three neonatal, surgery at 11 postnatal days; one adult) cats were tested when they were at least 6 months of age on a jumping-stand apparatus with stimuli that consisted of fields of different sized spots. If fine stereopsis was present, a significant difference in performance would be evident between the monocular and binocular testing conditions. The absence of fine stereopsis would be indicated by no such difference. The neonatal CC-sectioned cats showed that their fine stereopsis was normal; subsequently, the control cat received an adult corpus callosum section, and its fine stereoscopic ability was not diminished after surgery [Timney et al., 1985]. However, after the neonatal CC-sectioned cats had the optic chiasm sectioned as adults, fine stereopsis was eliminated [Timney et al., 1985]. Thus, the corpus callosum is one pathway, but not the exclusive pathway, in the visual system that provides the capability for fine stereopsis; the callosal role in fine stereopsis may be considered secondary. This is particularly interesting because stereoscopic abilities rely on binocular vision, and neonatal corpus callosum section has been shown to reduce significantly cortical binocularity in the striate cortex [Elberger, 1981] but not in the LS cortex [Elberger and Smith, 1983]. This suggests that either the cortical units mediating stereopsis are extrastriate, or else a small complement of binocular striate units are sufficient to mediate stereopsis.

Depth perceptions can be made using various visual cues, both monocular and binocular. When uniquely binocular cues are preselected for a visual discrimination of depth, the results indicate that the corpus callosum conveys information that is specifically beneficial for performing this task. The delayed ability for a simple depth preception task following neonatal CC section suggests either that fine stereopsis is not normally utilized early in development for such a task, or else that the ability for fine stereopsis may not be developed at the 1–2-month age that was tested. Evidently another visual cue or cues is utilized at that age which is exclusively mediated by the corpus callosum, and the disruption of this pathway forces an alternative decision-making strategy to be selected which accounts for the delay observed.

Interhemispheric Transfer

The role of the neonatal corpus callosum in the subsequently developed capacity for interhemispheric transfer was assessed in terms of performance on a variety of visual discriminations. Neonatal corpus callosum sectioned cats (two, surgery at 15 and 29 postnatal days) were monocularly trained as adults to perform seven different simultaneous visual discriminations between stimuli such as mirror-image and inverted stimulus pairs. One member of the pair was designated as positive and the cat was required to choose the randomly positioned positive stimulus. Immediately after making 90% correct responses with the initially trained eye, that same eye was covered with an opaque contact lens, and the other eye was tested to assess whether the learned information was present in the second hemisphere. Regardless of the difficulty of the task as determined by the number of trials required to achieve criterion, perfect interhemispheric transfer was observed in each case [Elberger, 1982b; unpublished data]. This indicates that during early development, the combining of information from the two eyes via the optic tract and optic chiasm pathways is sufficient to present learned visual information to each hemisphere. Corpus callosum section in the adult cat has also been shown to have no effect on interhemispheric transfer of visual information [discussed in Berlucchi, 1972]. Thus, either the reorganization of visual processing that occurs following neonatal corpus callosum section has no effect on the development of the capacity for interhemispheric transfer, or else the callosum has a secondary role in this visual function which might be observed if testing occurred at an earlier age.

EVIDENCE FOR A CORPUS CALLOSUM CRITICAL PERIOD IN VISUAL DEVELOPMENT
Extent of the Visual Field

Behavioral visual field perimetry testing was performed in order to determine whether the absence of corpus callosum inputs to visual cortex would affect the areas of the visual field that, when stimulated, could elicit a response. Since the callosum has been shown to interconnect a large extent of the visual field representation in the different visual cortical regions it was impossible to predict which, if any, regions would be affected. Control (6 normal) and CC-sectioned (13 neonatal, surgery at 13–22 days old; 3 adult, surgery at 9–20 months old) cats were tested both binocularly and monocularly when they were a minimum of 7 months old (12 for the adult CC group); the adult CC cats were also tested prior to the surgery when they were still normal [Elberger, 1979; Elberger and Spydell, 1985]. Cats were deprived of food for 23 hours prior to testing so that a food stimulus located at different positions in the visual field could be used. A positive response to a visual food stimulus at a given position was signified by a rapid approach to the object in order to consume it. A negative response was indicated by a failure to approach the food stimulus, or even to walk right past it without noticing it. The visual field was repeatedly sampled at 15° intervals both inside and outside of the normal extent of the visual field; when possible, the limits of the visual field were defined within a 5° interval [as in Elberger et al., 1983a]. The binocular testing condition does not distinguish between the separate response of either eye and the simultaneous response of both eyes, whereas the monocular testing condition is much more specific. Results from binocular testing for both control, neonatal CC-sectioned and adult CC-sectioned cats indicated that corpus callosum section had no effect on the total extent of the visual field represented by either eye. However, results from monocular testing of each eye indicated that neonatal CC section reduced the amount of overlap of the monocular visual fields by nearly eliminating the contralateral portion of the monocular visual field [Elberger, 1979; Elberger and Spydell, 1985]. Thus, the neonatal callosal input has a primary effect on reducing the extent of the binocular (the overlapping of the monocular) visual field. In contrast, the adult CC-sectioned cats had normal monocular visual fields, indicating that the binocular visual field was normal in extent [Elberger, 1979]. The difference in the results of the neonatal CC-sectioned versus adult CC-sectioned cats suggests that there is a critical period of time during which corpus callosum section has a permanent effect on the functions of the visual system. However, these studies do not pinpoint just what that limited time period is.

Visual evoked potential (VEP) analysis of the visual field extent was made to determine whether there was any physiological correspondence to the behaviorally determined perimetry results. Control (four normal) and CC-sectioned (ten, surgery at 15–29 postnatal days) cats were studied when they were a minimum of 9 months old. After being anesthetized, the extent of each cat's visual field was determined under monocular and binocular testing conditions using a periodically flashing light-emitting diode (LED) as a visual stimulus positioned at intervals throughout the normal binocular visual field extent. Responses were recorded using a gold disc scalp electrode located over the midpoint of the interaural line and were averaged over 128 trials. Using the first surface positive-negative-positive response at a visual field position to indicate the primary cortical event, the absence of this response or its appearance at less than 10% of the maximum amplitude observed for that same cat was interpreted as a nonresponsive visual field position. The data from each cat were recorded according to an assigned code by one investigator, and the other investigator determined when a positive response had occurred; thus, experimenter bias was ruled out. Under binocular testing conditions, no difference between the groups was found. Under monocular testing conditions, the control cats had a visual field extent (mean = 135; SD = 5.0) virtually identical [Elberger and Spydell, 1985] to the behaviorally determined extent of 135° [Elberger, 1979]. The CC-sectioned cats had monocular visual field extents (mean = 111.0; SD = 10.31) very similar [Elberger and Spydell, 1985] to the behaviorally determined extent of 95–105° [Elberger, 1979]. These physiologically derived results replicated the behaviorally determined results and provide further support for the conclusion that there is a restricted critical period of development during which the corpus callosum has a primary effect on the organization of the visual system.

Development of Visual Acuity

Behavioral determination of visual acuity development was made by measuring the visual acuity threshold at different ages. Control (8: 4 normal, 4 non-visual CC-sectioned) and CC-sectioned (20: three surgery during postnatal week 1, six during week 2, seven during week 3, three during week 4, one at week 29) cats were tested on a modified cat jumping stand [Elberger 1982a, 1984a] from 5 through 29 weeks of age. A simultaneous visual discrimination was made between a 95% contrast square-wave grating and a homogeneous gray of the same mean luminance. The grating was the positive stimulus, and a positive choice was made when the cat jumped onto a screen where the grating was projected. The spatial frequency of the grating was increased by 0.5 cycles per degree (cpd) steps from a 0.5 cpd start. The cat's threshold of acuity for that day was determined to be the highest spatial frequency at which the cat could perform at a 70% correct criterion level. Cats were tested monocularly and binocularly on a weekly basis, and the same results were obtained in both testing conditions. The cat with corpus callosum section at 29 weeks of age showed no effects of the surgery on its adult visual acuity threshold. The acuity thresholds of the 4-week CC-sectioned cats at 29 weeks of age were virtually identical to the acuity threshold of the 29-week CC-sectioned cat (Fig. 2); also, their visual acuity development was indistinguishable from that of the controls (F = 2.76; df = 1,22; P < .15) [Elberger, 1984a]. However, the 1-, 2-, and 3-week CC-sectioned cats showed significantly lower acuity thresholds throughout development as compared with the controls (P < .001 in each case). Furthermore, the difference was greatest in the 1-week CC-sectioned cats and least in the 3-week CC-sectioned cats [Elberger, 1984a] (Fig. 2). This indicates that there is a restricted time period for corpus callosum section to affect permanently the development of visual functions, and this critical period is completed by the end of the first postnatal month.

Development of Cortical Binocularity

Striate cortical binocularity was investigated in terms of the changes in the proportion of binocularly activated units as a result of corpus callosum section at different ages. Control (5 normal, 4 sham-operated) and CC-sectioned (31: 12 with surgery at 13–19 postnatal days, 19 with surgery at 21–168 postnatal days) cats were prepared for physiological recording when they were at least 7 months old, or when at least 8 weeks had elapsed after the callosal section in the case of the oldest operated cats. Striate cortical

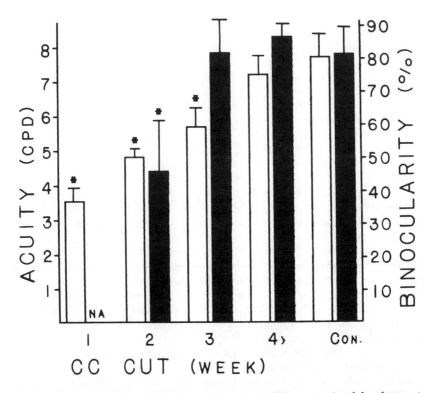

Fig. 2. The critical period for the role of the corpus callosum in visual development. Two visual functions are indicated by vertical scales on the left and right ordinates. The abscissa lists the different groups of cats, either as CC-sectioned at 1, 2, 3, or 4 and more postnatal weeks, or as control cats (Con.). The mean of the adult visual acuity threshold attained by these different groups is indicated by the height of the open bar, scaled to the left ordinate; the standard deviation is indicated by the height marked above the bar. The mean of the proportion of binocularly activated striate cortical units is indicated by the height of the solid bar, scaled to the right ordinate; the standard deviation is indicated by the height marked above the bar. NA means binocularity data for this group is not available. The asterisk above the bar indicates that performance was significantly different than that of the controls on the same function. The callosal role in these visual functions is direct, or primary. Neonatal section of the callosum by the fourth and third postnatal week has no effect on acuity and binocularity, respectively. Thus, the critical period for the corpus callosum role in these two visual functions is completed before the end of the first postnatal month.

regions representing the visual field from the vertical midline through more than 39° eccentricity were sampled in both hemispheres in the majority of the cats, with a mean of 27.7 units recorded from in each hemisphere [Elberger and Smith, 1985]. The results indicate that the proportion of binocularly activated cells for each group of cats was relatively consistent for cells with receptive fields throughout the entire region of the visual field that was examined, and was consistent for cells within the simple and complex classification categories [Elberger, 1981; Elberger and Smith, 1985]. For the cats with CC section at 21–168 postnatal days, the proportion of binocularly activated cells (80–97%) was consistently greater than or equal to the mean proportion of binocularly activated cells (range 64–90%) recorded for the controls (Fig. 2); thus corpus callosum section at 21 postnatal days or older has no effect on the proportion of binocularly activated striate cortical cells [Elberger, 1981; Elberger and Smith, 1985]. However, for the cats with CC section at 13–19 postnatal days, there was a smaller proportion of binocularly activated cells than was recorded for the controls, and the younger the age at CC section, the greater was the deficit (Fig. 2). Thus, neonatal callosal section has a primary effect on the development of striate cortical binocularity. The correlation between the age at surgery and the proportion of binocularly activated cells (r = −.88) was statistically significant (t = 5.86; df = 10; P < .001), indicating that this relationship was very consistent [Elberger and Smith, 1985]. The reduction in binocular activation was manifested as a decrease in the proportion of cells dominated by input from the eye ipsilateral to the cell being recorded [Elberger and Smith, 1985]. These data indicate that there is a critical period for corpus callosum section to affect striate cortical binocularity, and this critical period is restricted to less than the first three postnatal weeks. This definition of the endpoint of the callosal critical period is very similar to the endpoint suggested by the visual acuity study [Elberger, 1984a], thus providing strong evidence that when corpus callosum section has a primary effect on the development of a visual system function, the callosal effectiveness may only be present during the first postnatal month (Fig. 2).

Lateral suprasylvian (LS) cortical binocularity was studied in terms of whether there was a deficit in binocular activation of cortical units following section of the corpus callosum at different ages. Control (one normal) and CC sectioned (eight: three surgery at 15 postnatal days, five surgery at 21–22 postnatal days) cats were prepared for physiological recording when they were at least 10 months old. Cortical regions representing both central and peripheral regions of the visual field were sampled in the posteromedial or posterolateral edges of the suprasylvian sulcus. The results indicate that the proportion of binocularly activated units in the control cat (87%) was similar to the proportion obtained from the 15-day (94%) and 21,22-day CC-sectioned cats (98%) [Elberger and Smith, 1983]. Thus, section of the corpus callosum had no effect on the proportion of binocularly activated cells in the

LS cortex, even when surgery at the same age did alter this proportion in the striate cortex [Elberger, 1981; Elberger and Smith, 1985]. Alternatively, the callosum may have had a secondary effect on LS binocularity, which was later compensated for by other components of the visual system. This heterogeneity of callosal functions has previously been demonstrated in terms of the effect of lesioning different regions of the visual cortex on interhemispheric transfer of visual pattern discriminations [Berlucchi, 1972; Berlucchi et al., 1979]. In this case, the LS cortex was shown to have a different role than the striate cortex in interhemispheric transfer of visual pattern information. The connections of the striate cortex have been shown to change during development, from extensive interconnections throughout this area shortly after birth, to the restricted interconnections between the representations of the vertical midline seen in the adult by the end of the first postnatal month [Innocenti, 1978]. It is interesting to note that this period of critical morphological development of the corpus callosum closely corresponds to the critical period for the corpus callosum to affect striate cortical binocularity [Elberger and Smith, 1985]. Perhaps this suggests a mechanism by which the corpus callosum may be able to exert such a significant influence throughout the striate cortex. Conversely, the failure of the corpus callosum to exert an influence on lateral suprasylvian cortical binocularity during the same time period [Elberger and Smith, 1983] might suggest that either the morphological development of the callosal connections of LS cortex occurs prior to that for the striate cortex, or else the LS callosal connections do not undergo changes in distribution patterns during development. Assessment of the validity of such a speculation might provide further evidence for the potential mechanisms of the critical corpus callosum influence on visual development.

POSSIBLE ADDITIONAL FACTORS IN THE CORPUS CALLOSUM ROLE IN VISUAL DEVELOPMENT
Are Any Other Cerebral Commissural Fibers Involved?

One possible explanation for the conclusion that there is a callosal critical period for visual development is that there may be additional commissural fibers developing during the first postnatal month that restore the callosal functions after the effects of the neonatal surgery are demonstrated. This could be manifested in two ways: by additional corpus callosum fibers crossing from one hemisphere to another later on in order to interconnect the visual cortices, or by callosal fibers interconnecting visual cortices traveling in an indirect route through the intact anterior portion of the callosum. The first hypothesis was investigated using gross and histological examination of all of the brains of cats with neonatal corpus callosum section. The hypothesis was never supported in over 200 cases; thus it must be concluded that there is no secondary wave of callosal fibers migrating across the longitudinal fissure in order to interconnect the two hemispheres during the postnatal period of development. The second hypothesis was investigated by tracing the distribution of the cell bodies of callosal fibers located within the more anterior portion of the callosal bundle. Neonatal callosum-sectioned cats (6, surgery at 6–29 postnatal days) were reared to adulthood while several different measures (e.g., visuomotor performance, visual acuity, eye alignment) were used to confirm that the previously documented results of neonatal callosum section had occurred. When the cats were a minimum of 10 months old, the intact anterior portion of the callosum was sectioned and the severed ends of the callosal fibers were filled with the retrograde tracer horseradish peroxidase (HRP) as detailed previously [Elberger et al., 1983b; Elberger, 1984b]. The positions of the HRP-filled callosal cell bodies were located and none were found to be within the visual cortical areas 17–21 or the lateral suprasylvian group. This indicates that all callosally transmitted communication between visual cortical regions was interrupted as a result of the neonatal surgery. Thus there is no evidence to suggest that there is any direct communication between the visual cortices in each hemisphere following neonatal section of the posterior corpus callosum.

Are Any Other Components of the Visual Pathway Involved?

Some relatively small regions of the striate visual cortex were occasionally lesioned during the surgical section of the posterior corpus callosum. In all the cases where lesions occurred they were unilateral. Estimates were made of the extent of the lesion and this was correlated with the individual performance of each cat on a particular visual function measured after neonatal corpus callosum section. In sham-operated control cats, the frequency of occurrence of these lesions was similar in proportion to that observed in the callosum-sectioned cats [Elberger, 1981, 1984a; Elberger and Smith, 1985], indicating that the presence of such a lesion did not result in an alteration of a particular visual function after the surgery. In addition, there never was a detectable difference in any visual function within the groups of CC-sectioned cats related to the presence or absence of any such cortical lesion [Elberger, 1979–1981, 1982a, 1984a; Elberger and Smith, 1985]. The actual extent of these lesions were estimated to be a maximum of 6% of the unilateral striate cortical area [Elberger and Smith, 1985], so it is unlikely that such a small lesion would have produced an effect. Thus the evidence indicates that the interruption of corpus callosum fibers results in the observed changes in visual functions during development.

Are Secondary Conditions of Visual Input Involved?

Neonatal section of the posterior corpus callosum in cats has been shown to result in a permanent misalignment of the eyes known as strabismus. This misalignment is relatively small (3–11°) and divergent in direction when measured in the alert state using corneal reflex photography [Elberger, 1979; Elberger and Hirsch, 1982]. Experimental strabismus, whether surgically (cutting specific extraocular muscles) or optically (rearing with visual input only through prisms) induced, produces some visual alterations that are similar to those resulting from neonatal callosum section, such as reduced visual acuity [Jacobson and Ikeda, 1979] and reduced striate cortical binocularity [Levitt and Van Sluyters, 1982; Yinon, 1976]. It is therefore possible that the strabismus produced by the neonatal callosotomy might actually be the causal agent for the alterations in visual functions observed, rather than the disruption of interhemispheric communication being the causal agent. To explore this possibility the performances of neonatal callosum-sectioned versus strabismic cats were closely compared on the same, or similar, visual tasks to provide a measure as to how similar these two groups of cats actually are. Visual task performance will be discussed in the order presented for neonatal callosum sectioned cats.

Visuomotor behavior was assessed in cats with surgically produced divergent strabismus. When the surgery was performed in cats 3–7 postnatal weeks old, complete compensation for the misalignment occurred after approximately 2 weeks, but when the surgery was performed in a 4-month-old cat, compensation was not complete until almost 7 months after surgery [Olson, 1980]. This may be contrasted with the visuomotor performance of callosum-sectioned cats, where compensation as indicated by normal visuomotor behavior was completed in only 3–4 days [Elberger, 1982b]. Despite the similar divergent direction of the surgical strabismus, the performance of the callosum-sectioned cats was significantly different.

Stereopsis was measured in surgical strabismic cats using the same task described for the callosum-sectioned cats. The binocular and monocular conditions produced the same results, with the performance equivalent to the monocular condition in normals, indicating that no ability for fine stereopsis was present [cited in Mitchell et al., 1979]. In contrast, the callosum-sectioned cats showed binocular performance equivalent to that in normal cats [Timney et al., 1985]. Thus, surgical strabismic cats lose the ability for fine stereopsis while neonatal callosum-sectioned cats keep this ability intact.

Visual field extent was determined for both surgically and optically induced strabismic cats using similar perimetry tests. Under monocular testing conditions unilateral surgical strabismic animals had a normal visual field for the unoperated eye; however, the operated eye had a visual field loss in the contralateral portion that was graded in extent according to the amount the eye was deviated [Ikeda and Jacobson, 1977]. A cat with a photographically determined deviation of one eye of 10° showed visual responses of significant frequency out to 15°, and a reduced frequency of responses out to 30° in the contralateral portion of the monocular visual field; greater losses were noted with greater eye deviations [Ikeda and Jacobson, 1977]. In contrast, neonatal callosum-sectioned cats had a combined deviation for both eyes of 3–11° [Elberger, 1979, 1982b], yet the reduction in the extent of the visual field was greater than that with a larger surgical strabismus, and the visual field loss occurred for both eyes [Elberger, 1979]. In cats with optically induced strabismus, a reduction in the contralateral portion of the monocular visual field occurred for both eyes but was not as much [Elberger et al., 1983a] as occurred in the callosum-sectioned cats [Elberger, 1979]. In addition, half of these strabismic cats showed a unilateral reduction of the temporal portion of the visual field when tested with both eyes open [Elberger et al., 1983a]; this never occurred with callosum-sectioned cats [Elberger, 1979]. Thus the results of monocular and binocular visual field perimetry testing indicate that callosum-sectioned cats are dissimilar to surgically and optically induced strabismic cats.

Visual acuity thresholds were determined in cats with either divergent or convergent surgical strabismus. Cats were dark-reared until 40 postnatal days and then unilateral divergent strabismus of 20–26° was produced. The cats were tested on a jumping stand, the unoperated eye had normal acuity, and the operated eye had a 36–50% deficit [Von Grunau and Singer, 1980; as discussed in Elberger, 1982b]. Unilateral convergent strabismus was produced at 3, 6, and 8 postnatal weeks, with the unoperated eye having normal acuity, and the operated eye having a 70%, 49%, and 23% deficit in the 3-, 6-, and 8- week operated cats, respectively; surgery at 12 and 24 weeks resulted in normal acuity for both eyes [Jacobson and Ikeda, 1979; as discussed in Elberger, 1982b]. In contrast, callosum-sectioned cats had acuity deficits equal for both eyes, with a 52%, 38% and 28% deficit in the 1-, 2-, and 3-week sectioned cats, respectively; surgery at 4 and 29 weeks resulted in normal acuity [Elberger, 1984a]. Thus, strabismic cats differ from callosum-sectioned cats in terms of which eye had acuity deficits, in the age at which the surgical alteration could produce visual acuity deficits (at least 8 weeks for strabismic, and 3 weeks for callosum-sectioned cats), and in the amount of acuity deficit at the same age (with surgery at 3 weeks, a 70% deficit in strabismus and a 28% deficit with callosum section).

Striate cortical binocularity reduction can result from surgically or optically induced strabismus, but again, the age at which the surgical alteration results in loss of binocularity is different; this occurs when strabismus is induced through 11 postnatal weeks [Berman and Murphy, 1981; Levitt and Van Sluyters, 1982; Yinon, 1976] but occurs only when callosum section is within the first 3 postnatal weeks [Elberger and Smith, 1985]. In addition, with surgery at similar ages, the proportion of binocularity differs in the two groups. When divergent strabismus was produced at 12–43 days, only 24% binocularity remained [Berman and Murphy, 1981], yet in callosum section after 19 days normal binocularity resulted [Elberger and Smith, 1985].

Measures of eye alignment indicate that the strabismus of callosum-sectioned cats is only present in the awake state and disappears during paralysis [Elberger, 1979; Elberger and Hirsch, 1982]. This is in direct contrast to the misalignment that is present during paralysis for surgical strabismic cats [e.g., Berman and Murphy, 1981].

To summarize, neonatal CC-sectioned cats show substantial differences when compared with surgically or optically induced strabismic cats on every visual task measured for both groups of cats. It seems highly unlikely that the callosal results can be directly attributed to the strabismus that is produced. It is more likely that the strabismus is symptomatic of the alterations in the organization and processing of the visual system that results from neonatal corpus callosum section. If the eye misalignment that results from neonatal corpus callosum section is in any way thought to be involved in producing the visual alterations that follow the callosotomy, it would be most beneficial to consider this using a term other than strabismus in order to avoid any confusion because of the overwhelming differences between the consequences of these two conditions.

CONCLUSIONS AND SPECULATIONS

Several conclusions may be drawn from the evidence presented on the role of the corpus callosum in visual development:

1. There is a heterogeneity of callosal functions, with callosal input being necessary for the maximal development of some functions (primary role), or with callosal input being preferentially utilized for more efficient processing in other visual functions (secondary role). Furthermore, the callosum may not play a role in all binocular visual functions carried out in different regions of the visual cortex.

2. There is a critical period for the corpus callosum's primary roles in visual functions, and that critical period is completed before the end of the first postnatal month.

3. The alterations in visual functions that occur after neonatal corpus callosum section are most likely due to the interruption of callosal input to the visual cortices during the callosal critical period.

This leads to the speculation that the neonatal corpus callosum is heterogeneous either morphologically, physiologically, or neurochemically. This heterogeneity is expressed in terms of which callosal fibers survive to adulthood, and which are only present prior to the second postnatal month. These transitory callosal axons may be required in a two-step process initially to facilitate the binocular processing of visual information in the visual cortex, but once the callosal input has performed this function the callosal input is no longer necessary. At this point, visual experience becomes necessary in order to hard-wire, or make permanent, this function. The experiments detailed above indicate that normal visual experience is provided after the neonatal corpus callosum section, yet normal visual functions do not result. Therefore a normal, intact corpus callosum and normal visual experience are the two necessary ingredients for the visual system to develop normally, although each is necessary during different periods of development.

The mechanism for the significant role of the corpus callosum in visual development is yet to be determined, and there may be different mechanisms involved in different regions of the visual cortex. Most significantly, the traditional role of the corpus callosum in visual functions has been updated and expanded so that it now includes a critical role for the corpus callosum in visual development.

ACKNOWLEDGMENTS

This work was supported in part by National Institutes of Health grants MH36526 and NS20597 awarded to A.J.E., and by a University of Texas Biomedical Research Support Grant.

Thanks to James J. Aschberger for his assistance in executing the figures.

REFERENCES

Berlucchi G (1972): Anatomical and physiological aspects of visual functions of corpus callosum. Brain Res 37:371–392.

Berlucchi G, Gazzaniga MS, Rizzolatti G (1967): Microelectrode analysis of transfer of visual information by the corpus callosum. Arch Ital Biol 105:583–596.

Berlucchi G, Sprague JM, Antonini A, Simoni A (1979): Learning and interhemispheric transfer of visual pattern discriminations following unilateral suprasylvian lesions in split-chiasm cats. Exp Brain Res 34:551–574.

Berman N, Murphy EH (1981): The critical period for alteration in cortical binocularity resulting from divergent and convergent strabismus. Dev Brain Res 2:181–202.

Cornwell P, Overman W, Levitsky C, Shipley J, Lezynski B (1976): Performance on the visual cliff by cats with marginal gyrus lesions. J Comp Physiol Psychol 90:996–1010.

Elberger AJ (1979): The role of the corpus callosum in the development of interocular eye alignment and the organization of the visual field in the cat. Exp Brain Res 36:71–85.

Elberger AJ (1980): The effect of neonatal section of the corpus callosum on the development of depth perception in young cats. Vision Res 20:177–187.

Elberger AJ (1981): Ocular dominance in striate cortex is altered by neonatal section of the posterior corpus callosum in the cat. Exp Brain Res 41:280–291.

Elberger AJ (1982a): The corpus callosum is a critical factor for developing maximum visual acuity. Dev Brain Res 5:350–353.

Elberger AJ (1982b): The functional role of the corpus callosum in the developing visual system: A review. Prog Neurobiol 18:15–79.

Elberger AJ (1984a): The existence of a separate, brief critical period for the corpus callosum to affect visual development. Behav Brain Res 11:223–231.

Elberger AJ (1984b): The minimum extent of corpus callosum connections required for normal visual development in the cat. Hum Neurobiol 3:115–120.

Elberger AJ (1984c): Profound, short-term hypothermia is an effective adjunct to barbiturate anesthesia for surgery in feline neonates. Lab Anim 13:35–38.

Elberger AJ, Hirsch HVB (1982): Divergent strabismus following neonatal callosal section is due to a failure of convergence. Brain Res 239:275–278.

Elberger AJ, Smith ELS III (1983): Binocular properties of lateral suprasylvian cortex are not affected by neonatal corpus callosum section. Brain Res 278:295–298.

Elberger AJ, Smith ELS III (1985): The critical period for corpus callosum section to affect cortical binocularity. Exp Brain Res 57:213–223.

Elberger AJ, Smith ELS III, White JM (1983a): Optically induced strabismus results in visual field losses in cats. Brain Res 268:147–152.

Elberger AJ, Smith ELS III, White JM (1983b): Spatial dissociation of visual inputs alters the origin of the corpus callosum. Neurosci Lett. 35:19–24.

Elberger AJ, Spydell JD (1985): Visual field perimetry analysis using evoked potentials in normal and corpus callosum sectioned cats. Electroencephalogr Clin Neurophysiol 60:249–257.

Hubel DH, Wiesel TN (1967): Cortical and callosal connections concerned with the vertical meridian of visual fields in the cat. J Neurophysiol 30:1561–1573.

Ikeda H, Jacobson SG (1977): Nasal field loss in cats reared with convergent squint: Behavioural studies. J Physiol 270:367–381.

Innocenti GM (1978): Postnatal development of interhemispheric connections of the cat visual cortex. Arch Ital Biol 116:463–470.

Jacobson SG, Ikeda H (1979): Behavioural studies of spatial vision in cats reared with convergent squint: Is amblyopia due to arrest of development? Exp Brain Res 34:11–26.

Levitt FB, Van Sluyters RC (1982): The sensitive period for strabismus in the kitten. Dev Brain Res 3:323–327.

Mitchell DE, Kaye M, Timney B (1979): Assessment of depth perception in cats. Perception 8:389–396.

Myers RE (1956): Function of the corpus callosum in interocular transfer. Brain 79:358–363.

Olson CR (1980): Spatial localization in cats reared with strabismus. J Neurophysiol 43:792–806.

Segraves MA, Rosenquist AC (1982a): The distribution of the cells of origin of callosal projections in cat visual cortex. J Neurosci 2:1079–1089.

Segraves MA, Rosenquist AC (1982b): The afferent and efferent callosal connections of retinotopically defined areas in cat cortex. J Neurosci 2:1090–1107.

Shatz C (1977): Abnormal interhemispheric connections in the visual system of Boston Siamese cats. J Comp Neurol 171:229–246.

Timney B, Elberger AJ, Vandewater ML (1985): Binocular depth perception in the cat following early corpus callosum section. Exp Brain Res (In press).

Von Grunau MW, Singer W (1980): Functional amblyopia in kittens with unilateral exotropia. II. Correspondence between behavioural and electrophysiological assessment. Exp Brain Res 40:305–310.

Yinon U (1976): Age dependence of the effect of squint on cells in kittens' visual cortex. Exp Brain Res 26:151–157.

Two Hemispheres—One Brain:
Functions of the Corpus Callosum, pages 299–313
© 1986 Alan R. Liss, Inc.

Role of the Corpus Callosum for Binocular Coding in Siamese and Early-Strabismic Cats

C.A. MARZI, M. DI STEFANO, F. LEPORÉ, AND S. BÉDARD

Dipartimento di Psicologia Generale, Università di Padova, 35139 Padova (C.A.M.), Istituto di Fisiologia, Università di Pisa, 56100 Pisa (M.D.), Italy and Département de Psychologie, Université de Montréal, H3C 3J7 Montréal, Canada (F.L., S.B.).

In normal cats the vast majority of neurons in the visual cortex receive information from both eyes through the geniculocortical pathway. Congenital or acquired abnormalities can, however, cause a decrease of binocular neurons, either as a consequence of a misrouting of optic axons or as a result of surgical intervention on the eye muscles early in life. In this paper we shall present evidence that the corpus callosum plays a major role in compensating for an abnormally low convergence of inputs from the two eyes, and that such a compensation occurs only in visual areas beyond the striate and parastriate areas. In the first part of the paper we shall review evidence gathered in Siamese cats, and in the second part we shall report some preliminary results obtained in early-strabismic ordinary cats.

SIAMESE CATS

Following the initial observations of Guillery and Kaas [1971] and Hubel and Wiesel [1971], it is now widely known [see reviews in Guillery et al., 1974; Marzi, 1980] that Siamese cats, as well as albino mutants in general, have a reduced proportion of uncrossed optic axons as a consequence of an excessive decussation at the optic chiasma. Recently, Shatz and Kliot [1982], by using the axonal transport of intraocularly injected horseradish peroxidase or tritiated leucine, were able to demonstrate in fetal cats that this abnormality is present from the earliest stages of development of the retinogeniculate pathways. As a result of such a misrouting of optic axons, neurons in area 17, 18, and 19 [see Di Stefano et al., 1984, for recent findings on area 19] are driven through the contralateral eye only, and there is an unusual representation of a wide portion of the ipsilateral visual hemifield at the boundary between areas 17 and 18, where the abnormal contingent of misrouted geniculate fibers is housed in Boston Siamese cats [Hubel and Wiesel, 1971]. In this paper we shall not deal with the so-called Midwestern

Siamese cats [see Guillery et al., 1974] since all the Siamese cats used in our studies belonged to the Boston type only. In addition to the general contribution that it can provide to an understanding of the factors underlying the development of connections in the visual system, the study of the albino abnormality offers a unique opportunity to assess the correlation between abnormal neural structures and behavior in an otherwise intact animal. For example, one might expect the low proportion of binocular neurons in the striate and parastriate areas of Siamese cats to result in behavioral deficits of binocular vision. In agreement with such an expectation, it has been found that Siamese cats have a very poor stereopsis [Packwood and Gordon, 1975] and lack a binocular summation effect in contrast sensitivity [Von Grunau, 1982]. We reasoned that, in addition to the above deficits, the lack of central binocular coding might result in an impairment of an "higher-level" binocular function, such as perceptual generalization between the two eyes [Marzi, 1983]. To verify this prediction we tested intact Siamese cats for interocular transfer of monocularly learned form discriminations. In normal ordinary cats interocular transfer (IT) is almost perfect, in keeping with the very high proportion of binocular neurons in the visual cortex. To our surprise, however, we found that Siamese cats had an IT that was almost as good as that in ordinary cats [Marzi et al., 1976, 1979], (see Fig. 1), and only by using difficult discriminations were we able to show a slight impairment in the Siamese IT.

Thus it is clear from these results that the binocular neurons in visual areas 17 and 18 do not constitute an indispensable neuronal substrate for the interocular generalization of visual experience. Indeed, electrophysiological recordings from the same animals that were used for behavioral tests showed that they did lack binocular neurons in areas 17 and 18. It is likely however, that binocular neurons in those areas subserve stereopsis and binocular summation effects in acuity. Since it has been shown by Berlucchi et al. [1979] and by Ptito and Lepore [1983] that extrastriate areas such as the lateral suprasylvian visual areas (LSA), rather than the primary visual cortex, are critically involved in the IT of visual learning, we predicted that Siamese cats, even though they lack binocular neurons in area 17, 18, and 19, might still have a sufficiently high level of binocular interactions in such areas. To test this prediction we recorded from single cells in areas 17 and 18 of orthophoric Siamese cats (Siamese cats are often cross-eyed). Confirming our hypothesis, we found that although those cats lacked binocular neurons in areas 17 and 18, they had a high percentage of such neurons in the LSA. Such a percentage was essentially similar to that found in ordinary cats. Thus, the presence of binocular neurons in an area that has been shown to be involved in interhemispheric transfer of visual learning is well in keeping with the behavioral results in Siamese cats. A major question concerns the neural mechanisms underlying the sparing of binocularity in the LSA. There are in principle two possibilities to explain

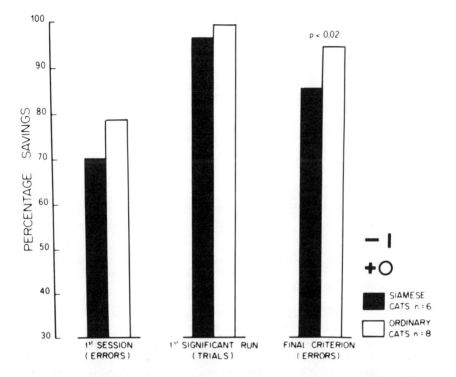

Fig. 1. Interocular transfer in intact ordinary and Siamese cats. Bar charts indicate the percentage saving between the first and second eye at three stages of learning: the first session, the first significant run, and the final criterion [from Marzi et al., 1979, with permission MacMillan Press, London, UK].

binocularity in the LSA of Siamese cats: one is that the contingent of normally routed fibers arising in the periphery of the temporal hemiretina might be sufficient to ensure, together with the normally crossed input from the nasal hemiretina, the observed level of binocular convergence. Such a possibility, however, can be excluded, since the normally projecting fibers in the temporal hemiretina of Siamese cats are very sparse especially in the central 20° of visual field representation [Marzi, 1980] (see Fig. 2); moreover, they have been shown to be unable to mediate spatial and form vision [Marzi and Di Stefano, 1978; Antonini et al., 1979] and to drive superior colliculus neurons [Antonini et al., 1979]. Notwithstanding this sparseness of uncrossed projections from the central temporal hemiretina, many of the cells in the LSA of our Siamese cats had both receptive fields (RFs) in the central portion of the visual field, and there were many cells with RFs extending considerably in the ipsilateral hemifield or lying entirely in it.

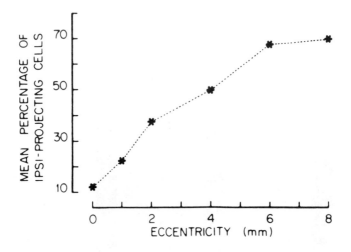

Fig. 2. Mean percentage of ipsilaterally projecting cells in temporal hemiretina of two Siamese cats as a function of eccentricity [from Marzi, 1980, with permission Elsevier Publications, Cambridge, UK].

Given that at least 20° of central temporal hemiretina and the whole nasal hemiretina project contralaterally, it follows that the only possibility for a cortical neuron to have a binocular RF in the ipsilateral visual field is to receive both a direct input from the contralateral eye and an indirect input from the ipsilateral eye via an interhemispheric commissural route. The same route must mediate the representation of the centralmost portion of the contralateral visual field through the ipsilateral eye. With these considerations in mind, we hypothesized that binocular interactions in LSA of Siamese cats are mainly mediated by the corpus callosum. Such an hypothesis was directly checked by sectioning the splenium and recording from LSA neurons both before and after surgery. Recordings were performed in some animals acutely and in other animals several weeks following surgery. The results were clear-cut in both acute and chronic conditions: the callosal transection resulted in a marked reduction or disappearance of responses mediated through the ipsilateral eye, while the visual field representation and the response properties of the cells driven by the contralateral eye were unaffected by callosal surgery. Such a result [Marzi et al., 1980, 1982a] is in complete agreement with findings obtained independently by Zeki and Fries [1980]. It is important to mention that a similar splenial section in ordinary cats resulted in no change in binocularity but determined a marked reduction of the ipsilateral visual field representation. These results prove that binocularity in the LSA of Siamese cats is subserved by a direct thalamic route for the contralateral eye and by an indirect commissural pathway for the ipsilateral eye. Such is not the case, however, in ordinary cats, where callosotomy does not affect binocularity in both striate and extrastriate areas.

DIFFERENCES BETWEEN CALLOSAL CONNECTIONS OF AREAS 17–19 AND LSA

One puzzling question is why in Siamese cats the callosal commissures are able to subserve binocularity in the LSA and not in areas 17–19, where there are essentially no binocular neurons, and the great majority of cells respond only to the contralateral eye. This question is even more puzzling when one considers that the callosal connections in Siamese cats are much more widespread than in ordinary cats and very often connect non-homotopic areas in the two hemispheres [Shatz, 1977a,b]. A possible answer to this question can be provided by taking into account the RF features and the response properties of the neurons in areas 17–19 on one hand and of neurons in the LSA on the other [see Orban, 1984, for a comprehensive review]. RFs of neurons in the striate and parastriate areas are considerably smaller than those in the LSA, and neuronal response properties, especially orientation selectivity, are much more specific in the former areas than in the latter. According to a well-known theory on the formation and maintenance of connections in the central nervous system, originally proposed by Hebb [1949] and subsequently extended by Hubel and Wiesel [1965] to the visual system [see also Stent, 1973], in order for a connection between two neurons to be maintained, the two cells have to be active together most of the time. When a presynaptic axon fails to excite the postsynaptic neuron while this in turn is being activated by other presynaptic axons, the synaptic efficiency of the former axon is decreased or annulled. In the visual cortex of common cats a binocular neuron is normally activated simultaneously through the two monocular subcortical inputs since the two monocular RFs are normally superimposed in the visual field and have identical response properties. Assuming that during the development of the visual system most cortical neurons receive an input from both eyes, it seems reasonable that a binocular input would be retained only by those neurons that have overlapping and functionally congruent RFs in the two eyes. On the contrary, the weaker monocular input would be lost by those cortical neurons that during development happen to receive spatially and/or functionally mismatched inputs from the two eyes. These developmental processes are likely to affect not only the interactions between the intrahemispheric pathways carrying information from both eyes to the cortex, but also those between intra- and interhemispheric monocular inputs to the cortex. In Siamese cats, during the development of functional central visual connections, the direct subcortical and the indirect callosal input are very unlikely to drive a cortical neuron in areas 17–19 together because the small size of RFs and the very strict requirements for various features of the stimulus, such as orientation or width, make unlikely the possibility of a spatial and functional overlap of the direct and interhemispheric inputs. Such is not the case, however, in the LSA, where RFs are very large and the response properties of the cells are rather loose. LSA neurons, for example, are not orientation-specific, and a precise correspondence between the orientation tuning of the direct and indirect inputs is not necessary. Furthermore, the large extension of RFs in LSA that very often include most of the central visual field of the animal, allows a spatial correspondence of the monocular inputs even if they originate from noncorresponding points in the two retinae. If LSA subserves IT in Siamese cats, it follows that section of the corpus callosum ought to impair IT since in LSA binocularity has a commissural basis. However, we found out [Marzi et al., 1979] that ortophoric Siamese cats with a section of the splenium of the corpus callosum still have a very good level of IT (see Fig. 3). On the contrary, strabismic Siamese cats show an impairment of IT following callosal section

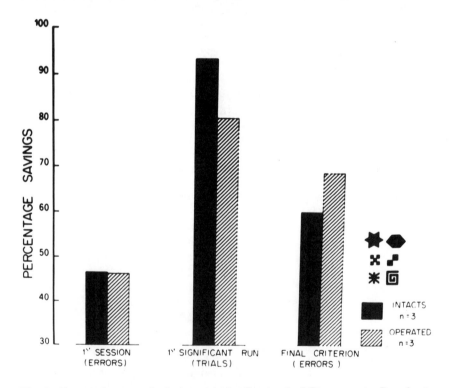

Fig. 3. Interocular transfer in intact and callosotomized Siamese cats. Bar charts indicate the percentage saving between the first and second eye at three stages of learning: the first session, the first significant run, and the final criterion [from Marzi et al., 1979, with permission MacMillan Press, London, UK].

[Lepore et al., 1983]. Thus, even though the results on strabismic Siamese cats are in accordance with the hypothesis that transfer is subserved by the binocular neurons of LSA, the positive IT found in ortophoric Siamese remains a puzzle. We reasoned, then, that there must be other areas that contain binocular neurons but in which binocularity is not totally dependent upon the corpus callosum. The superior colliculus (SC) was the major candidate since it has RFs almost as large as those of the LSA, and the response features of its cells are not as specific as in areas 17–19; therefore it is likely to retain binocularity in spite of the albino abnormality.

We recorded from the SC of Siamese cats and found that 86.7% of the cells were binocular, while only 17.8% of the neurons in areas 17 and 18 of the same animals could be driven from both eyes [Antonini et al., 1981]. Subsequent acute or chronic section of the corpus callosum severely reduced binocular interactions but did not abolish them, and therefore the SC might have been the structure underlying IT in callosum-sectioned Siamese cats. Although we lack direct evidence for it, it is likely that the strabismic cats tested by Lepore et al. [1983] may have undergone a total loss of binocular neurons after callosal section not only in LSA but in SC as well and this would explain the marked effect of commissurotomy. That the SC of strabismic Siamese cats might contain fewer binocular cells than in ortophoric Siamese cats is in agreement with the findings of Berman and Cynader [1972], who reported very few binocular neurons (20%) in the SC of Siamese cats with a convergent strabismus of 10° or more. A low percentage of binocular neurons compared to our own study has also been found by Lane et al. [1974] in cats of the Midwestern type. This type of Siamese cat is thought to adapt to its aberrant visual input by suppressing both the abnormally crossed and the uncrossed input from the temporal hemiretina of the ipsilateral eye. Such a suppression has been documented only for the geniculostriate system [Guillery et al., 1974] but it is possible that a similar suppression occurs in the SC of Midwestern but not Boston Siamese cats. Apart from the differences in percentage of binocular neurons in the SC of ortophoric and strabismic Siamese cats (a point that is worth further investigation because it seems to indicate that the effect of strabismus and of a genetically based excessive crossing of the visual pathways can add together to yield a most severe abnormality of the central visual system), the role of the SC in IT of Siamese cats seems to be an important one. Even though our evidence is still indirect (IT in Siamese cats should be tested following SC lesions), the possibility that the SC is involved in IT of visual discriminations is not surprising since such a structure has been shown to be critical for visual learning in the cat [Berlucchi et al., 1972].

ROLE OF THE CORPUS CALLOSUM FOR BINOCULARITY IN THE LSA OF EARLY STRABISMIC CATS

The above findings in Siamese cats have revealed an unusual function of the corpus callosum, namely, that of compensating for a lack of uncrossed visual input. Such a compensation, however, cannot take place in areas 17–19 because of a difficult matching between the direct subcortical input and the indirect commissural pathway, while it can occur in the LSA and SC because the matching of the inputs from the two eyes on cortical neurons is facilitated by the properties of the RFs in these two areas. A role of the corpus callosum similar to that in Siamese cats may be postulated for ordinary cats affected by strabismus. Various surgical or environmental procedures are known to disrupt binocularity in area 17 provided they are performed during the so-called critical period [see Berman and Murphy, 1982]. When adult, kittens that underwent surgically or optically induced artificial strabismus or alternate monocular occlusion do not generally present severe abnormalities in the response properties of cells in area 17 [see, however, Chino et al., 1983] but only lack binocularly activated neurons. Such an abnormality is somewhat different from that affecting Siamese cats because in early strabismic animals approximately equal numbers of neurons can be activated by each eye [Hubel and Wiesel, 1965] while in Siamese cats there is a strong predominance of the contralateral eye. In view of the results in the Siamese cats, one might expect in strabismic animals to find binocular cells in areas where neurons have RFs larger than the angle of strabismus. Therefore, as in Siamese cats, the LSA and SC should contain many binocular cells in spite of a lack of these cells in area 17. In agreement with such a prediction, Gordon and Gummow [1975] found a high percentage of binocular neurons in the SC of cats submitted to a section of the medial and lateral rectus of one eye during the second week of life, a procedure that was most effective in reducing binocular interactions in the primary visual cortex. Interestingly, binocularly driven cells were more numerous in the SC contralateral to the operated eye than in the SC ipsilateral to the operated eye, where there was instead a predominance of monocularly activated cells from the contralateral eye. Another important finding of Gordon and Gummow [1975] is that the decrease in binocularity is more marked for units with RFs medial border within $5°$ of the vertical meridian or in the ipsilateral hemifield than for more peripherally located cells. Such an effect might be related to the usually larger RF's size of peripheral units, and is in keeping with the hypothesis outlined above. In the light of the findings on SC, we decided to test whether common cats rendered strabismic before the end of the critical period also have many binocular cells in LSA. A summary of these findings has appeared elsewhere [Marzi et al., 1982b; Di Stefano et al., 1983].

Common kittens were rendered strabismic at 3–4 weeks of age by sectioning either the medial or the lateral rectus of one eye. They were then raised in the animal colony until they reached maturity, at which time they were used for single-cell recording. Recordings were carried out using tungsten microelectrodes and $N_2O:O_2$ anesthesia. Our usual procedure was to record in area 17, to make sure that most cells were monocular, and then to record in the LSA. RFs in the LSA were analyzed not only for ocular dominance but also for other characteristics, especially for RF size. The results obtained in strabismic cats were compared with results obtained in normal control cats. As could be expected, most cells in area 17 of normal cats were binocular, whereas those of strabismic cats were essentially (89%) monocular (Fig. 4). All cells in LSA of normal cats were binocular, whereas in strabismic animals there was a slight drop in binocularity, but the vast majority of cells (71%) were binocularly driven. A seven-point ocular dominance distribution was computed on our preliminary data and indicates that although the proportion of binocular cells is almost normal, the ocular dominance distribution is abnormal, being skewed in favor of the nonoperated eye.

Thus, in accord with our results in Siamese cats and those of Gordon and Gummow on the SC of strabismic ordinary cats [1975], the LSA retains a substantial amount of binocular activation even though binocular interaction is lost in the primary visual cortex. This result is in agreement with similar findings obtained independently by Von Grunau [1982].

Three possible mechanisms, working alone or in combination, can be held responsible for the preservation of binocularity in the LSA. First, RFs in the LSA are usually so large that even if the eyes are misaligned, the

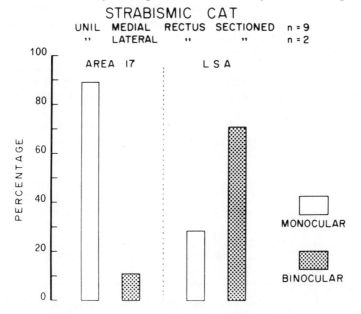

Fig. 4. Percentage binocular cells in areas 17 and lateral suprasylvian (LSA) in early-strabismic cats.

two monocular RFs can still overlap, and thus most cortical cells can be synchronously activated through both eyes. To test this possibility, we separated all cells into two groups: (a) cells whose RFs were smaller than the degree of divergence of the eyes (the available number of cells recorded in cats with a convergent squint was not sufficient to perform such an analysis) and (b) cells whose RFs were larger than the divergence of the eyes and that, therefore, could presumably still be synchronously activated in the strabismic cats. The results are presented in Table 1 and show that, although on the whole the majority of binocular cells had a RF larger than the angle of strabismus, there were many cells that retained their binocularity in spite of having a RF smaller than the angle of squint. Thus, a second possibility can be put forward, namely, that binocular cells in LSA may depend on a callosal route by virtue of a mechanism that is independent from an overlap of the two monocular inputs. A direct test of this hypothesis, i.e., recording from LSA before and after a section of the corpus callosum, is still in progress in our laboratory; however, the data gathered on a few cats in which we succeeded in splitting the posterior part of the corpus callosum showed a drop in binocular cells, although many cells still remained binocular. Figures 5 and 6 show the effects of callosum section on one cat with a convergent and one with a divergent strabismus, respectively. The effect of callosal section on binocularity is clearly much more severe in the esotropic than in the exotropic animal. Even though it is obviously premature to draw any firm conclusion, the existence of a difference between divergent and convergent strabismic cats on the effects of callosal section, would be in line with Berman and Murphy's results [1982] that in the visual cortex of early-strabismic cats, the overall percentage of binocular neurons is somewhat higher in exotropic (25%) than in esotropic (13%) animals.

Thus, the results of callosum section indicate that the commissural system does play a role in ensuring some degree of binocular convergence on LSA units, but that this role, at least in exotropic cats, is not as crucial as in Siamese cats. Further insights into the contribution of the corpus callosum will be provided by an analysis of the size of RFs before and after callosotomy and by a systematic investigation of the location in the visual field and of the response properties of the binocular cells that survive callosotomy.

TABLE 1. Relationship Between Degree of Exotropia and Receptive Field (RF) Sizes in Determining the Degree of Binocularity in LSA of Divergent Strabismic Cats

	Monocular	Binocular
RF < Exotropia	14	23
RF > Exotropia	4	24

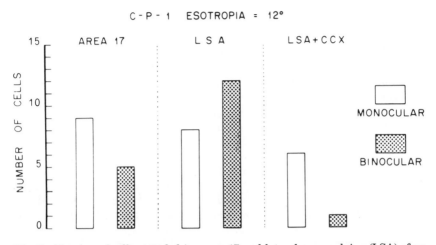

Fig. 5. Number of cells recorded in areas 17 and lateral suprasylvian (LSA) of an intact strabismic cat followed by acute transection of the corpus callosum and additional LSA recording.

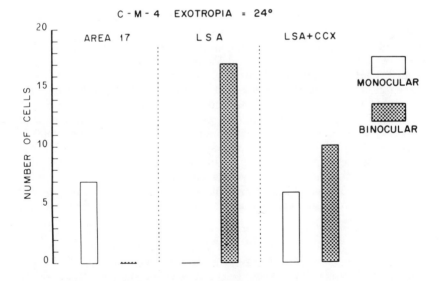

Fig. 6. Number of cells recorded in areas 17 and lateral suprasylvian (LSA) of an intact strabismic cat followed by acute transection of the corpus callosum and additional LSA recording.

Finally, a third possibility should be mentioned to explain the high degree of binocularity in the LSA of strabismic cats, namely, that LSA cells receive part of their input from other structures containing binocular cells, e.g., the SC. A direct answer to this question can be provided clearly only by lesion experiments in strabismic cats with a callosum section in which the residual binocularity in the LSA should be abolished by a SC ablation. However, in absence of such information, a reasonable guess is that it is the binocularity of the SC that depends upon LSA rather than vice versa. The SC is richly supplied with direct connections from this region [Heath and Jones, 1971; Kawamura et al., 1974; Holländer, 1974; Gilbert and Kelly, 1975], while ascending connections from SC to LSA are indirect through the thalamus (lateral posterior nucleus, posterior nucleus, and the C-laminae of the dorsal lateral geniculate nucleus; see summary diagram in Spear and Baumann [1979]). Moreover, removal of the SC does not influence the percentage of binocular cells in the LSA [Smith and Spear, 1979], which is instead markedly affected (loss of input from the ipsilateral eye) by a bilateral removal of areas 17 and 18 [Spear and Baumann, 1979].

In conclusion, the above results in Siamese cats and in strabismic common cats provide new evidence for a role of the callosal commissures in adapting to the consequences of an abnormal visual input. In keeping with our findings, there is anatomical evidence that the callosal connections in both Siamese cats [Shatz, 1977b; Berman and Payne, 1983] and in strabismic ordinary cats [Innocenti and Frost, 1979, 1980; Lund et al., 1978] are abnormally widespread. Whether this abundance of callosal connections represents a compensatory mechanism or is simply a consequence of an arrest of development [Berman and Payne, 1983], remains to be directly verified. Certainly, our evidence of a disruption of binocularity in LSA following callosum section hints at a functional role for the exuberant immature commissural connections. Finally, a general conclusion stemming from our findings is that the callosal compensation we have documented occurs in an area, such as LSA, that is implicated in higher-order perceptual processes [Marzi, 1983], while the primary visual cortex is not spared by the effects of an early alteration in binocular input. In keeping with this, both Siamese and strabismic ordinary cats are not impaired in IT of visual learning [see Berlucchi and Marzi, 1981 for a review], while they are impaired in binocular tasks presumably mediated by the primary visual cortex.

REFERENCES

Antonini A, Berlucchi G, Marzi CA, Sprague JM (1979): Behavioral and electrophysiological effects of unilateral optic tract section in ordinary and Siamese cats. J Comp Neurol 185:183–202.

Antonini A, Berlucchi G, Di Stefano M, Marzi CA (1981): Differences in binocular interactions between cortical areas 17 and 18 and superior colliculus of Siamese cats. J Comp Neurol 200:597–611.

Berlucchi G, Marzi CA (1981): Interocular and interhemispheric transfer of visual discriminations in cats. In Ingle D, Goodale M, Mansfield R (eds): "Advances in the Analysis of Visual Behavior." Cambridge: MIT Press, pp 719–750.

Berlucchi G, Sprague JM, Levy J, Di Berardino A (1972): Pretectum and superior colliculus in visually guided behavior and in flux and form discrimination in the cat. J Comp Physiol Psychol 78:123–172.

Berlucchi G, Sprague JM, Antonini A, Simoni A (1979): Learning and interhemispheric transfer of visual pattern discriminations following unilateral suprasylvian lesions in split-chiasm cats. Exp Brain Res 34:551–574.

Berman N, Cynader M (1972): Comparison of receptive-field organization of the superior colliculus in Siamese and normal cats. J Physiol (Lond) 224:363–389.

Berman N, Murphy EH (1982): The critical period for alteration in cortical binocularity resulting from divergent and convergent strabismus. Dev Brain Res 2:181–202.

Berman N, Payne BR (1983): Alterations in connections of the corpus callosum following convergent and divergent strabismus. Brain Res 274:201–212.

Chino YM, Shansky MS, Jankowski WL, Banser FA (1983): Effects of rearing kittens with convergent strabismus on development of receptive-field properties in striate cortex neurons. J Neurophysiol 50:265–286.

Di Stefano M, Bédard S, Tassinari G, Lepore F, Marzi CA (1982): Importance of the corpus callosum for binocularity in the lateral suprosylvian area of early strabismic cats. Behav Brain Res 8:279–280.

Di Stefano M, Bédard S, Marzi CA, Lepore F (1984): Lack of binocular activation of cells in area 19 of the Siamese cat. Brain Res 303:391–395.

Gilbert CD, Kelly JP (1975): The projections of cells in different layers of the cat's visual cortex. J Comp Neurol 163:81–106.

Gordon B, Gummow L (1975): Effects of extraocular muscle section on receptive fields in cat superior colliculus. Vision Res 15:1011–1019.

Guillery RW, Kaas JK (1971): A study of normal and congenitally abnormal retinogeniculate projections in cats. J Comp Neurol 143:73–100.

Guillery RW, Casagrande VA, Oberdorfer MD (1974): Congenitally abnormal vision in Siamese cats. Nature 252:195–199.

Hebb DO (1949): "Organization of Behavior." New York, John Wiley & Sons.

Heath CJ, Jones EG (1971): The anatomical organization of the suprasylvian gyrus in the cat. Ergebn Anat Entwickl 45:1–64.

Holländer H (1974): On the origin of corticotectal projections in the cat. Exp Brain Res 21:433–439.

Hubel DH, Wiesel TN (1965): Binocular interaction in striate cortex of kittens reared with artificial squint. J Neurophysiol 28:1041–1059.

Hubel DH, Wiesel TN (1971): Aberrant visual projections in the Siamese cat. J Physiol (Lond) 218:33–62.

Innocenti GM, Frost DO (1979): Effects of visual experience on the maturation of the efferent system to the corpus callosum. Nature 280:231–234.

Innocenti GM, Frost DO (1980): The postnatal development of visual callosal connections in the absence of visual experience or of the eyes. Exp Brain Res 39:365–375.

Kawamura S., Sprague JM, Niimi K (1974): Corticofugal projections from the visual cortices to the thalamus, pretectum and superior colliculus in the cat. J Comp Neurol 158:339–362.

Lane RH, Kaas JH, Allman J (1974): Visuotopic organization of the superior colliculus in normal and Siamese cats. Brain Res 70:413–430.

Lepore F, Samson A, Ptito M (1983): Le role du corps calleux dans le transfert interhémisphèrique d'apprentissage visuels chez le chat siamois. Rev Can Psychol 37:535–546.

Lund RD, Mitchell DE, Henry GH (1978): Squint-induced modification of callosal connections in cats. Brain Res 144:169–172.

Marzi CA (1980): Vision in Siamese cats. Trends Neurosci 3:165–169.

Marzi CA (1983): The neural basis of perceptual equivalence of visual stimuli in the cat. In Ewert JP, Capranica RR, Ingle DJ (eds): "Advances in Vertebrate Neuroethology." New York: Plenum Publ. Corp., pp 637–649.

Marzi CA, Di Stefano M (1978): Role of Siamese cat's crossed and uncrossed retinal fibres in pattern discrimination and interocular transfer. Arch Ital Biol 116:330–337.

Marzi CA, Simoni A, Di Stefano M (1976): Lack of binocularly driven neurones in the Siamese cat's visual cortex does not prevent successful interocular transfer of visual form discriminations. Brain Res 105:353–357.

Marzi CA, Di Stefano M, Simoni A (1979): Pathways of interocular transfer in Siamese cats. In Steele Russell I, Van Hof MW, Berlucchi G (eds): "Structure and Function of Cerebral Commissures." London: MacMillan Press, pp 299–309.

Marzi CA, Antonini A, Di Stefano M, Legg CR (1980): Callosum-dependent binocular interactions in the lateral suprasylvian area of Siamese cats which lack binocular neurons in areas 17 and 18. Brain Res 197:230–235.

Marzi CA, Antonini A, Di Stefano M, Legg CR (1982a): The contribution of the corpus callosum to receptive fields in the lateral suprasylvian visual areas of the cat. Behav Brain Res 4:155–176.

Marzi C, Lepore F, Bédard S, Di Stefano M (1982b): Binocular receptive fields of the lateral suprosylvian area (LSA), in strabismic cats: Importance of the corpus callosum. Invest Ophthal Vis Sci 22:88.

Orban GA (1984): "Neuronal Operations in the Visual Cortex." Berlin: Springer-Verlag.

Packwood J, Gordon B (1975): Stereopsis in normal domestic cat, Siamese cat, and cat raised with alternating monocular occlusion. J Neurophysiol 38:1485–1499.

Ptito M, Lepore F (1983): Effects of unilateral and bilateral lesions of the lateral suprasylvian area on learning and interhemispheric transfer of pattern discrimination in the cat. Behav Brain Res 7:211–237.

Shatz C (1977a): Abnormal interhemispheric connections in the visual system of Boston Siamese cats: A physiological study. J Comp Neurol 171:229–246.

Shatz C (1977b): Anatomy of interhemispheric connections in the visual system of Boston Siamese and ordinary cats. J Comp Neurol 173:497–518.

Shatz CJ, Kliot M (1982): Prenatal misrouting of the retinogeniculate pathway in Siamese cats. Nature 300:525–529.

Smith DC, Spear PD (1979): Effects of superior colliculus removal on receptive-field properties of neurons in lateral suprasylvian visual area of the cat. J Neurophysiol 42:57–75.

Spear PD, Baumann TP (1979): Effects of visual cortex removal on receptive-field properties of neurons in lateral suprasylvian visual area of the cat. J Neurophysiol 42:31–56.

Stent GS (1973): A physiological mechanism for Hebb's postulate of learning. Proc Natl Acad Sci USA 70:997–1001.

Von Grunau M (1982): Comparison of the effects of induced strabismus on binocularity in area 17 and the LS area in the cat. Brain Res 246:325–329.

Zeki S, Fries W (1980): Function of the corpus callosum in the Siamese cat. Proc R Soc Biol (Lond) 207:249–258.

Two Hemispheres—One Brain:
Functions of the Corpus Callosum, pages 315–333
© 1986 Alan R. Liss, Inc.

Localization of Visual Functions With Partially Split-Brain Monkeys

CHARLES R. HAMILTON AND BETTY A. VERMEIRE

Division of Biology, California Institute of Technology, Pasadena, California 91125

INTRODUCTION

In the 1950s Roger Sperry set the stage for the modern study of the functions of the cerebral commissures and of hemispheric specialization by developing with Ronald Myers the now classic split-brain preparation [Myers, 1961; Sperry, 1961]. Their original experiments with cats were the first to show convincingly that the corpus callosum transferred cognitively important information between the two cerebral hemispheres. Subsequently, the split-brain and related partially split-brain preparations were ingeniously exploited by Sperry and a number of colleagues to discover many of the capabilities and limitations of interhemispheric transfer of information in cats, monkeys, and other mammals [Doty and Negrao, 1973; Sperry, 1961, 1968]. Several chapters in this volume attest to the continuing vitality of this approach; in this chapter we will describe our recent attempts to separate and localize different components of visual perception by behavioral tests with partially split-brain monkeys.

While studying interhemispheric transfer through the cerebral commissures, Sperry and his colleagues made the correlated observation that cognitive functioning of the two separated hemispheres was independent: each side could perceive, learn, remember, and act on its own [Sperry, 1961]. This fascinating finding paved the way for later demonstrations with split-brain patients of specialized differences in cognitive functioning of the two halves of the human brain [Sperry et al., 1969; Sperry, 1982]. The influential hypothesis of complementary hemispheric superiorities based on fundamental differences in hemispheric processing that emerged from these studies [Bogen, 1969a,b; Levy, 1974; Sperry, 1974] provided a needed impetus and framework for interpreting the growing body of results from clinical studies of patients with unilateral brain damage. The ensuing explosion of research on lateralized processing in human beings, as indicated in several chapters of this book and in other recent reviews [Bradshaw and Nettleton, 1983;

Bryden, 1982; Corballis, 1983], is remarkable. We have summarized our split-brain studies that test for similar hemispheric specialization in monkeys in another book honoring Roger Sperry [Hamilton, 1985].

EXPERIMENTS WITH PARTIALLY SPLIT BRAINS

Many of the early split-brain studies with cats and monkeys showed that the corpus callosum was needed for interhemispheric transfer of learned visual pattern discriminations. Subsequent work established that the posteriormost 5–10 mm of the callosum in cats [Myers, 1959], 3–5 mm in monkeys [Hamilton and Brody, 1973; Hamilton unpublished], and approximately 10 mm in chimpanzees [Black and Myers, 1964] contain the critical fibers. In monkeys and chimpanzees, but not cats, the anterior commissure is also capable of transferring pattern discriminations interhemispherically [Doty and Negrao, 1973; Hamilton, 1982]. Visual discriminations based on brightness or movement in cats and primates also transfer via the forebrain commissures, although there is evidence that subcortical pathways may play a supporting role as we have discussed elsewhere [Peck et al., 1979].

The finding that interhemispheric transfer of visual discriminations may occur through more than one commissural pathway encourages looking for differences in the kinds of information that transfer through these different routes. Even within a pathway, such as the splenium of the corpus callosum, it may be possible to subdivide the fibers into functionally distinct groups that interconnect specific regions of the visual cortex. If so, then testing differential transfer through isolated bundles of fibers in partially split-brain monkeys should help reveal the functions of the visual areas they interconnect. This approach is especially intriguing now that over a dozen areas have been described, each with callosal connections and, presumably, specialized functions [Allman, 1977; Van Essen, 1985].

Anatomical Localization

It is well known that in monkeys the anterior commissure interconnects visual areas in the anterior inferotemporal cortex and the splenium interconnects visual areas in posterior inferotemporal and occipital cortices; this result has been repeatedly confirmed and refined with both anatomical [Pandya et al., 1971; Zeki, 1973; Jouandet and Gazzaniga, 1979; Van Essen, 1985] and physiological [Gross et al., 1976] techniques. However, neither the boundary between projections through the anterior commissure and the splenium nor the location in the splenium of fibers from different visual regions were known accurately when we initiated our behavioral studies of interhemispheric transfer in partially split-brain monkeys over a decade ago. Therefore, we also began to study the commissural location of fibers originating from several visual regions that interested us: the striate-prestriate border (V1/V2); the "movement area" in the superior temporal sulcus [Zeki, 1974], now usually termed MT; the "foveal prestriate cortex" [Gross et al., 1971], which was originally described behaviorally and presumably consists of the foveal portions of several more recently described areas (V3, V3a, VP, V4, VA); and the inferotemporal cortex (IT), containing at least two regions, TE and TEO [Iwai and Mishkin, 1969]. We used anterograde labeling with [^{3}H] proline or silver staining of degenerating fibers following discrete lesions to label the interhemispheric projections from these cortical visual regions. The commissural locations of the labeled fibers were determined by reconstructing the commissures from sections taken from the labeled hemisphere, and, where possible, by direct visualization of the label in sagittal sections of the commissures removed as a block from the unlabeled hemisphere. The locations of the injection sites or lesions were established with respect to recognizable histological features such as the V1/V2 border or the distinct myelination of MT. For label in less differentiated regions of the cortex, plots were made on a standard, flattened map of the visual cortex [Van Essen et al., 1982] and the area labeled inferred from the locations of visual areas in Van Essen's maps. This procedure worked surprisingly well in practice as judged by cross-checking these plots with those based on visible histological features. The results of these studies have appeared in brief format [Tieman et al., 1977; Hamilton, 1982; Hamilton et al., 1982].

The principal anatomical results are summarized in Figure 1. The location of the injection sites or lesion and the commissural location of the labeled fibers are depicted for 14 cases that were relatively clear-cut in their interpretation. Four other cases were less definitive because they had either complex labeling of several visual areas or did not produce any interhemispheric labeling. None of these cases, however, contradicted the results reported here, and each could be interpreted within the framework summarized next.

Three cases (V1/V2) showed that the fibers leaving the V1/V2 border on the lateral surface of the cortex pass through a very similar, restricted region in the ventral splenium. There is a suggestion of topographical mapping within this region, with fibers from more dorsal cortex passing slightly above those from more ventral cortex. One animal (VP) with an injection in the foveal portion of VP had label in the same splenial region. This was also true of a second monkey with label in VP (VP/VA), although its injection extended into foveal VA as well, presumably leading to the dorsal extension of the splenial label into the region characteristic of VA, as described below. For convenience, we use the designation VA to refer to the cortex subjacent to V4 as described by Van Essen [1985] and tentatively termed VA/V4 by him. The small area at the ventralmost part of the splenium that we did not label probably contains fibers from the V1/V2 border and and VP that lie in medial cortex. This is consistent with data reported by Pandya in this volume.

The V4 complex (V4 and VA) may well represent several areas [Van Essen, 1985]. Three monkeys labeled in this region sent fibers through the

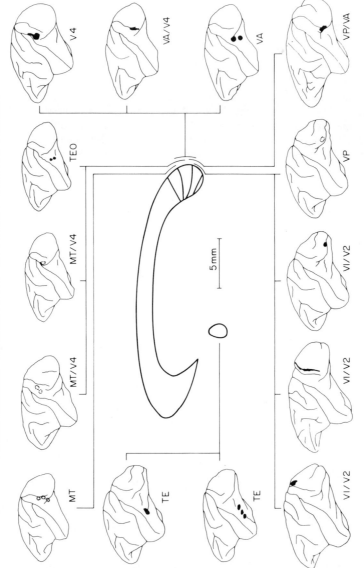

COMMISSURAL CONNECTIONS BETWEEN VISUAL AREAS

Fig. 1. Solid areas indicate injections of [³H] proline or lesions that were located on the exposed surface of the cerebral cortex. Dotted areas represent labeling in cortex buried in the sulci. The three segments indicated within the splenium contain, in descending order, fibers from MT, V4 + VA, and V1/V2 + VP. The anterior commissure contains fibers from TE.

splenium immediately dorsal to the V1/V2/VP segment. Label in VA appeared more ventral in the splenium than label in V4 proper. Two other monkeys that had label in V4 adjacent to and including part of area MT (MT/V4) sent fibers through the splenium dorsal and anterior to the preceding cases, again indicating some degree of topography within the V4/VA region of the splenium.

One monkey that had label restricted to MT showed label more dorsally than the two preceding cases that had label along the border of MT and V4. Taken together, they indicate that the fibers from MT cross anterior and dorsal to those from V4, which, in turn, are dorsal to VA.

Three monkeys had label confined to areas in the temporal lobe. One (TEO) that had an injection in the posterior IT within the transition zone TEO between TE and OA [Iwai and Mishkin, 1969] sent fibers through the splenium in essentially the same region as the two MT/V4 cases described above. If this single case is representative, then fibers from anterior TEO cross dorsal to those from adjacent VA, which includes the posterior portion of TEO. The other two monkeys (TE) were labeled in TE; they had commissural label only in the anterior commissure. Thus the ill-defined border between TE and TEO may be more easily definable by the separation of its commissural output than by cytoarchitecture. This line of demarcation appears to correspond well with the boundaries of the inferotemporal and foveal prestriate cortex defined behaviorally [Iwai and Mishkin, 1969; Gross et al., 1971].

For several of the cases described above, commissural projections to heterotopic areas were about as prevalent as those to homotopic areas. They were most dense to layer IV but often had periodic, columnar extensions throughout the cortical layers. In general, the heterotopic projections went to the next area in the cortical hierarchy, as described by Van Essen [Maunsell and Van Essen, 1983; Van Essen, 1985]; in no case did we observe commissural connections to preceding areas in the cortical hierarchy. Heterotopic projections were particularly striking from VA to TEO and TE and from MT to MST.

These anatomical findings have important implications for studying the interhemispheric transfer of visual information with behavioral techniques. First, the separation of splenial connections from different regions of the visual cortex is surprisingly systematic and seems sufficient to enable partial surgical disconnection of visual areas in the two hemispheres. Thus, for example, it should be possible to study interhemispheric transfer from V1/V2 and VP in the absence of transfer from other areas, or from MT and possibly anterior TEO without contributions to transfer from preceding visual areas. Of course, careful histological determination of the extent of innervation of the remaining splenial connections would be required for adequate interpretation of behavioral results, but this may be accomplished by labeling the surviving fibers before sacrifice.

Second, the anatomical results make it clear that interhemispheric transfer of pattern discriminations can originate from at least two different areas of visual cortex: the anterior IT cortex (TE) via the anterior commissure and the posterior IT (TEO) or before via the splenium. This extends an earlier suggestion that interhemispheric transfer of visual discriminations depends on transfer between the inferotemporal cortices [Seacord et al., 1979]. Furthermore, it again brings up the question of whether transfer of different types of visual discriminations may utilize pathways connecting other areas in the cortical hierarchy [Hamilton, 1982].

Third, transfer of pattern discriminations through the splenium need not involve a relay through the prestriate cortex of the receiving hemisphere in order to reach the contralateral IT cortex as is often suggested [Seacord et al., 1979; Ungerleider and Mishkin, 1982]. Heterotopic connections from the prestriate cortex (VA) to the IT cortex (TEO, TE) appeared sufficiently widespread in our cases and in those of others [Desimone et al., 1980] to support such transfer directly. In fact, heterotopic connections from several areas are so conspicuous that we wonder if they are not the principal route of communication in most cases of interhemispheric transfer. This possibility is independent of the question of whether interhemispheric transfer results from mechanisms of simple convergence of input from each hemisphere onto "bihemispheric" cells or whether more specialized mechanisms for transfer exist, a controversy we have discussed extensively elsewhere [Hamilton, 1982]. It would, however, relegate homotopic connections to wiring up receptive fields that straddle the vertical midline rather than to supporting interhemispheric transfer by convergence at that level. Experiments with combined unilateral cortical lesions and partial hemispheric disconnection could test these possibilities.

Behavioral Localization

Although we are now testing partially split-brain monkeys with different segments of the splenium intact, most of our data comes from subjects with coarser subdivision of the commissures. Specifically, we have tested transfer of several types of visual tasks through the commissures of the midbrain roof, the splenium of the corpus callosum, the anterior commissure, and the anterior third of the corpus callosum. The tasks included stereopsis along the vertical meridian of the visual field; interhemispheric transfer of tilt aftereffects; transfer of discrimination learning based on cues differing in pattern, orientation, direction of movement, or facial features; and transfer of learning sets. They were chosen because there is evidence for differential localization of their neural processing and, presumably, of their routes for interhemispheric transfer.

Stereopsis.

The perception of stereopsis requires a precise comparison of the images from each eye. Most binocular interactions occur intrahemispherically as would be expected from the overlapping, in-register projections from each eye, but along the vertical meridian of the visual field interhemispheric connections may play a role [Berlucchi and Rizzolatti, 1968; Bishop and Henry, 1971; Berlucchi, 1972]. Anatomical and physiological results show that the cortical representations of the vertical meridian are richly connected to the opposite side by callosal fibers [Berlucchi, 1972; Van Essen et al., 1982], and neurons along the vertical meridian have binocular properties based on callosal connections that are appropriate for stereopsis [Berlucchi and Rizzolatti, 1968]. A limited amount of behavioral data also suggests commissural participation in midline stereopsis [Blakemore, 1970; Mitchell and Blakemore, 1970; Timney and Lansdowne, 1981]. We decided to test for preservation of stereopsis in split-chiasm monkeys with the eventual goal of determining which commissural segments and, hence, which cortical areas were used. Conceivably, different regions would be involved in different types of stereopsis such as fine and coarse or local and global.

We first trained three normal monkeys to discriminate between two simple patterns seen as dynamic random-dot stereograms. After learning with a crossed disparity of about .5°, they easily generalized to crossed and uncrossed disparities between .1° and 1°. One monkey continued to perform well after section of its forebrain commissures. By contrast, the other two monkeys failed to distinguish the patterns following section of the optic chiasm despite heroic efforts to retrain them. It seems unlikely that this failure represents a basic inadequacy of the commissures to support midline stereopsis as split-chiasm cats appear successful at discriminating depth [Timney and Lansdowne, 1981]. Perhaps dynamic random-dot stereograms or the specific parameters used were not appropriate for revealing midline stereopsis. At any rate, we cannot test the sufficiency of different commissural segments until we can demonstrate stereopsis with split-chiasm monkeys.

To complement the previous approach, we have begun to look for deficits in midline stereopsis in subjects with the cerebral commissures sectioned. We used human patients rather than monkeys because control of eye fixation is necessary. In preliminary tests, three patients tested in free vision had no difficulty seeing stimuli presented as dynamic random-dot stereograms with either crossed or uncrossed disparities between 5' and 40'. For the experiments proper we chose a 2° hexagonal stimulus with 20' crossed disparity which was flashed for 100–200 msec at different positions on the horizontal meridian within the central 10° of the visual field. Because we did not want the patients to know in advance the position of the stimulus and because we did not want to overtax their patience, we measured the percent correct performance for a stimulus of constant duration rather than the relative thresholds at known positions. The subjects were asked to point to the position of the flashed stimulus if seen and to a dot well below the fixation point if not seen. The left hand was used to respond to stimuli presented to the left of center and the right hand for stimuli presented to the right in order to avoid verbal report, which would favor the left hemisphere.

Representative results for these patients and six normal subjects are shown in Figure 2. Two of the patients, N.G. and R.Y., showed a midline deficit consistent with that expected if commissural connections play a prominent role in stereopsis. Because small deficits in stereopsis with central vision have been reported for normal subjects [Richards, 1970; Breitmeyer et al., 1975] we confirmed that deficits also were present 5° above

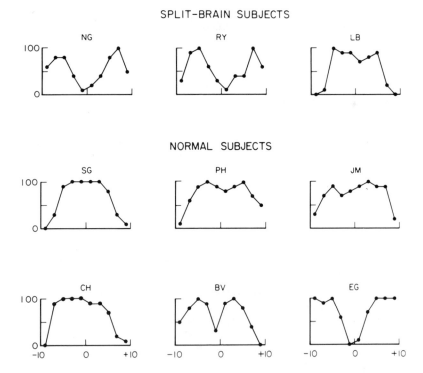

PERCENT DETECTION OF A SMALL FLASHED STIMULUS
vs. POSITION IN THE VISUAL FIELD (DEGREES)

SPLIT-BRAIN SUBJECTS

NORMAL SUBJECTS

Fig. 2. The relative performance for detecting dynamic random-dot stereograms, flashed for less than 200 msec and subtending 2° (split-brain patients) or 1.5° (normal subjects), is plotted for different eccentricities along the horizontal meridian.

and below the horizontal meridian. Furthermore, no midline scotomata were observed with monocular control tests using similar, non-stereoscopic stimuli. The third subject, L.B., did not show a comparable midline loss. Although L.B. has frequently shown less severe split-brain symptoms than the other patients, this result was unexpected because he had apparently shown a central deficit when tested with simple line stimuli and large 2° disparities [Mitchell and Blakemore, 1971]. Conceivably, only coarse stereopsis depends on commissural connections [Bishop and Henry, 1971; Berlucchi, 1972] and the 20' disparity we used may have been within L.B.'s limits for fine stereopsis and therefore not affected by commissural section. Conversely, the 20' disparity may have represented coarse stereopsis for N.G. and R.Y. and therefore may have been affected by severing the commissures. This argument assumes there is some meaning to the concepts of fine and coarse stereopsis when applied to viewing random-dot stereograms, which is not obvious. Alternatively, N.G. and R.Y. may be stereo-anomalous independent of their surgery as has been reported for a surprisingly large proportion of "normal" subjects [Richards, 1971]. In fact, one of our normal subjects (E.G.) showed a midline deficit rather like that of N.G. and R.Y. Tests with different amounts and directions of disparity and additional types of stimuli should determine if the split-brain subjects are truly different from the normal population. Despite these qualifications we feel that, overall, our results favor a participation of the commissures in stereopsis, accompanied by considerable variability in the extent to which the commissures are normally used for midline stereopsis.

Tilt aftereffects.

After viewing a field of lines tilted about 10° from vertical, an objectively vertical line appears tilted a degree or two in the opposite direction. This illusion is referred to as the tilt aftereffect. For subjects with normal vision a monocularly induced tilt aftereffect transfers to the unadapted eye with an efficiency of about 70%. Because stereoblind subjects usually fail to show such interocular transfer, it has been proposed that the binocular neurons in V1 or V2 thought to be responsible for stereopsis are also responsible for transfer of tilt aftereffects [Movshon et al., 1972; Mitchell and Ware, 1974]. For monkeys with section of the optic chiasm, any interocular transfer would require the cerebral commissures. Furthermore, if the proposed dependency on binocular neurons in V1 or V2 is correct, then the ventral splenium should be crucial for transfer. We have begun to study this possibility.

We first had to develop a means for convincing our monkeys to look at a grating of lines for many minutes in order to establish an aftereffect and maintain it throughout the testing session. This was accomplished by requiring the monkeys to monitor a screen filled by the grating for the appearance of a blank field that unpredictably replaced the grating at 5–15-

second intervals. If the monkey then pressed the screen quickly, a line oriented somewhere between $\pm$ 10° from vertical was briefly flashed. The monkey had previously learned to push this line if vertical and avoid it if tilted in order to receive a food reward. An aftereffect was indicated by systematic choices of an appropriately tilted line as vertical after adapting to a tilted grating but not after viewing a vertical grating. This method was successful, as indicated by preliminary experiments with binocular adaptation in five monkeys as shown in Figure 3. The average aftereffect of .72° was significant (P < .005) and was about half the magnitude of that measured for human subjects tested with the same apparatus and procedures. We attribute the reduced magnitude to the fact that the monkeys only watched the grating about 75% of the time, while the human subjects watched nearly 100% of the time.

To test for interhemispheric transfer of the aftereffect, four of the partially split-brain monkeys adapted to a tilted grating monocularly and were tested for aftereffects with either the adapted or unadapted eye in a series of 32 sessions that balanced various extraneous variables. These aftereffects are also shown in Figure 3. The average aftereffect for the adapted eye was .55° (P < .005) and for the unadapted eye .51° (P < .005). These results show that good interocular transfer was present and that both the anterior

TILT AFTEREFFECTS IN DEGREES FOR FIVE PARTIALLY SPLIT-BRAIN MONKEYS

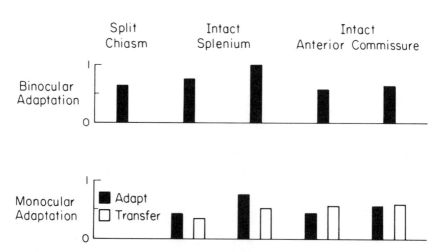

Fig. 3. The magnitude in degrees of the tilt aftereffect is shown following binocular adaptation in the upper plot. The magnitude of the aftereffect measured separately with the adapted and unadapted eyes following exposure of the adapted eye is shown in the lower plot.

commissure and the splenium can mediate interhemispheric transfer of the aftereffect.

Because interhemispheric transfer of the tilt aftereffect may occur through the anterior commissure as well as through the splenium, it does not appear that the generation and transfer of the aftereffect is restricted to binocular neurons in V1 and V2. Presumably binocular neurons from later levels of visual processing such as TE can also participate. We cannot infer that the neuronal populations involved in tilt aftereffects differ from those involved in stereopsis, however, because we do not yet know the capabilities of different commissural pathways for supporting midline stereopsis. These questions should be answerable with the procedures we have developed.

Discrimination learning.

In contrast to the experiments just described, the ones discussed next involve learning to distinguish two stimuli and therefore may involve additional regions of the cerebral cortex that, in turn, may utilize additional routes for interhemispheric transfer. It must be recognized, however, that learning or memory per se need not transfer, for transfer of basic sensory information could be sufficient for both hemispheres to learn the discriminations independently [Berlucchi, 1972]. In fact, it has been our position that this more parsimonious mechanism of sensory-perceptual transfer is sufficient to account for most of the existing behavioral data and therefore should be preferred until convincing counterexamples are reported [Hamilton, 1982]. If differential transfer of learned discriminations occurs through specific commissural pathways, then, it presumably reflects basic specializations in the cortical processing of the sensory information being discriminated rather than transfer of learning.

We have tested partially split-brain monkeys with either the splenium or the anterior commissure intact for interhemispheric transfer of discriminations based on several submodalities of vision. Other preparations, such as normal or split-chiasm monkeys, which should transfer, and split-brain monkeys, which should not transfer, were tested for comparison. The specific stimulus categories were chosen because physiological or behavioral data suggested their processing might depend on different regions of the cerebral cortex. The discriminations were based on (1) *patterns*, presented as two-dimensional geometrical shapes subtending about 5°–7° of visual angle; (2) *orientation*, made by inverting one of a pair of asymmetric patterns to give up-down differences, or by tilting one of two grids of lines by 45°; (3) *direction of movement*, produced by rotating a logarithmic spiral subtending about 30° clockwise or counterclockwise, or by changing the direction by 90° or 180° that a small field of dots moved; and (4) *facial features*, presented as sets of photographs of different monkeys' faces, or as different facial expressions made by an individual monkey. Most of these stimuli are pictured in other reports [Hamilton and Tieman, 1973; Hamilton, 1985]. The surgical and training procedures are the same as those routinely used at Caltech [Sperry, 1968; Hamilton and Tieman, 1973]. In brief, the monkeys were taught with one eye to discriminate stimuli for a food reward and then were tested with the other eye for transfer of training. The amount of transfer was expressed as a percentage of savings based on the errors-through-criterion made by the first and second eyes, 100 (1st − 2nd)/(1st + 2nd), and as a difference in initial transfer between the two eyes based on the percentage of correct responses made on the first 40 trials with each eye (2nd − 1st). The results for the savings measure are shown in Figure 4.

The most general finding is an ability of either the splenium or the anterior commissure to transfer information critical to the discriminations tested irrespective of the category of visual stimulus that was learned. The magnitude of transfer was often less than that for normal or split-chiasm monkeys but greater than the near-zero transfer of split-brain monkeys. This confirms several earlier studies that used patterns [Hamilton, 1982] and extends the conclusion to additional submodalities of vision. The approximate equivalence of transfer through the two commissural routes is initially rather surprising because it seems to imply that the anterior inferotemporal cortex has access to all the categories of visual information that we tested in contrast to our expectations based on separation of functions in the cortex. However, this approximate equivalence may result from a common role of the inferotemporal cortex in the learning of any visual discrimination. If so, the specific category of visual stimuli being processed may be indicated by more subtle differences in the relative efficiency of transfer through the two routes. For example, the ratio of transfer by the anterior commissure to that by the splenium is greatest for discrimination of facial features (.93), an ability that may involve processing by areas in the superior temporal sulcus [Perrett et al., 1982] that appear richly interconnected by the anterior commissure [Jouandet and Gazzaniga, 1979] as well as the splenium [Pandya et al., 1971]. By contrast, the ratio for transfer of discriminations based on orientation is much lower (.47), which suggests that the anterior commissure has poorer access to this kind of information. This is in keeping with other behavioral data that suggest less participation of inferotemporal cortex in learning [Gross, 1978] and transfer [Butler, 1979] of discriminations of orientation. The other categories had ratios ranging from .73 to .76, perhaps indicating an intermediate level of temporal lobe involvement. More data are needed before further pursuing this argument, but at least these tentative findings of differential transfer are encouraging to our goal of fractionating interhemispheric transfer into more basic components.

Another finding of interest is the significant transfer of the discrimination of a rotating spiral through the commissures of the midbrain. Distinguishing an expanding from a contracting spiral showed about 30% savings

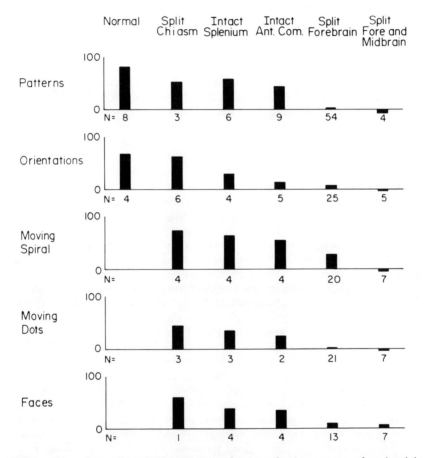

Fig. 4. The average magnitude of interocular transfer (percentage of savings) is indicated for six groups of monkeys with different amounts of hemispheric disconnection. Five categories of visual discriminations were learned by monkeys from the experimental groups. The number of subjects tested to date is indicated below each bar.

(P < .01) in the split-forebrain monkeys but no transfer in the monkeys with additional section of the commissures of the midbrain roof. This extends the original findings of Tieman [1974] and provides a baseline against which transfer via the forebrain commissures may be evaluated. It should be noted that it is not simply movement that recruits the midbrain, as shown by the lack of transfer in split-forebrain monkeys of discriminations between fields of moving dots. Rather, a more specific feature, perhaps the larger size of the spiral and the resulting increase in peripheral stimulation, invokes midbrain mechanisms.

In summary, some interpretable division of labor in transfer by the interhemispheric commissures is indicated by these results. More specific conclusions await results from our experiments that are in progress with monkeys that have partial disconnection of the splenium. Preliminary results from these subjects are already tantalizing and suggest that differential transfer will occur through different splenial segments in accord with the presumed specializations of the cortical regions they connect.

Learning sets.

The experiments with stereopsis and tilt aftereffects tested for transfer of visual information thought to be processed early in the visual hierarchy; the discrimination experiments tested for transfer of several kinds of visual information that should depend on processing at later levels and included the possibility of transfer of learning or memory per se. In most experiments it is hard to identify or separate sensory transfer from mnemonic transfer and, therefore, it is difficult to determine if learning and memory as such can transfer across the commissures [Hamilton, 1982]. One possible way to test this is to examine the interhemispheric transfer of learning sets. Learning sets are often thought to represent the learning of rules or strategies for solving problems. They are manifested as the increased ease with which successive problems in a series are learned, culminating in one or few trial learning after extensive practice with a particular type of discrimination. We expected that learning sets would show transfer through the splenium or the anterior commissure because the individual problems can themselves transfer. At minimum, this should allow each hemisphere to develop its own learning set. We also expected that split-brain monkeys would not show transfer because of the presumed cortical nature of this ability. Because the frontal cortex is thought to be involved in this higher-order process [Mishkin, 1964], we felt that the anterior portions of the corpus callosum might allow significant transfer of learning sets even though individual discriminations leading to their formation could not transfer. This would permit a separation of sensory transfer from transfer of learning and memory. These experiments were originally designed and undertaken by Sullivan [1971] and continued by others in our laboratory; similar experiments with object learning sets were independently performed by Noble [1973].

We chose to study the development and transfer of reversal learning sets because of the ease with which training could be accomplished. To establish a reversal set, the monkeys were first taught a simple pattern discrimination through one eye. After a 90% criterion was reached, the reward values were reversed and the subject learned to choose the previously unrewarded stimulus. This was repeated until fifty such reversals were trained to ensure that the reversing strategy was well established before the second eye was trained in the same manner.

These results are summarized in Figure 5. It is apparent that the split-brain subjects showed no consistent transfer of the learning set when the second side was tested; the pattern of progressive reduction of trials taken to reverse is similar for both sides. By contrast, the monkeys with the anterior commissure left intact showed a substantial advantage when tested with the second eye, indicating that a learning set transferred to or was developed independently by the second side. We expect that similar results

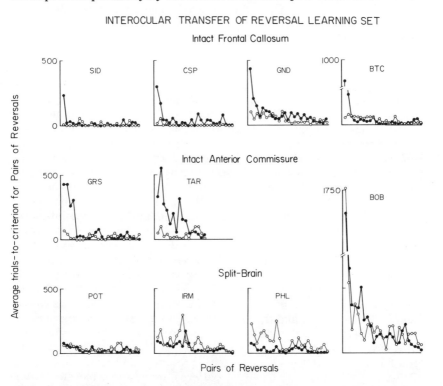

Fig. 5. The development of reversal learning sets by the eye trained first (filled circles) and the eye trained second (open circles) is depicted for three groups of monkeys with differing degrees of brain bisection.

will be found with monkeys having an intact splenium, but these data are not yet available. Most importantly, the monkeys with the anterior one-third to one-half of the corpus callosum left intact also showed a significant advantage when the second hemisphere was tested. This was in marked contrast to their inability to transfer a variety of individual discriminations that were tested in control experiments.

We conclude that learning sets formed in one hemisphere can transfer through or are otherwise made available to the other hemisphere by the anterior corpus callosum. The possibility that the second side independently develops a learning set is contraindicated by the lack of transfer through the frontal callosum of the individual sensory discriminations necessary for such development. At present, the transfer of learning sets represents the only convincing example of interhemispheric transfer of higher-order cognitive information in nonhuman animals. Despite interpretations to the contrary, all other cases of transfer of learning, memory, or other higher-order processes can be explained more parsimoniously in terms of sensory transfer accompanied by independent learning by the indirectly trained hemisphere [Hamilton, 1982].

CONCLUSIONS

To summarize, we have shown with anatomical methods that commissural connections between visual areas are quite well localized within the splenium of the corpus callosum and the anterior commissure of macaque monkeys. These commissural regions correspond well with those that are known from behavioral experiments to be necessary and sufficient for inter-hemispheric transfer of a variety of visual discriminations. Furthermore, the localization of connections is distinct enough to allow selective surgical disconnection of designated visual areas while leaving others interconnected. Thus by determining behaviorally what kinds of visual information can transfer in monkeys with different commissural segments intact, we can make inferences about the functions of the visual regions that connect through these segments. Our experiments with this method so far have produced the following results: (1) The cerebral commissures appear to be used for midline stereopsis produced by dynamic random-dot stereograms. (2) Contrary to expectation, interhemispheric transfer of tilt aftereffects, a sensory adaptation, can occur through the anterior commissure as well as through the splenium and therefore appears to involve mechanisms in the anterior inferotemporal cortex as well as mechanisms prior to that level. Thus sites of binocular convergence in V1 or V2 are not necessary for transfer of the aftereffect as is frequently presumed. (3) Transfer of a variety of visual discriminations based on patterns, orientation, movement, and facial features can transfer through the anterior commissure as well as the splenium. This suggests that many if not all forms of visual discrimination learning utilize the inferotemporal cortex, with gradations in the magnitude of transfer through the anterior commissure probably reflecting the more cortically localized aspects of specialized stimulus processing. Preliminary experiments with monkeys having more precise disconnection of the splenium have given hints of separation of function for categories of visual stimulation such as orientation, movement, and facial features. (4) Discriminating direction of movement in some cases utilizes midbrain mechanisms as well as cortical ones. (5) The ability to learn rules or strategies for solving visual problems involves mechanisms in the frontal cortex as shown by the transfer of learning sets through the anterior corpus callosum. Taken together, these results support a hierarchical organization of visual processing that is analyzable without cortical lesions by behavioral tests with partially split-brain monkeys.

ACKNOWLEDGMENTS

We thank S.B. Tieman and M.V. Sullivan for initiating and performing some of the experiments discussed in this chapter and R.W. Sperry for his continuing support and criticism. Most of the research was supported by MH-35323.

REFERENCES

Allman J (1977): Evolution of the visual system in the early primates. In Sprague JM, Epstein AN (eds): "Progress in Psychobiology and Physiological Psychology." San Francisco: Academic Press, Vol 7, pp 1–53.

Berlucchi G (1972): Anatomical and physiological aspects of visual functions of corpus callosum. Brain Res 37:371–392.

Berlucchi G, Rizzolatti G (1968): Binocularly driven neurons in visual cortex of split-chiasm cats. Science 159:308–310.

Bishop PO, Henry GH (1971): Spatial vision. Ann Rev Psychol 22:119–160.

Black P, Myers RE (1964): Visual function of the forebrain commissures in the chimpanzee. Science 146:799–800.

Blakemore C (1970): Binocular depth discrimination and the optic chiasm. Vision Res 10:43–47.

Bogen JE (1969a): The other side of the brain. I: Dysgraphia and dyscopia following cerebral commissurotomy. Bull LA Neurol Soc 34:73–105.

Bogen JE (1969b): The other side of the brain. II: An appositional mind. Bull LA Neurol Soc 34:135–162.

Bradshaw JL, Nettleton NC (1983): "Human Cerebral Asymmetry." Englewood Cliffs, NJ: Prentice Hall.

Breitmeyer B, Julesz B, Kropfl W (1975): Dynamic random-dot stereograms reveal up-down anisotropy and left-right isotropy between cortical hemifields. Science 187:269–270.

Bryden MP (1982): "Laterality: Functional Asymmetry in the Intact Brain." New York: Academic Press.

Butler SR (1979): Interhemispheric transfer of visual information via the corpus callosum and anterior commissure in the monkey. In Russell IS, van Hof MW, Berlucchi G (eds): "Structure and Function of Cerebral Commissures." Baltimore: University Park Press, pp 343–357.

Corballis MC (1983): "Human Laterality." New York: Academic Press.

Desimone R, Fleming J, Gross CG (1980): Prestriate afferents to inferior temporal cortex: An HRP study. Brain Res 184:41–55.

Doty RW, Negrao N (1973): Forebrain commissures and vision. In Jung R (ed): "Handbook of Sensory Physiology." Berlin: Springer, Vol VII/3, part B.

Gross CG (1978): Inferior temporal lesions do not impair discrimination of rotated patterns in monkeys. J Comp Physiol Psychol 92:1095–1109.

Gross CG, Bender DB, Mishkin M (1976): Contributions of the corpus callosum and the anterior commissure to visual activation of inferior temporal neurons. Brain Res 131:227–239.

Gross CG, Cowey A, Manning FJ (1971): Further analysis of visual discrimination deficits following foveal prestriate and inferotemporal lesions in rhesus monkeys. J Comp Physiol Psychol 76:1–7.

Hamilton CR (1982): Mechanisms of interocular equivalence. In Ingle DJ, Goodale MA, Mansfield RJW (eds): "Analysis of Visual Behavior." Cambridge, MA: MIT Press, pp 693–717.

Hamilton CR (1985): Hemispheric specialization in monkeys. In Trevarthen CB (ed): "Brain Circuits and Functions of the Mind: Festschrift for RW Sperry." Cambridge: Cambridge University Press (in press).

Hamilton CR, Brody BA (1973): Separation of visual functions within the corpus callosum of monkeys. Brain Res 49:185–189.

Hamilton CR, Tieman SB (1973): Interocular transfer of mirror image discriminations by chiasm-sectioned monkeys. Brain Res 64:241–255.

Hamilton CR, Tieman SB, Vermeire BA, Meyer RL (1982): Localization of interhemispheric visual connections in macaques. Soc Neurosci Abst 80:628.

Iwai E, Mishkin M (1969): Further evidence on the locus of the visual area in the temporal lobe of the monkey. Exp Neurol 25:585–594.

Jouandet ML, Gazzaniga MS (1979): Cortical field of origin of the anterior commissure of the rhesus monkey. Exp Neurol 66:381–397.

Levy J (1974): Psychobiological implications of bilateral asymmetry. In Dimond SJ, Beaumont JG (eds): "Hemispheric Dominance and the Human Brain." London: Elek Science, pp 121–183.

Maunsell JHR, Van Essen DC (1983): The connections of the middle temporal visual area (MT) and their relationship to a cortical hierarchy in the macaque monkey. J Neurosci 3:2563–2586.

Mishkin M (1964): Perseveration of central sets after frontal lesions in monkeys. In Warren JM, Akert K (eds): "The Frontal Granular Cortex and Behavior." New York: McGraw-Hill, pp 219–241.

Mitchell DE, Blakemore C (1970): Binocular depth perception and the corpus callosum. Vision Res 10:49–54.

Mitchell DE, Ware C (1974): Interocular transfer of a visual aftereffect in normal and stereoblind humans. J Physiol 236:707–721.

Movshon JA, Chambers BEI, Blakemore C (1972): Interocular transfer in normal humans and those who lack stereopsis. Perception 1:483–490.

Myers RE (1959): Localization of function in the corpus callosum. Arch Neurol 1:44–47.

Myers RE (1961): Corpus callosum and visual gnosis. In Fessard A (ed): "Brain Mechanisms and Learning." Oxford: Blackwell, pp 481–505.

Noble, J (1973): Interocular transfer in the monkey: Rostral corpus callosum mediates transfer of object learning set but not of single-problem learning. Brain Res 50:147–162.

Pandya DN, Karol EA, Heilbroun D (1971): The topographical distribution of interhemispheric projections in the corpus callosum of the rhesus monkey. Brain Res 32:31–43.

Peck CK, Crewther SG, Hamilton CR (1979): Partial interocular transfer of brightness and movement discrimination by split-brain cats. Brain Res 163:61–75.

Perrett DI, Rolls ET, Caan W (1982): Visual neurones responsive to faces in the monkey temporal cortex. Exp Brain Res 47:329–342.

Richards W (1970): Stereopsis and stereoblindness. Exp Brain Res 10:380–388.

Richards W (1971): Anomalous stereoscopic depth perception. J Opt Soc Am 61:410–414.

Seacord L, Gross CG, Mishkin M (1979): Role of inferior temporal cortex in interhemispheric transfer. Brain Res 167:259–272.

Sperry RW (1961): Cerebral organization and behavior. Science 133:1749–1757.

Sperry RW (1968): Mental unity following surgical disconnection of the cerebral hemispheres. Harvey Lect 62:293–323.

Sperry RW (1974): Lateral specialization in the surgically separated hemispheres. In Schmitt FO, Worden FG (eds): "The Neurosciences Third Study Program." Cambridge MA: MIT Press, pp 5–9.

Sperry RW (1982): Some effects of disconnecting the cerebral hemispheres. Science 217:1223–1226.

Sperry RW, Gazzaniga MS, Bogen JE (1969): Interhemispheric relationships: the neocortical commissures; syndromes of hemisphere disconnection. In Vinken PJ, Bruyn GW (eds): "Handbook of Clinical Neurology." Amsterdam: North Holland, vol 4, pp 273–290.

Sullivan MV (1971): Interhemispheric transfer of visual discriminations and learning sets via anterior commissure and anterior corpus callosum in monkeys. Ph.D. dissertation, Stanford University, Stanford, CA.

Tieman SB (1974): Interhemispheric transfer of visual information in partially split-brain monkeys. Ph.D. dissertation, Stanford University, Stanford, CA.

Tieman SB, Hamilton CR, Meyer RL (1977): Commissural connections of visual areas in the macaque. Anat Rec 187:731.

Timney B, Lansdowne G (1981): Preservation of stereopsis in cats following neonatal section of the optic chiasm. Soc Neurosci Abst 7:674.

Ungerleider LG, Mishkin M (1982): Two cortical visual systems. In Ingle DJ, Goodale MA, Mansfield RJW (eds): "Analysis of Visual Behavior." Cambridge, MA: MIT Press, pp 549–586.

Van Essen DC (1985): Functional organization of primate visual cortex. In Jones EG, Peters AA (eds): "Cerebral Cortex." New York: Plenum Press (in press).

Van Essen DC, Newsome WTN, Bixby JL (1982): The pattern of interhemispheric connections and its relationship to extrastriate visual areas in the macaque monkey. J Neurosci 2:265–283.

Zeki SM (1973): Comparison of the cortical degeneration in the visual regions of the temporal lobe of the monkey following section of the anterior commissure and the splenium. J Comp Neurol 148:167–176.

Zeki SM (1974): Functional organization of a visual area in the posterior bank of the superior temporal sulcus of the rhesus monkey. J Physiol 236:549–573.

Two Hemispheres—One Brain:
Functions of the Corpus Callosum, pages 335–350
© 1986 Alan R. Liss, Inc.

Neural Mechanisms for Stereopsis in Cats

MAURICE PTITO, FRANCO LEPORÉ, MARYSE LASSONDE,
CAROLE DION, AND DOM MICELI

Groupe de Recherche en Neuropsychologie, Université du Québec à Trois-Rivières (M.P., M.L., C.D., D.M.), Centre de Recherche en Sciences Neurologiques (M.P., F.L.), and Département de Psychologie (F.L.), Université de Montréal, Québec, Canada

"The neural mechanisms that have recently been proposed as a basis for stereopsis have relied almost entirely on evidence obtained from the cat. It is a serious criticism for this work that there is as yet no behavioral evidence for stereopsis in this animal. The application of the random-dot technique to the cat should resolve this criticism" [Bishop and Henry, 1971].

INTRODUCTION

Perception of depth depends upon monocular and binocular depth cues. With the invention by Wheatstone in 1838 of the stereoscope, the monocular cues to depth perception were eliminated and it was shown that retinal image disparity was the one essential requirement to see depth. Indeed, in most mammals, including man, the horizontal separation of the eyes is such that each eye receives a slightly different image of the three-dimensional visual world. The difference between the retinal images (horizontal retinal disparity) is used by the brain during the fusion process to provide the sense of depth. This binocular extraction of the depth dimension is called stereopsis. We owe to Julesz [1960] the demonstration that stereoscopic depth perception is possible not only without monocular or binocular cues except retinal image disparity but also without monocular form perception. Julesz [1960] developed computer-generated random-dot stereograms that, when viewed monocularly, appear uniform and do not have any recognizable feature or form. The two random-dot patterns are identical except for a central region that is displaced laterally in one of them with respect to the same region in the other. When viewed through a stereoscope, binocular fusion produces a strong impression of depth with the central configuration appearing in front of or behind its surround. Presumably, this process might depend upon (1) a local stereopsis mechanism by which the depth information is first extracted on the basis of a dot-by-dot comparison and (2) a global mechanism which is needed to select among different possible sets of corresponding retinal pairs, one set of matched pairs that, by their depth value, can provide the recognition of the 3-D form [Julesz, 1971]. When considering the spatial range over which stereopsis operates for a given fixation point, the local stereoscopic mechanism may be further subdivided into two levels of stereoscopic perception. One, referred to as patent or fine stereopsis, operates over a narrow range of spatial disparities (.5°), while the other, referred to as qualitative or coarse stereopsis, corresponds to the perception in depth of images that are separated by a much larger range of retinal disparities (up to 7–10°) [Bishop, 1981]. Any comprehensive neural theory of stereopsis must thus take into account the existence of these different processes as well as the fact that stereoscopic depth perception may precede and be independent of neural mechanisms underlying form perception.

PHYSIOLOGICAL SUBSTRATES

In the late sixties, disparity-sensitive cells were found in the striate cortex of cats [Barlow et al., 1967; Nikara et al., 1968] that could well subserve stereopsis depth perception. The presence of these "depth cells" was later confirmed and their properties specified not only in the cat [Pettigrew et al., 1968; Joshua and Bishop, 1970; Bishop et al., 1971; Hubel and Wiesel, 1973; Von der Heydt et al., 1978; Fisher and Krueger, 1979; Ferster, 1981] but also in the monkey [Hubel and Wiesel, 1970; Poggio and Fisher, 1977; Poggio and Talbot, 1981; Poggio, 1984]. Initially, Hubel and Wiesel [1970, 1973] had reported these disparity-sensitive neurons to be present only in area 18 (V2) of both species' cortex, which led them to conclude that the elaboration and processing of stereoperception happens outside the primary visual cortex. However, studies carried out in the alert monkey under conditions of normal binocular vision have shown the presence of disparity sensitive cells not only in the parastriate (V2) cortex but also in the primary visual area (V1) [Poggio and Fisher, 1977; Poggio and Talbot, 1981; Poggio, 1984]. The authors were able to distinguish several types of stereoscopic neurons, which they grouped into two categories. In the first, they included cells that were disparity sensitive over a limited range and whose responses to stimuli could be differentiated into two classes: tuned excitatory and tuned inhibitory neurons. The second category comprised neurons sensitive to a wide range of retinal disparities having a reciprocal selectivity for crossed and uncrossed disparities (the far and near neurons). The properties of the tuned and reciprocal cortical cells make them appropriate to mediate, respectively, fine and coarse stereopsis mechanisms [Bishop, 1981; Poggio, 1984]. Furthermore, some of these cells could have their responses elicited by random-dot stereograms [Poggio, 1984]. While tuned and reciprocal cells showed no functional relationship with the simple complex classification, cells sensitive to random-dot stereograms were all of the complex type [Poggio, 1984]. It thus seems that complex cells have the unique capacity of solving the global correspondence problem by responding to the "correct" binocular matches over the receptive field in the two eyes. These neurophysiological data obtained on monkeys have yet to be verified in cats.

NEURAL STRUCTURES
Pathways

Cortical binocular cells that are considered to be responsible for depth perception receive their input either via the optic chiasma or via the trans-callosal route. Section of the chiasm substantially reduces the number of binocularly driven cells in areas 17 and 18 [Berlucchi and Rizolatti, 1968], and the residual binocular cells are assumed to receive their input via the corpus callosum [Berlucchi et al., 1967; Hubel and Wiesel, 1967; Berlucchi and Rizzolatti, 1968; Innocenti, 1980; Lepore and Guillemot, 1982; Minciacchi and Antonini, 1984]. However, the contribution of the corpus callosum to binocularity is somewhat a matter of debate, some authors reporting a significant decrease in the number of binocular cortical cells following callosal section [Payne et al., 1980], while others found a slight or no change in binocularity [Lepore et al., 1983; Minciacchi and Antonini, 1984]. Independently of the controversy regarding the callosal involvement in binocularity, the fact remains that a combined section of the optic chiasm and the corpus callosum abolishes cortical binocularity, while lesion of either structure separately does not [Antonini et al., 1983].

Since absence of cortical binocularity generally results in stereoblindness [Packwood and Gordon, 1975; Blake and Hirsh, 1975; Mitchell and Timney, 1982], it is reasonable to suggest that the interruption of either or both pathways should interfere with stereopsis. Attempts to verify this assumption have come mostly from human studies, but their conclusions are rather equivocal. Performance on Julesz patterns was reported to be normal in commissurotomized patients and in isolated cases of callosal agenesis [Ettlinger et al., 1972], but binocular perception of distance was found to be impaired in the same type of patients [Lassonde, this volume]. Furthermore, deficits in midline stereopsis evaluated with a haploscope were found in these patients [Mitchell and Blakemore, 1970; Jeeves, 1979] but not in chiasmatomized ones [Blakemore, 1970]. In animals, few studies have been carried out to test the effects of chiasmatomy and callosotomy on depth perception. Recently, Timney et al. [1985] have reported that stereoacuity evaluated with the jumping-stand technique was greatly affected by the section of the optic chiasm and to a much lesser extent by the callosal split. However, their conclusions are somewhat limited by the fact that the method used in their study was not devoid of monocular cues. A more direct appraisal of the relative effects of callosotomy and chiasmatomy on binocular depth perception still needs to be done.

CORTICAL MECHANISMS

Areas 17 and 18 being the main recipient of the retinothalamic pathway, it is reasonable to assume that these regions play an important role in visual processing. This assumption proved to be true in man and monkeys, who show profound deficits in various visual functions following striate cortex lesions [Lepore et al., 1976; Pasik and Pasik, 1971; Miller et al., 1980] but not in cats, which display normal postoperative behavior [Sprague et al., 1977; Berkley and Sprague, 1979; Ptito et al., 1982]. Concerning stereoscopic depth perception, the electrophysiological studies reported in the previous section seem to indicate the presence in the cortex of neurons tuned to horizontal retinal disparity that could mediate stereopsis. In fact, lesions of areas V1 and V2 of the macaque monkey greatly elevate stereoacuity thresholds while leaving intact global stereopsis [Cowey and Wilkinson, in Cowey and Porter, 1979]. On the other hand, removal of the inferotemporal cortex impairs global stereopsis, as measured with random-dot stereograms [Cowey and Porter, 1979]. This dissociation between local and global stereopsis with regard to the cortical areas involved has not been reported in man. Indeed, most studies have shown that both types of stereopsis are affected by posterior lesions [Ross, 1983]. In the cat, Kaye et al. [1981] have demonstrated that ablations of areas 17–18 resulted in very poor binocular thresholds, as measured with the jumping-stand technique and concluded that binocular depth perception, at least in this species, is dependent upon the integrity of the primary visual cortex. However, the effect of cortical removal on global stereopsis has not yet been assessed in these animals.

Although appropriate evaluation of global stereopsis using random-dot stereograms proved to be feasible in the monkey [Bough, 1970; Cowey et al., 1975], no behavioral technique has yet been devised to evaluate this function in the cat. Mitchell and Timney [1982] mention that the main problem in the use of anaglyphic presentation of stimuli concerns the fact that cats have to wear goggles or contact lenses so as to permit separate control of the visual stimuli to the two eyes. A variety of techniques were thus devised to evaluate depth perception in this species, such as the shadow-casting [Packwood and Gordon, 1975], the visual cliff [Walk and Gibson, 1961; Cornwell et al., 1976], the jumping-stand [see Mitchell and Timney, 1982], and the line stereograms [Fox and Blake, 1971]. These various behavioral methods offer, however, only an assumption that cats indeed have stereopsis because the discriminations in some cases are not totally free of monocular cues (visual cliff and jumping-stand experiments), while in others the stimuli used had a configuration or form (shadow casting and line stereograms). A more direct assessment of stereoscopic functions in the cat appears to be particularly important, since our knowledge of the neural mechanisms involved in stereopsis has relied heavily on evidence obtained in this species.

In the present series of experiments, we therefore describe a behavioral technique that makes use of the Julesz random-dot stereograms and has been successful in assessing global stereopsis in normal cats. We also report data concerning the relative contribution of the optic chiasm, the corpus callosum, and the primary visual cortex in the operation of this specific stereoscopic mechanism.

METHODS
Surgery and Histology

Surgery was carried out on 15 cats using halothane anesthesia under conditions of partial asepsis. The splitting of the chiasma was performed using the transbuccal approach described by Myers [1956], whereas the section of the posterior third of the corpus callosum was done according to the method described by Ptito and Lepore [1983a]. Resection of areas 17–18 bilaterally was performed by subpial aspiration under microscopic viewing. Following the lesions, the animals were given antibiotics and other postoperative care for at least 2 weeks.

After completing their behavioral training, they were anesthetized and perfused through the heart with isotonic saline followed by 10% formalin. The brains were removed, blocked in paraffin, and cut into coronal sections 10 μm thick. For most of the brain, only one slice every 200 μm was retained, whereas in that portion of the block containing the optic chiasm, every second slice was kept. The retained sections were stained using the Kluver-Barrera [1953] method.

Apparatus and Procedure

A Thompson-like two-choice discrimination box was used. It consisted of three compartments: a holding section, a runway, choice section at the end of which were two doors (8.5 cm apart) hinged at the top and carrying the discriminanda; these two doors gave access to the third section (reinforcement chamber). The stereoscopic stimuli were random-dot stereograms of the type developed by Julesz [1960]. The stereograms consisted of a matrix of squares each assigned a brightness value at random. The two matrices were identical except that one of them had a rectangular region at its center in which the pattern was displaced uniformly to one side. The stereograms were generated by a computer (MINC), photographed from a short persistence screen using a 35-mm camera, and the resulting negatives were mounted on slides. Two sets of stereotargets were obtained: one which produced a vertical rectangle and the other an horizontal one. The disparity in each stereopair was 20' of arc when viewed from the start of the choice section and was well within the range of stereoacuity thresholds reported by Packwood and Gordon [1975] using the shadow casting technique. To the naked eye or in monocular vision, the two matrices looked identical. However, under appropriate viewing conditions (through red and green lenses), the horizontal and vertical rectangles appear to float out in space in front of the observer (crossed stereopsis). The stereotargets were projected onto the door-plaques by means of two pairs of 35-mm projectors mounted vertically above each other. All four projector lenses were covered with colored filters (red and green) and calibrated so as to produce perfect register of the matrices.

Sets of corneal lenses of various sizes were constructed. Each lens was made of plexiglas and its curvature fitted the eyeball of each cat. It had at its center a round aperture on which the red and green filters could be mounted. These lenses were easy to place and were well tolerated by the animals. Great care was taken to eliminate possible infection by washing the lenses after each use in an ophthalmic solution. Figure 1 illustrates one cat wearing the corneal lenses.

All cats were familiarized with the test box for a period of 1 week. They were taught to leave the starting chamber promptly, to approach the trans-illuminated doors, to push one of them, and to exit from the box to get a food reward. They were then trained on a simple light-dark discrimination (the dark panel being the positive stimulus) followed by two pattern discriminations. The first was a vertical vs. a horizontal bar on a white background followed by the same stimuli on a surround made out of random-dots iden-

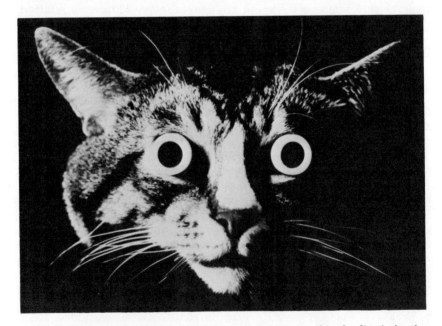

Fig. 1.   Photograph of one cat wearing the contact lenses used in the discrimination of the random-dot stereograms.

tical to the configuration used for the stereoscopic stimuli (termed the pseudostereoscopic condition). In this situation cats were allowed 1,000 trials overtraining in order to maximize the consolidation of learning and to give them adequate preparation for the stereoscopic condition. It was also during this period that the cats were familiarized with the placing and wearing of the lenses.

A session consisted of 40 trials, and the animals were tested 6 days a week. The stimuli were presented at random on the two doors according to the Gellerman tables [1933] so that the positive stimulus was 20 times on the right and 20 times on the left. The learning criterion was set at 36 correct responses (90% correct) for two consecutive days. After criterion was reached in the stereoscopic task, a number of control tests were used to ensure that the animals were using only disparity cues and no other strategies to account for their performance. In each control session, cats were subjected to the stereopairs in stereoscopic conditions and monocular trials were interspersed in the sequence. Thus, in a 40-trials session, the first 10 were carried out with the colored lenses, the next 10 with the occlusion of one eye (left or right), the next 10 with the colored lenses, and the last 10 in monocular vision. This procedure was used for 10 sessions in order to get 100 trials for each eye. Other controls included binocular testing in the absence of the colored lenses and conditions where the stimuli had a null disparity.

After completing the preoperative phase of testing, the cats were randomly assigned to three groups. Subjects in group 1 (N = 5) had their optic chiasma (OC) sectioned, and those in group 2 (N = 5) underwent a transection of their corpus callosum (CC). Following the postoperative evaluation, some animals in group 1 received an additional section of the callosum and some cats in group 2 had their optic chiasm cut. These subgroups were pooled together to form a split-brain group (N = 6). The fourth group was composed of cats (N = 4) that received a bilateral removal of cortical areas 17–18.

Operated animals were retested on the same preoperative paradigm. However, in the stereoscopic condition, only 24 sessions were allowed to the animals to solve the random-dot problem, after which testing was discontinued.

Ocular Alignment

The photographic method described by Sherman [1971] to measure ocular alignment was used in all cats. Subjects were hand-held by a familiar experimenter while facing a black cardboard screen bearing a hole into which the camera's lens could be fitted. The camera was set on a tripod behind the screen, and right above its lens at its center a point source of light produced by an optic fiber system served as a fixation target. The experimenter positioned himself behind the screen out of view of the animal.

When the subject gazed at the light source, the latter produced a corneal reflection in each eye, which was captured by the photographic film. Using appropriate calibration measures, photographs were enlarged to life-size, and the distance of each spot of light to the center of the corresponding pupil was evaluated. Data were pooled and averaged from a great number of measurements taken by two different observers.

RESULTS
Histological Results

A microscopic examination of the Kluver-Barrera-stained material indicated that the optic chiasma and the corpora callosa were completely transected in all animals. The cortical areas 17–18 were largely destroyed, including parts of area 19.

Behavioral Results

Preoperative testing.

Learning was assessed using the total number of correct responses to reach criterion. At the preoperative level, all cats resolved quite rapidly the light-dark discrimination task. They also performed well in the pattern discrimination task. In the semistereoscopic condition, however, learning was somewhat prolonged, but criterion was achieved for all cats. Learning was even slower in the stereoscopic condition, but criterion was reached after an average number of 865 trials. Data were pooled, averaged, and plotted according to the method of number of trials to successive criteria. This type of presentation gives the number of trials needed by the animals to reach successively more difficult criteria, thereby indicating higher levels of discriminative abilities.

Figure 2 depicts the average learning curve for all cats, showing in the abscissa the various criteria and in the ordinate the number of trials needed by the animals to attain each of them.

This figure indicates that all subjects could solve the random-dot problem using solely disparity cues. This conclusion was reinforced by the results obtained in the control tests. Indeed, when monocular trials were interleaved with regular binocular trials (inset in Figure 2), performance on the random-dot stereograms dropped to chance levels.

Postoperative testing.

Postoperative testing revealed that the chiasmatomy, the callosotomy, or both combined left unaffected the learning and retention of the light-dark, the pattern, and the pseudostereoscopic discriminations. However, following section of the optic chiasm, stereopsis appeared to be impaired, in that after 1,000 trials cats never reached the preestablished learning criterion. Their performance was, however, better than chance, averaging during the last five sessions 68% correct responses; this is higher than the performance obtained in the control situations (Fig. 3B).

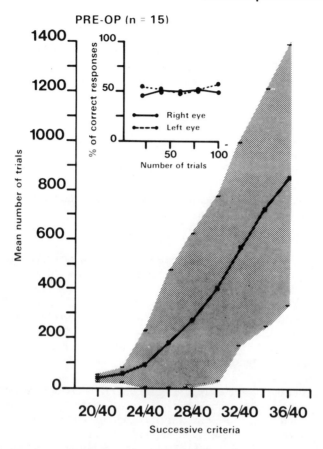

Fig. 2. Preoperative average performance for all cats in the stereoscopic condition.

Following callosotomy, the cats had no problem reattaining the learning criterion in the stereoscopic task. Their final performance was comparable to that of normals, indicating that the callosal section did not interfere with stereopsis (Fig. 3A).

When both the optic chiasm and the corpus callosum were sectioned, stereopsis was abolished. The performance of these split-brain animals remained at chance levels, comparable to that obtained in the control situations (Fig. 3C).

Cortical Lesions

The light-dark, the pattern, and the pseudostereoscopic discriminations were not impaired by the removal of areas 17 and 18 of each hemisphere. In the stereoscopic condition, however, performance was poor and none of the animals could reach criterion even after 1,000 trials. Results depicted in Figure 3D indicate that the average performance during testing was comparable to that of the control situations. Moreover, the results obtained following the cortical lesions resemble those found in the split-brain animals.

Eye Alignment

The average ocular deviations derived from normal, split-chiasma, split-callosum, split-brain, and visual-cortex-lesioned cats are depicted in Figure 4.

It appears from this figure that all deviations observed following the various lesions were well within the range of those obtained for normal cats that learned the stereoscopic discrimination. These results rule out the possibility that the deficits observed in stereopsis could be due to strabismus induced by the surgical manipulations.

DISCUSSION

Our results offer convincing evidence that cats indeed have stereopsis, which confirms and extends previous reports that suggested the presence of this function in this species [Walk and Gibson, 1961; Fox and Blake, 1971; Packwood and Gordon, 1975; Cornwell et al., 1976; Mitchell and Timney, 1982]. Our results further demonstrate that cats can perceive depth on the sole basis of stimulus disparity. This finding is of importance, since it provides a behavioral correlate to the numerous electrophysiological studies that have indicated the existence of disparity-tuned cells in the cat's visual cortex.

This parallel between electrophysiological and behavioral results is further strengthened when considering the consequences of sectioning the pathways known to mediate binocularity, and hence stereopsis in the cat. Indeed, the stereoscopic impairment found following our lesions seems proportionately related to the quantitative loss in binocularity reported in similar preparations. In effect, chiasmatomy induces a drastic reduction in the number of cortical binocular cells in the primary visual areas, while leaving a small proportion of units that can still be driven by both eyes [Berlucchi and Rizzolatti, 1968]. At the behavioral level, we were also able to show a strong, albeit incomplete, impairment in stereopsis following section of the chiasmatic route. The remaining binocular cells, which are thought to depend upon the callosal input, could account for the residual capacity of the chiasmatomized cats to perform the stereoscopic task. On the other hand, lesion of the callosum alone does not alter to any great extent the stereoscopic process, a result that reflects the small change in binocularity that occurs following callosotomy [Minciacchi and Antonini, 1984]. Nonetheless, it would be difficult to deny the callosal contribution to such a process, since only the combined sections of the two pathways produce a complete loss of binocularity [Antonini et al., 1983] as well as the

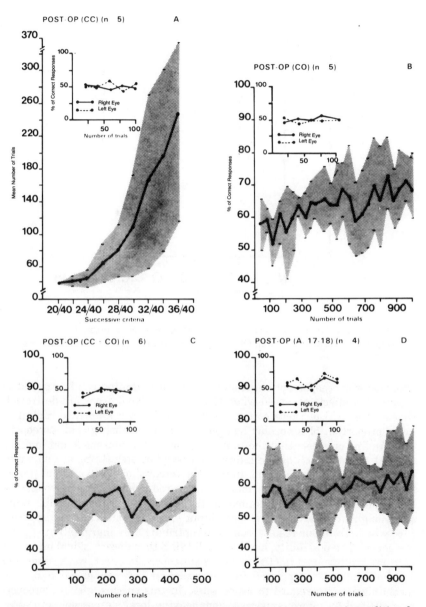

Fig. 3. Postoperative average performance curves in the stereoscopic condition for cats with A. Section of the corpus callosum (CC). B. Section of the optic chiasm (CO). C. Section of both commissures (CC + CO). D. Bilateral ablation of cortical areas A.17–18 (VC).

OCULAR ALIGNMENT

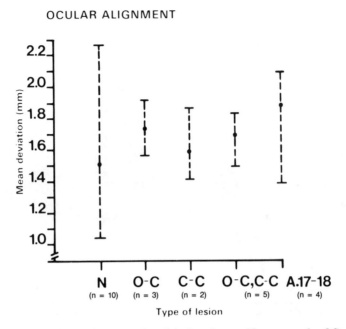

Fig. 4. Eye alignment for normal and lesioned cats. N = normals. OC = optic chiasma; CC = corpus callosum; OC, CC = split-brain; A. 17–18 = cortical lesions.

abolition of stereoperception. A similar line of reasoning can be applied to explain the effects observed when the primary visual areas are destroyed. Indeed, removal of these cortical regions, which are known to contain a large proportion of binocular neurons, seems to abolish global stereopsis. This finding suggests that the remaining binocular neurons found in other cortical regions, such as the lateral suprasylvian area (LSS), are not sufficient to mediate this function. In fact, the removal of 17–18 afferent projections to LSS induces in the latter a large reduction in the proportion of binocular cells [Spear and Baumann, 1979]. The remaining binocular units are thought to receive part of their input via the corpus callosum, a structure which, from our results, seems to contribute only marginally to global stereopsis. The possibility, however, still exists that these residual binocular neurons are involved in other types of stereopsis. In effect, work conducted on the monkey has pointed to a dissociation between global and local mechanisms with regard to lesion sites. In this species, global stereopsis was affected by inferotemporal lesions leaving local stereoscopic processes intact, while the reverse was found after striate lesions [Cowey and Porter, 1979].

However, these conclusions may be somewhat limited by the fact that local stereopsis has always been studied using a narrow range of spatial disparities, thus restricting the conclusions to the fine local stereoscopic mechanism. Before definite statements can be made concerning the relative contribution of various pathways or cerebral areas to the different stereoscopic functions, studies of coarse stereopsis must be undertaken.

Such studies are certainly justified when considering the recent dissociation of binocular units into three main categories (tuned, far-near, and global cells) whose differences in properties would indicate that they may subserve respectively the fine, coarse, and global stereopsis mechanisms [Poggio and Poggio, 1984]. Coarse stereopsis could very well be mediated by cortical regions other than those implicated in fine and global stereopsis. In fact, the suggestion has been made that cortical areas having binocular cells with large receptive fields (such as LSS) would be ideally suited to analyze stimuli with large disparity values. On the other hand the relative contribution of the two pathways to binocularity (the optic chiasma and the corpus callosum) may vary in terms of which mechanism (fine, coarse, or global) is under study. Evidence from human studies [Jeeves, 1979; Lassonde, this volume] would indicate that the contribution of the corpus callosum in coarse stereopsis far exceeds its participation in global stereopsis.

CONCLUSIONS

Our results clearly demonstrate that global stereopsis is subserved in the cat by the geniculostriate system. Furthermore, the finding that lesions of the primary visual areas abolish global stereopsis while leaving other visual functions intact supports Julesz's original conclusion [1960] that the neural mechanisms for stereopsis must come into play before, and operate independently of, those responsible for form perception. Finally, it also appears that the callosum involvement in such stereoprocessing is minimal. Its role in other types of stereopsis still needs to be investigated.

REFERENCES

Antonini A, Berlucchi G, Lepore F (1983): Physiological organization of callosal connections of a visual suprasylvian cortical area in the cat. J Neurophysiol 49:902–921.

Barlow HB, Blakemore C, Pettigrew JD (1967): The neural mechanisms of binocular depth discrimination. J Physiol Lond 193:327–342.

Berkley MA, Sprague JM (1979): Striate cortex and visual acuity functions in the cat. J Comp Neurol 187:679–702.

Berlucchi G, Rizzolatti G (1968): Binocularly driven neurons in visual cortex of split-chiasm cats. Science 159:308–310.

Berlucchi G, Gazzaniga MS, Rizzolatti G (1967): Microelectrode analysis of transfer of visual information by the corpus callosum. Arch Ital Biol 105:583–596.

Bishop PO (1981): Binocular vision. In Moses RA (ed): "Adler's Physiology of the Eye." St. Louis: Mosby, p 575–649.

Bishop PO, Henry GH (1971): Spatial vision. Annu Rev Psychol 22:119–160.

Bishop PO, Henry GH, Smith CJ (1971): Binocular interaction fields of single units in the cat striate cortex. J Physiol 216:39–68.

Blake R, Hirsh HVB (1975): Deficits in binocular depth perception after alternating monocular deprivation. Science 190:1114–1116.

Blakemore C (1970): Binocular depth perception and the optic chiasm. Vision Res 10:43–47.

Bough EW (1970): Stereoscopic vision in the macaque monkey: A behavioral demonstration. Nature 225:42.

Cornwell P, Warren JM, Nonneman AJ (1976): Marginal and extra marginal cortical lesions and visual discriminations by cats. J Comp Physiol Psychol 90:986–995.

Cowey A, Porter R (1979): Brain damage and global stereopsis. Proc R Soc Lond [Biol] 204:399–407.

Cowey A, Parkinson AM, Warwick L (1975): Global stereopsis in rhesus monkeys. Q J Exp Psychol 27:93–109.

Ettlinger G, Blakemore CB, Milner AD, Wilson J (1972): Agenesis of the corpus callosum: A behavioral investigation. Brain 95:327–346.

Ferster D (1981): A comparison of binocular depth mechanisms in areas 17 and 18 of the cat visual cortex. J Physiol 311:623–655.

Fisher B, Krueger J (1979): Disparity tuning and binocularity of single neurons in the cat visual cortex. Exp Brain Res 35:1–8.

Fox R, Blake RR (1971): Stereoscopic vision in the cat. Nature 233:55–56.

Gellerman LW (1933): Chance orders of alternating stimuli in visual discrimination experiments. J Genet Psychol 42:207–208.

Hubel DH, Wiesel TN (1967): Cortical and callosal connections concerned with the vertical meridian of visual field in the cat. J Neurophysiol 30:1561–1573.

Hubel DH, Wiesel TN (1970): Cells sensitive to binocular depth in area 18 of the macaque monkey cortex. Nature 225:41–42.

Hubel DH, Wiesel TN (1973): A reexamination of stereoscopic mechanisms in the cat. J Physiol 232:290–309.

Innocenti GM (1980): The primary visual pathway through the corpus callosum: Morphological and functional aspects in the cat. Arch Ital Biol 118:124–188.

Jeeves MA (1979): Some limits to interhemispheric integration in cases of callosal agenesis and partial commissurotomy. In Russel IS, Van Hof MW, Berlucchi G (eds): "Structure and Function of the Cerebral Commissures." London: McMillan, p 449–474.

Joshua DE, Bishop PO (1970): Binocular single vision and depth discrimination. Receptive fields disparities for central and peripheral vision and binocular interaction on peripheral units in cat striate cortex. Exp Brain Res 10:389–416.

Julesz B (1960): Binocular depth perception of computer generated patterns. Bell Syst Techn J 39:1125–1162.

Julesz B (1971): "Foundations of Cyclopean Perception." Chicago: University of Chicago Press.

Kaye M, Mitchell DE, Cynader M (1981): Selective loss of binocular depth perception after ablation of cat visual cortex. Nature, 293:60–62.

Kluver H, Barrera E (1953): A method for the combined staining of cells and fibers in the nervous system. J Neuropathol Exp Neurol 12:400–403.

Lassonde MC (1986): The facilitatory action of the corpus callosum. (This volume).

Lepore F, Ptito M, Cardu B, Dumont M (1976): Effects of colliculectomy and striatectomy on achromatic differential thresholds in the monkey. Physiol Behav 16:285–291.

Lepore F, Guillemot JP (1982): Visual receptive field properties of cells innervated through the corpus callosum in the cat. Exp Brain Res 46:413–424.

Lepore F, Samson A, Molotchnikoff S (1983): Effects on binocular interaction of cells in visual cortex of the cat following the transection of the optic tract. Exp Brain Res 50:392–396.

Miller M, Pasik P, Pasik T (1980): Extrageniculostriate vision in the monkey. VII. Contrast sensitivity functions. J Neurophysiol 43:1510–1526.

Minciacchi D, Antonini A (1984): Binocularity in the visual cortex of the adult cat does not depend on the integrity of the corpus callosum. Behav Brain Res 13:183–192.

Mitchell DE, Timney B (1982): Behavioral measurement of normal and abnormal development of vision in the cat. In Ingle DJ, Goodale MA, Mansfield JW (eds): "Analysis of Visual Behavior." Cambridge: The MIT Press, p 483–523.

Mitchell DE, Blakemore C (1970): Binocular depth perception and the corpus callosum. Vision Res 10:49–54.

Myers RE (1956): Function of the corpus callosum in interocular transfer. Brain 118:358–363.

Nikara T, Bishop PO, Pettigrew JD (1968): Analysis of retinal correspondence by studying receptive fields of binocular single units in cats striate cortex. Exp Brain Res 6:353–372.

Packwood J, Gordon B (1975): Stereopsis in normal domestic cat, siamese cat and cat raised with alternating monocular occlusion. J Neurophysiol 38:1485–1499.

Pasik P, Pasik T (1971): The visual world of monkeys deprived of striate cortex: Effective stimulus parameters and the importance of the accessory optic system. Vision Res 11:419–435.

Pettigrew JD, Nikara T, Bishop PO (1968): Binocular interaction on single units in cat striate cortex: Simultaneous stimulation by single moving slits with receptive fields in correspondence. Exp Brain Res 6:391–410.

Payne BR, Elberger AJ, Berman N, Murphy EH (1980): Binocularity in the cat visual cortex is reduced by sectioning the corpus callosum. Science 207:1097–1099.

Poggio GF (1985): Processing of stereoscopic information in primate visual cortex. In Edelman G, Cowan WM, Gall WE (eds): "Dynamic Aspects of Neocortical Function." New York: Wiley.

Poggio GF, Poggio T (1984): The analysis of stereopsis. Annu Rev Neurosci 7:379–412.

Poggio GF, Talbot WH (1981): Mechanisms of static and dynamic stereopsis in foveal cortex of the rhesus monkey. J Physiol 315:469–492.

Poggio GF, Fisher B (1977): Binocular interaction and depth sensitivity of striate and prestriate cortical neurons of the behaving rhesus monkey. J Neurophysiol 40:1392–1405.

Ptito M, Lepore F (1983a): Interocular transfer in cats with early callosal transection. Nature 301:513–515.

Ptito M, Lepore F (1983b): Effects of unilateral and bilateral lesions of the lateral suprasylvian area on learning and interhemispheric transfer of pattern discrimination in the cat. Behav Brain Res 7:211–227.

Ptito M, Lepore F, Lassonde M, Miceli D (1982): Effects of selective lesions of visual cortical areas on pattern discrimination in the split-brain cat. Neurosci Lett 10:395.

Ross JE (1983): Disturbance of stereoscopic vision in patients with unilateral stroke. Behav Brain Res 7:99–112.

Sherman SM (1971): Role of visual cortex in interocular transfer in the cat. Exp Neurol 30:34–45.

Spear PD, Baumann TP (1979): Effects of visual cortex removal on receptive field properties of neurons in lateral suprasylvian area of the cat. J Neurophysiol 42:31–56.

Sprague JM, Levy J, Di Berardino A, Berlucchi G (1977): Visual cortical areas mediating form discrimination in the cat. J Comp Neurol 172:441–488.

Timney B, Elberger AJ, Vandewater ML (1985): Binocular depth perception in the cat following early corpus callosum section. Exp Brain Res (in press).

Von der Heydt R, Adorjany C, Hanny P, Baumgartner G (1978): Disparity sensitivity and receptive field incongruity of units in the cat striate cortex. Exp Brain Res 31:423–545.

Walk RD, Gibson JJ (1961): A comparative and analytical study of visual depth perception. Psychol Monogr 75:1–44.

Wheatstone C (1838): Contributions to the physiology of vision. I. On some remarkable, and hitherto unobserved, phenomena of binocular vision. Philos Trans R Soc Lond 128:371.

Two Hemispheres—One Brain:
Functions of the Corpus Callosum, pages 351–357
© 1986 Alan R. Liss, Inc.

Visual Discrimination Learning and Interhemispheric Transfer in the Cat, as Affected by 6-Hydroxydopamine

JAMES M. SPRAGUE, ALAN C. CHURCH, C.N. LIU, W.W. CHAMBERS, AND LOUIS B. FLEXNER

Department of Anatomy and Institute of Neurological Sciences, University of Pennsylvania, Philadelphia, Pennsylvania 19104

Interhemispheric transfer of learning is of great interest for several reasons: it allows us to study the movement of the memory trace, or engram, from one area of the brain to another using a known commissural pathway; and in a more general sense it allows us to learn something of the interaction between the two hemispheres in the mediation of learning and memory. This approach to function of the brain is the legacy of the pioneering research of Roger Sperry, whom we are honoring in this volume.

In an effort to work out the contributions of the various visual areas of the cortex to different aspects of vision, Berlucchi and Sprague [1981] found that no retention of preoperatively learned form discriminations was present after selective removal of the suprasylvian gyri in the cat. Furthermore, this lesion placed unilaterally in the split-chiasm animal resulted in prolonged learning using the eye on the lesioned side and blocked interhemispheric transfer to the lesioned hemisphere [Berlucchi et al., 1979]. Both effects were specific to a lesion in this area, in that comparable deficits were not found after removal of the striate and peristriate cortices, areas 17+18 [Berlucchi et al., 1978; Berlucchi and Sprague, 1981].

We used these findings as the basis for study of the role of cortical norepinephrine (NE) and dopamine (DA) in learning, memory and interhemispheric transfer of pattern and form discriminations. In a series of cats, 6-hydroxydopamine (6-OHDA) was applied selectively to the same area of the suprasylvian gyrus of one hemisphere as was ablated by Berlucchi et al. [1979], a procedure that destroys the nerve terminals containing these

Alan C. Church is now with the Drug Enforcement Administration, Washington, D.C. 20537.

transmitters. In three animals sacrificed 14 days after 6-OHDA, samples taken from comparable sites in the two hemispheres were analyzed using high performance liquid chromatography (HPLC) [Felice et al., 1978]. This sensitive technique revealed no detectable amounts of NE and DA in the suprasylvian gyrus previously treated with 6-OHDA; adjacent gyri in the same hemisphere had transmitter levels not significantly different (t-test) than those in three untreated control animals. However, the opposite side of the brain showed significant increases in both transmitters (Table 1). The phenomenon of compensatory change in transmitter activity levels on the two sides of the brain has been studied extensively by Glowinski and his collaborators [see Nieoullon et al., 1977].

Table I also shows the results of HPLC analysis in three cats used for behavioral studies and sacrificed 24–39 months after the same treatment with 6-OHDA. Levels of NE had undergone substantial alteration from those present at 14 days and were not significantly different from controls. DA levels also showed considerable change over this period of time but were more variable than NE and were still significantly increased on the untreated side.

The data presented in Table 1 indicate that the destructive effects of 6-OHDA on NE and DA were limited to the suprasylvian gyrus, but led to

TABLE 1. Data Showing the Levels of NE and DA Using the High Performance Liquid Chromatography Technique in Three Control Cats, Three Cats 14 Days After Treatment of the Left Suprasylvian Gyrus (LSS) With 6-OHDA, and Three Cats 2–3 Years After 6-OHDA.[1]

	LSS	LES	LL	RSS	RES	RL
NE (μg)						
Controls (N=3)	.24±.08	.20±.07	.24±.06	.16±.01	.20±.07	.20±.04
6-OHDA, 14 days (N=3)	0*	.49±.21	.18±.03	.76±.10**	.60±.12*	.65±.08**
6-OHDA, 2–3 yrs (N=3)	.09±.04	.17±.06	.19±.08	.29±.08	.25±.05	.22±.08
DA (μg)						
Controls (N=3)	.07±.01	.04±.01	.07±.01	.05±.01	.04±.03	.07±.02
6-OHDA, 14 days (N=3)	0**	.17±.08	.36±.25	.40±.04**	.13±.13	.58±.05***
6-OHDA, 2–3 yrs (N=3)	.12±.09	.15±.05	.28±.12	.23±.06*	.15±.04	.30±.06*

[1]Samples taken from left suprasylvian (LSS), left ectosylvian (LES) and left lateral (LL) gyri; comparable samples taken from the right gyri (RSS, RES, RL). Readings are means ± SE; significance is expressed as treated animals compared with controls.
*P < 0.05.
**P < 0.01.
***P < 0.001.

widespread increases on the opposite side of the brain. The restitution of NE and DA means that the behavioral testing over periods of several years was conducted against gradually shifting concentrations of these transmitters on both sides of the brain.

Our initial prediction, on the basis of the ablation experiments cited above, was that learning as well as transfer might be adversely affected on the side of the brain with reduced levels of NE and DA in the cortex. This prediction was not realized and in fact the opposite was true.

The basic plan of the experiments was as follows:

1. The test apparatus and methods of testing have been described in detail by Sprague et al. [1977]; briefly the apparatus consisted of a holding chamber and an approach alley at the end of which were two top-hinged doors carrying glass panels, on which the discrimanda were rear-projected. The door bearing the negative stimulus was locked, and the animal was trained to push open and pass through the positive door to obtain a food reward on a platform behind the doors. The positive and negative stimuli were alternated from side to side according to a modified Gellerman schedule. Performance was measured by (a) the number of trials needed to achieve a significant run of correct choices with only one error [Runnels et al., 1968; Sprague et al., 1977], using a probability of .01, and (b) the number of errors in reaching a criterion of 90% or better correct choices on two successive days. The first evaluation was considered a reliable measure of the beginning of learning, while the second indicated the cat had achieved a stable, high level of discrimination.

2. Three cats were trained binocularly to a simple flux discrimination, using dark as the positive stimulus, followed by monocular training until performance reached criterion using either eye.

3. All surgical procedures were carried out under nembutal anesthesia, using sterile precautions. The optic chiasm was first split by aspiration using the transbuccal approach described by Myers [1955]. Completeness of the surgery was confirmed using a perimetry test [Sprague and Meikle, 1965; Sherman, 1973], which showed a bitemporal hemianopsia. In order to prove that each eye had an adequate visual field, the animals were retested monocularly on the previously learned flux discrimination. Following this each cat was trained monocularly in a pattern discrimination (square-wave gratings), and in some cases also in a form task ($\triangle \ \nabla$ or $+0$); after performance reached criterion, transfer to the untrained eye was tested and training was continued until criterion was achieved.

4. After discrimination performance was clearly established and stable using either eye, a craniotomy was made over the middle and posterior suprasylvian gyri of one hemisphere. A solution of tranylcypromine, 5 mg/ kg (a monoamine oxidase inhibitor), was injected intramuscularly, 1 hour before the dura and arachnoid were excised and a fitted plastic chamber

was placed directly over the cortex; contact of the chamber with the gyrus was sealed with vasoline to prevent leakage. The chamber was next filled with a solution of 6-OHDA (1 mg/ml) containing 0.5 mg/ml ascorbic acid as an antioxidant; after 15 minutes this solution was replaced by a fresh one so that exposure totaled 30 minutes. This solution was then withdrawn and replaced for 30 minutes with saline to reduce residual 6-OHDA. Two to three weeks later the cats were returned to the test box.

BEHAVIORAL RESULTS

The experiment was designed so that it would be possible to test the effects of transmitter imbalance on (a) retention of discriminations learned before treatment with 6-OHDA, (b) rate of learning, and (c) interhemispheric transfer of discriminations learned after 6-OHDA.

1. Retention of the previously learned discriminations was tested monocularly. The gratings were retained at criterion in each eye; the form discrimination ($\triangle$ $\triangledown$) was either retained or relearned with a savings.

Summary: Good performance after treatment with 6-OHDA was found in discriminations learned before 6-OHDA.

2. New gratings and new form discriminations were next taught to the cats, using the eye on the untreated side of the brain, followed by testing of interhemispheric transfer to the side with the chemical lesion. The new grating was learned normally (i.e., within the range of trials/errors of a series of split-chiasm controls); initial transfer within the first block of trials was not present, but criterion was achieved with considerable savings. Subsequent presentation of a reversal of sign of these gratings resulted in a comparable performance.

In contrast, new forms were not learned using the eye on the untreated side (testing was discontinued after reaching the number of trials equal to twice the standard error of a population of controls). After shifting to the eye on the lesioned side, learning occurred at a rate wihin the range of controls; once learned these discriminations were transferred back to the first hemisphere at a high level (Fig. 1). When reversals of these forms were presented, in the same monocular sequence, performance was the same as that just noted. These changes were present in one animal 1 month after 6-OHDA, but in two other cats the deficit on the untreated hemisphere appeared only after a delay of 9 and 15½ months, respectively.

Summary: No deficit in learning and transfer of new flux and pattern (gratings) tasks was found after treatment with 6-OHDA. Form discriminations in contrast showed a paradoxical result in that no significant learning occurred in the untreated hemisphere. However, normal learning was possible using the eye of the chemically lesioned hemisphere and this learning was transferred back to first side. In other words, the untreated or "intact"

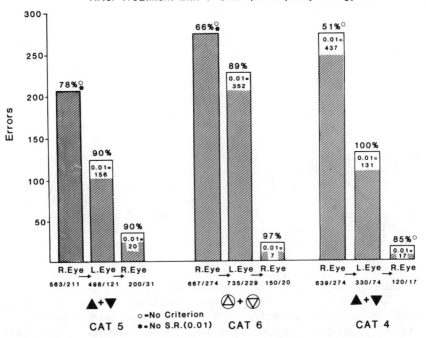

Fig. 1. Bar graphs showing monocular performance in visual discriminations, three cats using in sequence the right (R) eye (untreated cortex) and left (L) eye (cortex treated with 6-OHDA). The percentage above the bars is the final level of correct discrimination. ○, no criterion was reached; *, no significant run was achieved. Number of trials of first significant run is indicated within the bar. Below the bars is shown the number of trials/errors performed.

side did not learn using direct visual input, but showed learning at a high level using indirect input via the callosal commissure.

3. In two animals, after extensive retesting in which all discriminations were brought to criterion performance using either eye, the posterior two-thirds of the callosum was split. The cats were then retested on all discriminations using each eye on alternate days; the results were very clear in that performance mediated by the two sides of the brain was markedly altered. Discrimination using the eye on the side of the treated hemisphere was then deficient and in many cases remained at chance, while that on the untreated side, which had previously been defective, was greatly improved and was superior to that of the other brain half.

Summary: The asymmetric, and seemingly paradoxical performance after unilateral treatment with 6-OHDA, in which the treated side was superior to the untreated, was reversed by severance of the corpus callosum.

CONCLUSIONS

These results are based on a relatively small population of animals and in that sense must be reviewed as something less than a final statement. Nonetheless, we feel justified in presenting them because of the considerable uniformity among the cats and in the unexpected nature of the behavioral findings.

Our rather simple method of applying the neurotoxin to the cortical surface was successful in that no detectable NE and DA were found by biochemical assay (HPLC) in the specific area of the cortex exposed to 6-OHDA, and this loss was limited to the suprasylvian gyrus.

The HPLC analysis of our material confirmed the general principle discovered and elucidated by others of the dynamic lability of certain transmitters, in that diminishment of their rate of release on one side of the brain is followed by increase on the other side [Nieoullon et al., 1977]. The compensatory shift in NE and DA concentrations was well established in our material by 14 days, but the results of others [Nieoullon et al., 1977] indicate that such changes in other brain sites can occur within an hour.

Our experiments were directed to the suprasylvian gyrus by the previous work of Berlucchi et al. [1979], because ablation of this area alone caused major deficits in both learning and interhemispheric transfer in split-chiasm cats. Our behavioral results compared with those of Berlucchi et al. [1979] indicate the great difference between total ablation of this gyrus and the chemical destruction of two transmitters, which in contrast to ablation left visual discrimination intact.

This selective chemical lesion did, however, seriously affect certain aspects of discrimination mediated by the hemisphere contralateral to that treated with 6-OHDA. Tasks based on the perception of differences in total luminous flux and of low spatial frequencies in the form of square-wave gratings presented no problem. Discriminations based on forms (shapes), however, were not learned when the eye on the nontreated side was used, but showed a high degree of transfer from the lesioned hemisphere. This finding stands in contradiction to the accepted generalization that learning by direct retinal input is more efficient than by indirect visual input via the callosum [see Lepore et al., 1982].

Whether the increase in NE and DA levels in the contralateral cortex is related to the defect in form discrimination by this hemisphere is unknown, and the problem needs further study. That the callosum played a significant role in this seemingly paradoxical asymmetry of learning appears to be clear in that its severance resulted in a reversal of the asymmetry so that the deficit occurred on the lesioned side and the intact side appeared normal.

Also unknown is whether the callosum is responsible for the increase in transmitters in the hemisphere opposite to that treated with 6-OHDA. These problems are now under study.

ACKNOWLEDGMENTS

This research was supported in part by USPHS Research Grant EY-00577 and S07 RR05415-23. We wish to thank Drs. Eliot Stellar and Thomas Rainbow, and Mrs. Jeanne Levy for help in various aspects of this work.

REFERENCES

Berlucchi G, Sprague JM, Lepore F, Mascetti GG (1978): Effects of lesions of areas 17, 18 and 19 on interocular transfer of pattern discriminations in split-chiasm cats. Exp Brain Res 31:275–297.

Berlucchi G, Sprague JM, Antonini A, Simoni A (1979): Learning and interhemispheric transfer of visual pattern discriminations following unilateral suprasylvanian lesions in split-chiasm cats. Exp Brain Res 34:551–574.

Berlucchi G, Sprague JM (1981): The cerebral cortex in visual learning and memory, and in interhemispheric transfer in the cat. In Schmitt FO, Worden FG, Adelman G, Dennis JG (eds): "The Organization of the Cerebral Cortex." Cambridge, Mass.: The MIT Press, pp 415–440.

Felice LJ, Felice JD, Kissinger PT (1978): Determination of catecholamines in rat brain parts by reverse-phase ion-pair liquid chromatography. J Neurochem 31:1461–1465.

Lepore F, Phaneuf J, Samson A, Guillemot J-P (1982): Interhemispheric transfer of visual pattern discriminations: Evidence for a bilateral storage of the engram. Behav Brain Res 5:359–374.

Myers RE (1955): Interocular transfer of pattern discriminations in cats following section of crossed optic fibres. J Comp Physiol Psychol 48:470–473.

Nieoullon A, Cheramy A, Glowinski J (1977): Interdependence of the nigrostriatal dopaminergic systems on the two sides of the brain in the cat. Science 198:416–418.

Runnels LK, Thompson R, Runnels P (1968): Near-perfect runs as a learning criterion. J Math Psych 5:362–368.

Sherman SM (1973): Visual field defects in monocularly and binocularly deprived cats. Brain Res 49:25–45.

Sprague JM, Meikle Jr TH (1965): The role of the superior colliculus in visually guided behavior. Exp Neurol 11:115–146.

Sprague JM, Levy J, DeBerardino A, Berlucchi G (1977): Visual cortical areas mediating form discrimination in the cat. J Comp Neurol 172:441–488.

SECTION V
HUMAN NEUROPSYCHOLOGY I

Two Hemispheres—One Brain:
Functions of the Corpus Callosum, pages 361–368
© 1986 Alan R. Liss, Inc.

Effectiveness of Corpus Callosotomy for Control of Intractable Epilepsy in Children

GUY GEOFFROY, MARYSE LASSONDE, HANNELORE SAUERWEIN AND MICHEL DÉCARIE

Division of Neurology and Neurosurgery, Hôpital Sainte-Justine, Université de Montréal, Montréal (G.G., M.D.) and Groupe de Recherche en Neuropsychologie, Université du Québec à Trois-Rivières, Québec (M.L., H.S.) Canada

INTRODUCTION

The functional properties of the corpus callosum may be unfavorable to patients with epilepsy since this commissure seems to promote the interhemispheric propagation of epileptic discharges [Erickson, 1940; Musgrave and Gloor, 1980]. As a result of this propagation, a primary focalized or lateralized epileptogenic abnormality may become generalized, and the clinical expression may be more dramatic, more dangerous, and, especially, more difficult to control with medication.

Epilepsy is a very frequent symptom, affecting 0.5% to 1% of the general population. About 75% of epileptic patients are children. More than 80% of these are perfectly controlled with medication, and in a large number of cases there is a reasonable hope for a complete cure. About 5% of affected children, however, have intractable epilepsy. Conventional surgery (resection of a focus or a lobectomy) may be considered if the epileptogenic focus is unique and so localized that its resection will not cause any permanent neurological dysfunction. But some children have severe generalized seizures (convulsive or akinetic) with diffuse EEG abnormalities and are thus not candidates for conventional surgery. Their seizures are frequent, life-threatening, and require many hospital admissions. Furthermore, in attempting to control their attacks, the dosage of the medication often has to be raised close to toxic levels. This diminishes the patients' alertness and responsivity and renders interventions of parents and educators useless. The patients reported here were not candidates for conventional surgery for the following reasons:

1. The primary epileptogenic abnormality (responsible for the generalization) involved the entire hemisphere (hemispherectomy is not considered unless a contralateral chronic motor deficit is present).

2. There were independent discharges over the other hemisphere.

3. The primary focus was located in the motor area.

The long-term effects of commissurotomy in adult patients are well documented [Gazzaniga et al., 1962; Bogen and Vogel, 1975]. On the clinical level, "split-brain" operations, involving the corpus callosum, the anterior and hippocampal commissures, and the massa intermedia [Bogen and Vogel, 1962; Luessenhop, 1970; Wilson et al., 1977] have generally resulted in improvement. However, neuropsychological studies [e.g., Zaidel and Sperry, 1974, 1977; Campbell et al., 1981] have shown that complete commissurotomy may cause lasting deficits in higher (cognitive) and lower (sensorimotor) functions. For this reason, we decided to follow Wilson et al. [1978], who showed that sectioning of the corpus callosum alone is an easier and safer surgical procedure, causes fewer deficits, and seems to be as effective as commissurotomy in the management of intractable seizures. The following is a brief account of our first 15 patients.

METHODS

Nine girls and six boys, aged 3–16, were selected for callosotomy by the following criteria [Geoffroy et al., 1983]:

1. They had generalized and frequent attacks (more than three a day).

2. They had received medical treatment for more than 3 years, using conventional or experimental medication including steroids and ketogenic diet in most cases.

3. They were not considered candidates for conventional surgical resections.

4. They were severely handicapped and unable to lead a normal life, and they needed frequent hospital admissions or even institutionalization.

All children had a standard neuroclinical examination, complete neuroradiological studies, and many electroencephalograms. Each patient was submitted to extensive pre- and postoperative psychological examination and continues to be followed by a team composed of a neurologist, a neurosurgeon, and clinical and experimental neuropsychologists.

The operations were performed between October 1978 and April 1983 using a modified version of the technique of Wilson et al. [1978] as described before [see Geoffroy et al., 1983]. In all patients, the entire corpus callosum was sectioned. The effectiveness of the surgery was evaluated in terms of degree of postoperative improvement. Improvement was considered:

1. *Slight* when the frequency of seizures was somewhat reduced, "status epilepticus" abolished, and/or a better medical management and fewer readmissions were achieved;

2. *Notable* when previous generalized seizures changed to partial ones or when there was a reduction of at least 50% in the frequency of the convulsions, resulting in an improvement of the quality of life; and

3. *Remarkable* when a significant reduction of the number of seizures to not more than 2–3 per month had occurred.

Psychological evaluations varied from observation and simple manipulations in the more seriously handicapped cases to complete assessment of cognitive, perceptual, sensory and motor functions, employing the Neuropsychological Battery of Trois-Rivières. This battery consisted essentially of a combination of the Battery of Michigan, excerpts of the Healstead-Reitan Battery, and a number of other selected standardized tests. These were complemented by specially devised "split-brain" examinations. Detailed accounts of the clinical and experimental methods and findings are the subject of separate papers [Geoffroy et al., 1985; Lassonde et al., 1985].

RESULTS

Out of the 15 patients, only two failed to show any substantial improvement. Both had severe epileptogenic encephalopathy with diffuse multifocal EEG abnormalties. However, no deterioration was observed. Thirteen chil-

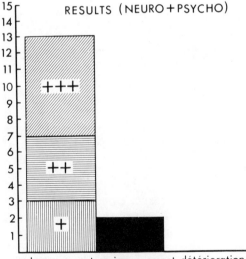

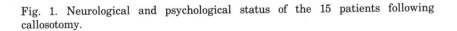

Fig. 1. Neurological and psychological status of the 15 patients following callosotomy.

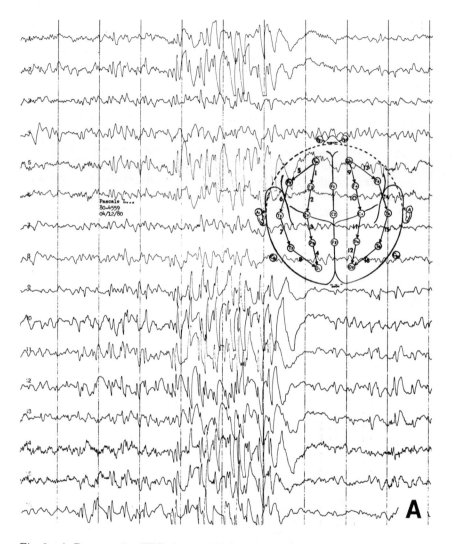

Fig. 2. A. Preoperative EEG of case 1. Right frontoparietal epileptogenic focus with secondary bilateral synchrony (from Geoffroy et al. [1983]; reproduced by permission). B. Postoperative record of the same patient. Right centroparietal focus with occasional synchronous low-voltage spikes over the left hemisphere but without a well-organized "generalized burst" (from Geoffroy et al. [1983]; reproduced by permission).

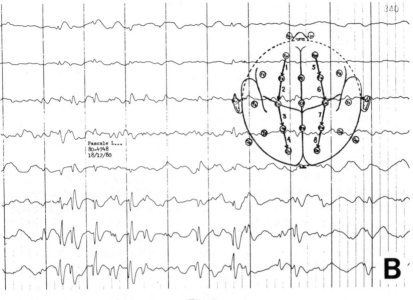

Fig. 2

dren (87%) showed improvement; it was "slight" in three, "notable" in four and "remarkable" in six (Fig. 1). The case reports of two of the six latter patients will be presented here.

Case 1

This young girl was 7 years old at the time of surgery. She had a ventriculoperitoneal shunt early in life for congenital hydrocephaly. Her first seizure occurred at age 3. She received all types of anticonvulsive medication, including ketogenic diet, without showing any improvement. Preoperatively, she had akinetic seizures with a 5-minute interval between attacks and, less frequently, tonic-clonic and "absence" seizures. EEG records from this period revealed the presence of an active epileptogenic abnormality over the centroparietal area of the right hemisphere with frequent bilateral synchronization (Fig. 2A). Since surgery, she has had only one left focal convulsion despite an important reduction of medication, and EEG abnormalities remain confined to the right centroparietal focus, except for occasional synchronous low-voltage spikes over the left hemisphere (Fig. 2B). Although the callosotomy did not result in noticeable changes on the intellectual level (IQ Leiter: 70), her memory and posture improved considerably. Moreover, behaviorally, this previously anorexic patient has shown a significant increase in appetite accompanied by a more positive attitude toward her family and social contacts. Her improvement is remarkable. (Part of this case report is reprinted from Geoffroy et al. [1983], by permission of *Neurology*.)

Case 2

This boy was 6 years 10 months old at the time of callosotomy. The operation was performed because of severe intractable seizures (tonic-clonic, absences, akinetic and myoclonic) of unknown cause that began at age 3 and developed frequently into "status epilepticus." He was treated with all known regimens including adrenocorticotropin (ACTH), ketogenic diet, and taurine. Before surgery, the daily medication of this patient consisted of 1.5 mg clonazepam, 375 mg valproic acid, 125 mg phenitoin, and 60 mg phenobarbital. His preoperative EEG (Fig. 3A) showed a very active epileptogenic abnormality over the right centroparietal region with frequent secondary generalization. He was also hyperkinetic and moderately retarded (Mental age: 3½ years; IQ 50). Since the callosotomy, he has not had a single seizure, although the medication has been importantly reduced (500 mg carbamazepine per day). Recent EEG recordings show only occasional seizure discharges over the right temporal region (Fig. 3B). Moreover, 1 year postoperatively, this child has gained approximately 2 years of mental age (IQ 70) and continues to show substantial improvements in all psychological functions. He is also considerably less agitated, which enables him to concentrate more adequately on various tasks. His improvement is truly remarkable.

DISCUSSION

Children with intractable generalized epilepsy, especially those with initially lateralized EEGs, may be successfully treated by corpus callosotomy. The surgical technique is simple and without complication [Wilson et al., 1978; Geoffroy et al., 1983]. No permanent neurological nor psychological deficits were observed in our patients. On the contrary, 87% of the patients improved, 46% of them dramatically.

These results indicate that surgical section of the corpus callosum prevents the propagation of epileptogenic discharges to the opposite hemisphere; seizure activity remains essentially lateralized and responds more favorably to medication. Moreover, callosotomy appears to reduce the frequency and severity of seizure discharges in the original focus (e.g., Fig. 3B). This observation points to the corpus callosum as the most important pathway by which each hemisphere excerts a facilitatory influence on its counterpart (see also Lassonde in this issue). In fact, the facilitatory influence of callosal influx on the activation of contralateral cortical neurons has been experimentally demonstrated by the electrophysiological studies of Bremer [1967] in the cat. These experiments have shown that evoked responses to electrical stimulation of various areas of the visual cortex are

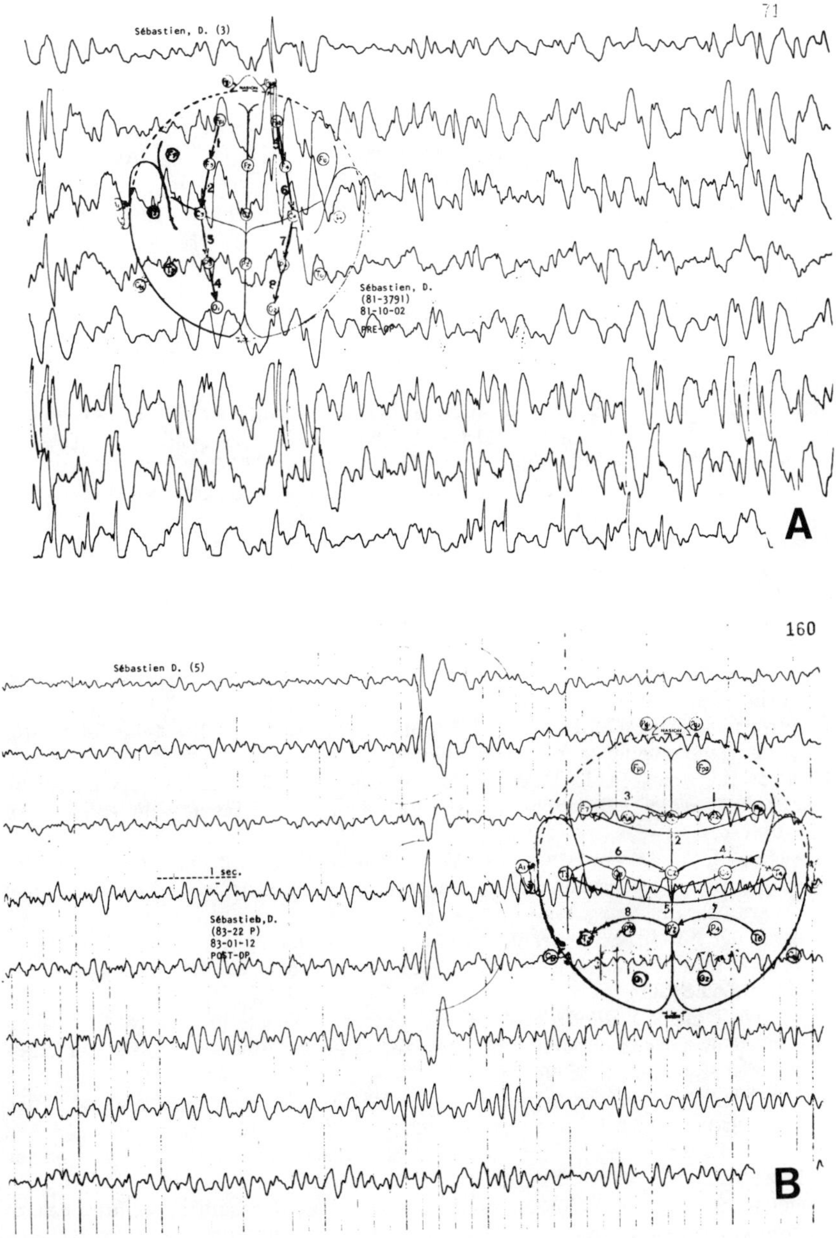

Fig. 3. A. Preoperative EEG of case 2, showing a very active epileptogenic abnormality over the right centroparietal region with frequent secondary generalization. B. Postoperative record of the same patient. A few spikes over the right anterior and mid-temporal regions.

augmented when they are preceded by stimulation of homotopic zones in the opposite hemisphere. This facilitatory effect is abolished by sectioning the corpus callosum.

Thus, the functional properties of the corpus callosum seem to be disadvantageous to the epileptic patient in more than one way, and surgical division of this commissure may not only help to arrest interhemispheric spreading of seizure discharges but could also prevent the healthy hemisphere from potentiating abnormal neural activity in the lesioned hemisphere that might otherwise remain subliminal.

REFERENCES

Bogen JE, Vogel PJ (1962): Cerebral commissurotomy in man. Bull Los Angeles Neurol Soc 27:169–172.

Bogen JE, Vogel PJ (1975): Neurologic status in the long-term following complete cerebral commissurotomy. In Michel F, Schott B (eds): "Les syndromes de disconnexion calleuse chez l'homme." Lyon: Hop Neurol pp 227–251.

Bremer F (1967): Le corps calleux à la lumière de travaux récents. Lav Med 38:835–843.

Campbell AL, Bogen JE, Smith A (1981): Disorganization and reorganization of cognitive and sensori-motor functions in cerebral commissurotomy. Brain 104:493–511.

Erickson TC (1940): Spread of the epileptic discharges. Arch Neurol Psychiatr 43:429–452.

Gazzaniga MS, Bogen JE, Sperry RW (1962): Some functional effects of sectioning of the cerebral commissures in man. Proc Natl Acad Sci USA 48:1765–1769.

Geoffroy G, Lassonde M, Delisle F, Décarie M (1983): Corpus callosotomy for control of intractable epilepsy in children. Neurology 33:891–897.

Geoffroy G, Sauerwein H, Lassonde M, Décarie M (1985): A further report on the effectiveness of callosotomy in the management of intractable epilepsy in children.

Lassonde M, Sauerwein H, Geoffroy G, Décarie M (1985): Effects of early and late transection of the corpus callosum in children: A study of tactual and tactuomotor transfer and integration.

Luessenhop AJ (1970): Interhemispheric commissurotomy: (the split-brain operation) as an alternate to hemispherectomy for control of intractable seizures. Am Surg 36:265–268.

Musgrave J, Gloor P (1980): The role of the corpus callosum in bilateral interhemispheric synchrony of spike and wave discharge in feline generalized penicillin epilepsy. Epilepsia 21:369–378.

Wilson DH, Reeves A, Gazzaniga M, Culver C (1977): Cerebral commissurotomy for the control of intractable seizures. Neurology 27:708–715.

Wilson DH, Reeves A, Gazzaniga M (1978): Division of the corpus callosum for incontrollable epilepsy. Neurology 28:649–653.

Zaidel D, Sperry RW (1974): Memory impairment after commissurotomy in man. Brain 97:263–272.

Zaidel D, Sperry RW (1977): Some long-term motor effects of cerebral commissurotomy in man. Neuropsychologia 15:193–204.

Two Hemispheres—One Brain:
Functions of the Corpus Callosum, pages 369–383
© 1986 Alan R. Liss, Inc.

The Role of Vision in the Patterning of Prehension Movements

M. JEANNEROD

Laboratoire de Neuropsychologie Expérimentale, INSERM-Unité 94, 69500 Bron, France

INTRODUCTION

Prehension movements directed at visual objects involve two clearly different (although superimposed) segmental components. One of these two components corresponds to transportation of the hand as a whole at vicinity of the target object (reaching, or transportation component). It involves proximal joints and muscle groups and reflects computation by the visual system of spatial location of the object with respect to the body. The second component corresponds to an adjustment of the hand posture and the respective position of the fingers (grasping, or manipulation component). It involves distal joints and muscles and reflects visual computation of shape, size, and weight of the object [Jeannerod, 1981].

In normal subjects prehension movements are highly accurate in spite of being relatively fast. In addition to precise computation of the target-related parameters, this accuracy requires coordination of the different segmental components. Different possible mechanims may account for motor coordination during prehension. According to one conception, movements are patterned centrally by way of representations of programs and subsequently executed in a ballistic fashion, that is, with no or little intervention of sensory feedbacks. Lashley proposed that motor patterns should be considered as independent of sensory control for both initiation and timing of muscle contractions as well as for the intensity and duration of these contractions, because he believed that tactile, kinesthetic, and visual inputs triggered by a movement had latencies too long to account for feedback regulation [see Lashley, 1951].

This view was substantiated by the results of experiments in deafferented animals. Provided these animals are allowed sufficient postoperative time to learn how to use their deafferented limb, they can perform precise movements, including those involving the fingers [Bossom, 1974; Taub et al, 1975; Gilman et al, 1976].

Another conception holds that movements are guided by feedback loops after they have been initiated. These feedback loops originate from both visual and somatosensory information generated by the ongoing movement. Logically the only way to disentangle these two opposite conceptions would be to exclude movement-generated sensory information. In that event the observed performance would reflect directly the content of the program. Although visual information can be easily manipulated in experimental conditions, this is not the case for somatosensory information. In this chapter, we take advantage of pathological conditions in one patient with a lesion in the parietal lobe. This lesion had created a disconnection between somatosensory input and motor areas at the cortical level, thus producing effects similar to those produced by peripheral deafferentation of somatosensory feedback. Such a situation was of a particular interest since, when visual feedback from the movements was also suppressed experimentally, it allowed observation of motor patterns that could only be the expression of central mechanisms activated in anticipation to the movement.

METHODS

Subjects sat in front of a box divided horizontally by a semireflecting mirror into two equal compartments. They looked through a window within the upper compartment and placed their right or left arm below the mirror, that is, within the lower compartment (Fig. 1). Small solid objects (e.g, a small sphere) were placed in the lower compartment in the subjects' sagittal plane at 20 cm to 40 cm from the body. A cinecamera running at 50 frames/ s was placed on one side of the box in order to film the radial aspect of the hand under study. Two different conditions of visual feedback from the hand movements were used: (1) complete visual feedback in which the subjects could see the lower compartment through the mirror, and had continuous vision of their hand and the target prior to and during their movement; (2) no visual feedback, in which the view of the moving hand was masked throughout the movement, although the target remained visible permanently. This was obtained by inserting a mask below the mirror between the two compartments. Thus, the subject could see in the mirror the virtual image of an object placed at the top of the upper compartment and projecting in the lower compartment. This protocol is commonly used in eye-hand coordination experiments [Held and Gottlieb, 1958].

The subjects were instructed to place their hand under study on a starting block near the body axis, with the forearm in the prone position and the fingers semiflexed. They were required to reach for, and to grasp the target object as fast and precisely as possible, and to carry it near the starting block. No formal time constraint was given for movement execution.

Prehension movements were analyzed from the film. For each single frame, the hand position in space (transportation component) and the size of the finger grip (manipulation component) were measured and the corre-

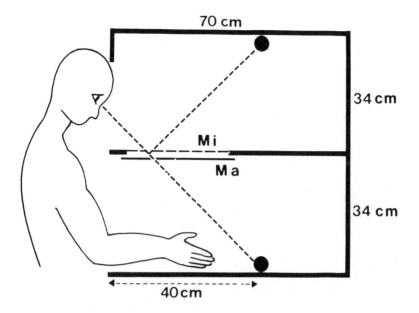
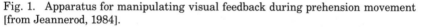

Fig. 1.   Apparatus for manipulating visual feedback during prehension movement [from Jeannerod, 1984].

sponding trajectories reconstructed graphically with the help of a MINC 11 computer. The following parameters were used for data analysis: T, total movement duration; V, peak tangential velocity of the transportation component. Two additional parameters were found to be of interest for matching the two components of prehension. The late part of the transportation component was consistently marked by a breakpoint where the velocity tended to reincrease. The position in time of this breakpoint (parameter A) was measured on the acceleration graph. Similarly, the late part of the manipulation component was marked with a reversal of finger movements from extension to flexion. The position in time of this event (parameter B) was measured as the point of maximal grip aperture.

RESULTS
Normal Subjects

Data were obtained from seven normal young right-handed subjects [see Jeannerod, 1984]. Prehension movements will be first described as they appear in the no-visual-feedback condition. In a further section the changes produced by the introduction of visual feedback during the movement will be mentioned.

Transportation component.

Duration (T) of the movements was found to vary across subjects. For movements directed at targets located at 40 cm, mean duration ranged from about 674 ms in one of the subjects up to about 1,013 ms in another one. This large variability can be explained by the fact that no time constraints were given. However, intrasubject variability was relatively low since coefficients of variation were around 10% in most subjects.

The general pattern of the arm trajectory was that of a reverted U-shaped form. The hand was first raised from the resting position and subsequently lowered down to the object. The profile of tangential velocity of this trajectory was asymmetrical. It was consistently marked by a sharp rise up to a peak, followed by a less steep deceleration. Mean peak velocity ranged between 56 cm/s and 82 cm/s for 40-cm movements, with peak velocities over 100 cm/s in individual examples. The peak in tangential velocity was reached within 308 ms on the average (Fig. 2).

Peak velocity appeared to be poorly correlated to movement duration over the all sample of movements. However, when this was studied in individual subjects, a clear correlation appeared in three out of the seven subjects (the shorter the movement duration, the higher the peak velocity). No such correlation was observed in the other four subjects.

Correlation of peak velocity to target distance was tested in three subjects (subjects 5–7). Correlation coefficients were found to be as high as 0.91, 0.93, and 0.92, respectively ($P < .001$).

The position on the time axis of the change in tangential velocity during deceleration (parameter A) was measured for each individual movement. Figure 3 shows the repartition of A values as a function of total duration (T) of the corresponding movements. It can be see that the breakpoint occurs at a time that corresponds to 70% to 80% of total movement duration (Fig. 2 shows an individual example). The correlation $A = f(T)$ was found to be significant at the .01 or the .001 level in six of the seven subjects. As a consequence of the relatively invariant position of A on the time axis, the duration $T - A$ (i.e., the duration of the secondary movement) can be considered as a relatively constant ratio of total movement duration.

Manipulation component.

The resting position imposed on the subjects' hand before performing the movements implied semiflexion of the fingers. As the arm displacement started, the fingers began to stretch and the grip size increased rapidly up to a maximum aperture. At a later stage, the fingers flexed again and the grip size was reduced in order to match the size of the target object. The size of the maximum grip aperture was a function of the anticipated size of the object; i.e., it was larger when the movement was directed at a large object [Jeannerod, 1981].

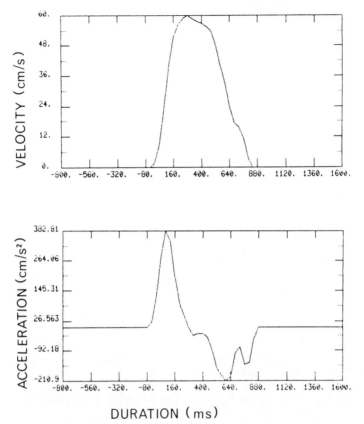

Fig. 2. Velocity and acceleration profiles of the arm during a single prehension movement. Subject 6, target placed at 32 cm from body. No-visual-feedback condition. Total movement duration, 800 ms; time to velocity peak, 280 ms, onset of reacceleration (parameter A), 600 ms. Curves have been smoothed by using a least-square polynominal approximation. Frequency cutoff: 5 Hz.

The average position on the time axis of parameter B (the point where grip aperture is maximum) appeared to be within 74% to 81% of total movement duration in six of the seven subjects. In the remaining subject, it occurred earlier. In addition the time value corresponding to B for each given movement was found to be very close to that corresponding to A for the same movement. Figure 4 demonstrates this fact in subjects 6 and 7 in showing that the point of maximum grip aperture corresponds to the onset of reacceleration of the arm. A strong positive correlation was found between the values of A and B for each subject: in six subjects the coeff-

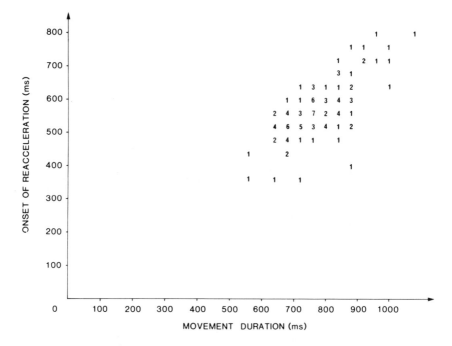

Fig. 3. Onset of reacceleration of the arm as a function of total duration of prehension movements. Digits indicate number of occurences.

icients of correlation ranged between 0.76 and 0.89. In one subject, r was .49 (P < .1).

Influence of vision on prehension movements.

Movements performed under visual control had a significantly longer duration. In addition, the value of parameter A was less than in the no visual feedback condition. The decrease in the value of A together with the increase in movement duration resulted in increase of the value T − A of the secondary movement.

Clinical Observation

Case report.

This case has been fully reported by Jeannerod et al. [1984]. Only the aspects relevant to the present problem are reported here. The patient, R.S., was a 48-year-old right-handed woman who suffered several episodes of meningeal hemorrhage for a left-occipital dural angioma. In September 1976, an embolization treatment had been undertaken with the aim of occluding the occipital artery, the main afferent to the angioma. Pieces of

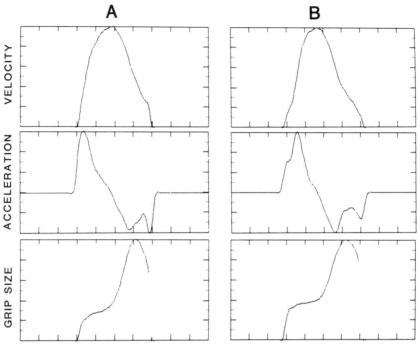

Fig. 4. Averaged prehension movements. Nineteen and 20 movements have been averaged in subjects 6 and 7, respectively. Upper two curves are averaged velocity and acceleration profiles as a function of time for the transportation component. Lower curve is averaged finger grip size as a function of time (manipulation component) from the corresponding movements.

Gelfoam were introduced successfully into the angioma via the external carotid artery. When the catheter was pulled back, however, a fragment of Gelfoam was unfortunately released into the internal carotid artery, which occluded a branch of the sylvian artery. This produced infarction of a large zone of the parietal lobe of the left hemisphere. The postoperative arteriogram showed complete occlusion of the posterior parietal branch, which was intact on the preoperative arteriogram. The artery to the angular gyrus was also blocked but appeared to be filled back through a cortical anastomosis. The CT scan revealed a clear-cut hypodensity of the whole postcentral gyrus, except for its mesial part, and of the supramarginal gyrus. The precentral gyrus was apparently spared. The thalamus seemed to be intact, although the thalamic parietal radiations were likely to be destroyed.

Following this cerebral insult, R.S. presented a complex syndrome with a right hemianopia and a right hemianesthesia. Aphasia was present with alexia and agraphia. Ideational apraxia was also present, but cleared rapidly. No signs of posterior parietal involvement, such as unilateral neglect or optic ataxia, were present at any stage. The "body image" was never perturbed.

At the time of testing, the somatosensory deficit appeared to be stable since little or no change was observed over the past 3 years. Sensory loss was virutally complete for the right hand and wrist. At the level of the right arm and shoulder, tactile anesthesia was less severe, since strong stimuli were detected and grossly localized. Sensitivity to cold, warm, as well as vibratory stimuli was impaired with the same distribution as for the tactile stimuli. Sensations evoked by passive movements were abolished at the right fingers and wrist. At the right elbow the direction of passively induced movements could not be consistently detected. In the absence of visual control, R.S. made frequent errors whenever she indicated the direction of passive movements verbally or she tried to match the angle of her right elbow with her other arm. The level of detection was influenced by the velocity of the movement. Better detection was achieved when movements were applied briskly, whereas slow movements were never detected. Finally, at the right shoulder, the direction of passive movements could be detected with less error and matching with the other arm was reasonably good.

Repeated neurological examination never revealed any clinically detectable pure motor deficit. Tendon reflexes were found to be symmetrical in both arms and legs. Plantar reflexes were flexor on both sides. Muscle tone in the right upper limb was normal. In the early stages of recovery, R.S. would not use her right hand spontaneously; later, she used her right hand in everyday life for many types of action, provided she could control her movements visually. Without visual control, however, movements with her right upper limb became awkward and inefficient. Independent and rapid finger movements, such as in drumming or tapping, were performed more proficiently under visual control. In the absence of vision, the rate of tapping with the right index finger could not be sustained and rapidly degraded. However, an almost normal tapping rate could be sustained when the taps were made audible.

Finally, R.S. was tested for her ability to make distal sequential gestures under visual control and without vision. Under visual control, she was able to touch accurately with the tip of her thumb any part of the palmar surface of her four other fingers. Without vision, however, she was unable to do so. In her attempts, movements were clumsy and spatially disoriented. This observation is contradictory to that made by Volpe et al. [979] in their patients with severe hemianesthesia. Our patient was found to be able to draw in the air figures or letters without difficulty under visual control.

Without vision, the same movements could not be executed. In her attempts, R.S. described verbally what she thought she was doing, but her fingers appeared to move randomly and with a very limited amplitude. Looking at the videotape recording of these gestures a naive observer would probaly term the impairment a "melokinetic" apraxia.

Simple reaction time was studied by monitoring the depression of a key with either index finger in response to an acoustic or visual stimulus. In both conditions, reaction time was longer when the right index was used. Response to a visual stimulus took 332 (51) ms with the left and 367 (49) ms with the right index. Response to an acoustic stimulus took 223.5 (52) ms with the left and 353.8 (81) ms with the right index.

Prehension Movements

R.S.'s prehension movements were analyzed separately for each hand. Only a few trials were made for the left (normal) hand. A total of 50 trials in different conditions of visual feedback were obtained with the right (affected) hand. In addition to the two conditions already described for the normal subjects (complete-visual-feedback and no-visual-feedback conditions), a third contition was used. In that condition, vision of the hand was masked before the onset and during the early part of the movement but became available in its later part (terminal visual feedback condition).

With her normal (left) arm, R.S. behaved like a normal subject. In the no-visual-feedback condition (the most restrictive condition), movements performed with that arm were fast and accurate. Total movement duration was 552 (39.1) ms on the average. The trajectory of the transportation component had the usual reverted U-shaped profile. Its peak tangential velocity was 90 (12.2) cm/s on the average. This peak was reached within 272 (29.9) ms (Fig. 5A). The manipulation component was also normal.

Prehension movements performed with the arm contralateral to the lesion were in no way similar to those performed with the normal arm. In all conditions, the shape of the trajectory of the transportation component was different from that of the normal arm. The right hand was usually swept toward the target, sometimes without loosing contact with the table. Under those circumstances the hand was raised at a later stage when near the object. Furthermore, the quality of execution of prehension movements by the right hand was closely dependent upon the availability of visual feedback from the moving hand.

In the complete-visual-feedback condition mean total movement duration was 813.3 (62.7) ms and thus much longer than with the normal arm. This increase in movement time was not due to a slowing in the early phase of the transportation component, since peak tangential velocity was reached, on the average, after 226.6 (18.8) ms. Peak velocity was 74.8 (12.4) ms. Inspection of the velocity profile of these movements revealed that the increase in movement time was due to the contribution of the low-velocity

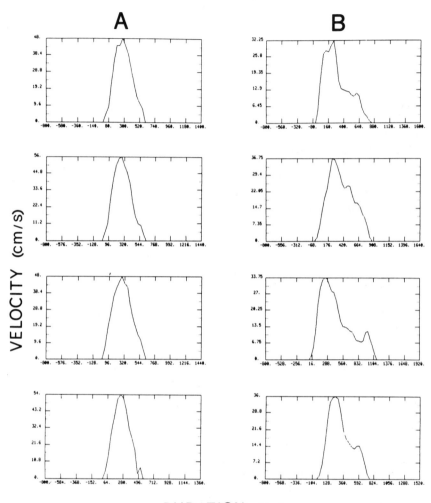

DURATION (ms)

Fig. 5. Velocity profiles of individual arm movements during reaching in the patient. A. Left (normal) arm in the no-visual-feedback condition. B–D. Right (affected) arm in the complete-visual-feedback, no-visual-feedback, and terminal-visual-feedback conditions, respectively. Four movements are represented in a row for each condition. Notice different time scales.

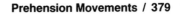

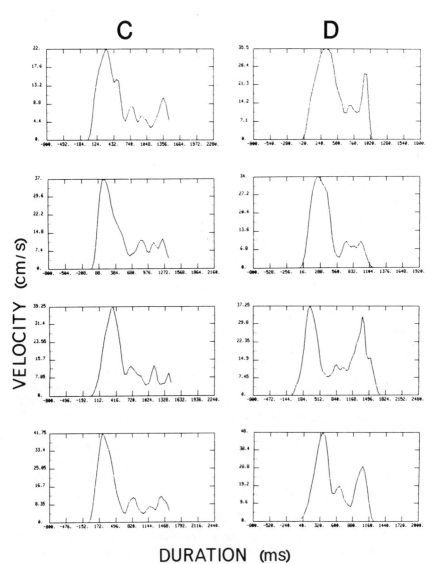

C

D

VELOCITY (cm/s)

DURATION (ms)

Fig. 5

phase of the trajectory (Fig. 5B). This was confirmed in the terminal-visual-feedback and no-visual-feedback conditions. In these conditions the initial phase of transportation was only slightly modified with respect to the complete-visual-feedback condition: peak velocity was reached after 248 (100.8) ms in the terminal-visual-feedback condition and 296 (74.1) ms in the no-visual-feedback conditions. Peak velocity, however, was rather low: 64.8 (11.6) cm/s and 63.6 (14) cm/s, respectively. By contrast, the late phase of transportation was severely affected by visual deprivation. In the no-visual-feedback condition, the low-velocity plateau had a virtually infinite duration. The hand kept endlessly "searching" above the object location without making the final grasp. Obviously in such cases movement duration could not be measured (Fig. 5C). In the terminal-visual-feedback condition, the peak of tangential velocity was followed by a long-lasting, low-velocity plateau until a second high-velocity peak occurred. As a consequence, the movement ended with a brisk grasping of the object (Fig. 5D). It seems that, in the absence of visual feedback, the low-velocity phase cannot be ended and no grasp occurs; when visual feedback becomes available again, a new ballistic movement with a high-velocity peak is generated and eventually yields to grasping of the object. Total movement duration in this situation was 1,032 (226) ms.

The manipulation component of prehension movements was found to be severely impaired in all conditions tested. Basically the anticipatory finger posturing so clearly observed in movements with the normal hand was lacking. Extension of the fingers could be seen after the onset of the movement, but then the hand was kept outstretched without anticipatory flexion of the fingers. In the no-visual-feedback condition the fingers remained spread out during searching for the object. After some time, extension tended to become exaggerated, and this posture was maintained until the end of the trial.

In the complete- and terminal-visual-feedback situations, some late and incomplete visual posturing was observed. This resulted in awkward prehension in which the whole palmar surface of the hand was involved in the grasp, rather than fingertips only.

DISCUSSION

One of the main conclusions to be drawn from this study is that prehension movements have a relatively fixed temporal structure. Movement duration tends to be invariant for each given subject and is poorly correlated with movement amplitude. Instead, different amplitudes of the same movement are achieved by changing peak velocity. Temporal invariance is commonly observed in many types of goal-directed movements [Viviani and Terzuolo, 1980]. In the case of prehension, this characteristic affects not only total movement duration, but also the internal repartition of the changes in velocity during the trajectory. Thus, coupling of the two components can be maintained in different movement amplitudes by keeping a relatively constant position in movement time for the reacceleration of transportation and the concomitant closure of the finger grip [see Jeannerod, 1984].

Another conclusion to be drawn from the above results in normal subjects is that temporal structure of prehension is largely independent of visual feedback generated by the moving limb. Thus, the initial pickup of information by the visual system could account for precise computation of maximum velocity of the transportation component as well as for the maximum grip aperture. Those are the two critical parameters for transferring the spatial aspects of the target into a temporally defined movement. This does not mean that visual feedback is not involved in the control of movements such as prehension. On the contrary, vision is an essential factor in movement control but it acts principally at the anticipatory stage and in conjunction with the reafferent inputs generated by the movement [Jeannerod and Prablanc, 1984].

Contribution of proprioceptive input to the regulation of movement can only be determined from animal experiments and clinical observation in man. Our patient, who was devoid of conscious cutaneous sensation and position sense from her affected arm, was severely impaired in almost all aspects of movement generation when visual information was no longer available to her. First, movement initiation was delayed. Muscular contraction could not be sustained in order to produce a constant level of force. Only very simple, monoarticular tasks could be performed, although more complex tasks involving coordination between fingers could not be executed. This fact was particularly apparent during prehension movements where grasping and manipulation of the object could not be achieved with the right hand in the absence of vision. Restoration of visual feedback only partly improved the performance, since accurate prehension remained impossible. These results indicate that our patient, unlike normal subjects, had to use vision to substitute for the control normally exerted by proprioceptive input to the cortex. They also indicate that visual feedback alone is not sufficient for achieving the normal movement pattern. The main limitation of vision is the relatively long delay needed for visual input to transfer to motor commands and to alter an ongoing movement. Visuomotor delays range between 130 ms and 250 ms according to authors [e.g., Keele and Posner, 1968; Carlton, 1981], that is, much longer than those measured for the somatosensory loop (ca. 90 ms, according to Marsden et al. [1978]). Also, visual feedback may carry information as to position of the whole limb with respect to the target, but not about coordination between segments.

Although the role of vision seems to be limited to the spatial aspects of the movement (direction of the hand at target location and terminal accuracy), the role of somatosensory feedback would be to determine the timing of coordination. In our patient, the situation created by the lesion has revealed a clear dissociation between the mechanisms generating the spatial and the temporal aspects of the movement. In the absence of visual feedback, the computation of final hand position was preserved, although the timing responsible for intersegmental coordination was lost. This conception is not in contradiction with that implying preprogrammation of the movement. It only indicates that motor programs have a limited capacity in the time domain and that information as to execution of the initial part of a program is needed in order to start the subsequent part of the movement.

Finally, one point specifically concerning our patient deserves comment in the context of this book, namely, incompleteness of hemianesthesia. Although sensations from the patient's right distal segments of the upper limb appeared to be completely abolished, sensations from more proximal segments of the same limb appeared to be relatively preserved. This finding has been previously reported following parietal lesions [see Critchley, 1953]. In our patient, preservation of cutaneous and kinesthetic sensations was paralleled by preservation of the ability to control movements executed with proximal segments. Figure 5B–D clearly shows that the initial part of transportation components was normal (i.e., time to peak velocity with that arm was the same as the normal arm), although the final part (corresponding to approach of the target-object and closure of the finger grip) was deeply affected. This difference in movement control can thus be attributed to different degrees of sparing of somatic sensory function in proximal and distal segments of the affected limb.

Several anatomical pathways might account for this difference. First, one has to postulate existence of ipsilateral projections transferring somatic sensory information from proximal part of the right arm to the right hemisphere. In man, existence of an isilateral somatic sensory representation at the cortical level seems to be attested by observations in hemidecorticated patients. These patients report sensation from their arm contralateral to the ablated hemisphere [Kohn and Dennis, 1974]. In our patient, output from the right somatic sensory cortex could reach the motor cortex on the same side and from there participate in the control of proximal segments of musculature of the right arm [Brinkman and Kuypers, 1973].

An alternative route for somatic sensory information to influence movements of the right arm would be a callosal route transferring this information to the damaged hemisphere. The problem with this hypothesis is repartition of cortical areas, which would both receive somatic sensory information and be connected with the opposite hemisphere. According to Pandya and Seltzer [this volume], posterior parietal areas in each hemisphere are widely connected to each other. As we have seen that in our patient these areas were likely to be intact [Jeannerod et al., 1984], they could represent a possible relay for somatic sensory information coming from homologous areas on the right side. Finally, one has to postulate that intrahemispheric transfer between posterior parietal areas and premotor areas [Jones and Powell, 1970] could still be possible within the left hemisphere.

ACKNOWLEDGMENTS

I thank C. Prablanc for allowing me to use his computer program for processing movement kinematics.

REFERENCES

Bossom, J (1974): Movement without propioception. Brain Res 71:285–296.

Brinkman J, Kuypers HGJM (1973): Cerebral control of contralateral and ipsilateral arm, hand and finger movements in the split-brain rhesus monkey. Brain 96:653–674.

Carlton LG (1981): Processing visual feedback information for movement control. J Exp Psychol Hum Percept Perf 7:1019–1030.

Critchley M (1953): "The Parietal Lobes." London; Arnold.

Gilman S, Carr D, Hollenberg J (1976): Kinematic effect of deafferentiation and cerebellar ablation. Brain 99:311–330.

Held R, Gottlieb N (1958): Technique far studying adaptation to disarranged hand eye coordination. Percept Mot Skills 8:83–86.

Jeannerod M (1981): Intersegmental coordination during reaching at natural visual objects. In: Long, J. Baddeley A (eds): "Attention and Performance IX." Hillsdale: Erlbaum, pp 153–168.

Jeannerod M. (1984): The timing of natural prehension movements. J Mot Behav 16:235–254.

Jeannerod M, Prablanc C (1983): The visual control of reaching movements. In Desmedt J (ed): "Motor Control Mechanisms in Man." New York: Raven Press, pp 13–29.

Jeannerod M, Michel F, Prablanc C (1984): The control of hand movements in a case of hemianaesthesia following a parietal lesion. Brain 107:899–920.

Jones EG, Powell TPS (1970): An anatomical study of converging sensory pathways within the cerebral cortex of the monkey. Brain 93:793–820.

Keele SW, Posner MI (1968): Processing of visual feedback in rapid movements. J Exp Psychol 77:155–158.

Kohn B, Dennis M (1974): Somatosensory functions after cerebral hemidecortication for infantile hemiplegia. Neuropsychologia 12:119–130.

Lashley KS (1951): The problem of serial order in behavior. In: Jeffrees LA (ed): "Cerebral Mechanisms and Behavior." New York: Wiley.

Marsden CD, Merton DA, Morton HB, Adam JER, Hallet M (1978): Automatic and voluntary responses to muscle stretch in man. In: Desmedt JE (ed): "Cerebral Motor Control in Man: Long Loop Mechanims." Prog Clin Neurophysiol, Basel: Karger, Vol. 4, pp 167–177.

Taub E, Goldberg IA, Taub P (1975): Deafferentation in monkeys: Pointing at a target without visual feedback. Exp Neurol 46:178–186.

Viviani P, Terzuolo C (1980): Space-time invariance in learned motor skills. In:Stelmach, GE, Requin J (eds): "Tutorials in Motor Behavior." North-Holland, Amsterdam, 1980, pp 525–533.

Volpe BT, Ledoux JE, Gazzaniga MS (1979): Spatially oriented movements in the absence of proprioception. Neurology 29:1309–1313.

Two Hemispheres—One Brain:
Functions of the Corpus Callosum, pages 385–401
© 1986 Alan R. Liss, Inc.

The Facilitatory Influence of the Corpus Callosum on Intrahemispheric Processing

MARYSE LASSONDE

Groupe de Recherche en Neuropsychologie, Université du Québec à Trois-Rivières, and Hôpital Sainte-Justine de Montréal, Canada

Sperry's reappraisal of the consequences of callosal transection on interhemispheric transfer has marked the end of a long speculative period regarding the function of this cerebral commissure. As early as 1925, Bykoff had shown that division of the corpus callosum in the dog abolished the transfer of an unilaterally acquired response. Yet few attempts had been made to reconcile this finding with clinical accounts of the effect of callosal lesions that were already indicative of a disconnection syndrome. Furthermore, owing to the fact that Akelaitis's study [1941] of the callosotomized patients of Van Wagenen and Herren [1940] had failed to demonstrate any permanent neurobehavioral changes following callosal section, symptoms, such as alexia in the left visual half-field [Déjerine, 1892; Trescher and Ford, 1937; Maspes, 1948; Thiébaut, 1955] and left-sided ideomotor apraxia [Liepmann and Maas, 1907; Bonhoeffer, 1914], continued to be ascribed to the presence of extracallosal pathology [e.g., Rohmer et al., 1959]. It was not before the development by Myers and Sperry [1953,1958] of tests specifically designed to assess interhemispheric transfer in the split-brain animal, and their later adaptation by Sperry and collaborators [e.g., Sperry and Gazzaniga, 1967; Sperry et al., 1969] to the study of the commissurotomized patients of Bogen and Vogel, that these earlier described symptoms became associated with the interruption of information flow between the two hemispheres, each specialized for its own set of functions.

Since then, an impressive amount of research has been carried out to define the functional characteristics of the cerebral hemispheres. Much of this work stems from the study of information processing in the isolated hemisphere of split-brain patients [e.g., Gazzaniga and Sperry, 1967; Sperry, 1974; Levy, 1974]. Research conducted on patients with unilateral brain lesions [e.g., Milner, 1974] as well as on normal subjects [Bryden, 1982] have further contributed to elucidate the functional properties of the hemispheres. The results have confirmed the earlier notion [e.g., Jackson, 1874] that the left hemisphere is predominantly specialized for linguistic functions while the right is more proficient in processing perceptual information. However, the origin and development of hemispheric specialization is still a matter of controversy.

Several authors take the position that the corpus callosum plays a crucial role in the establishment of hemispheric asymmetry by providing the pathway by which each hemisphere may exert an inhibitory action on its counterpart in order to prevail in a given function [e.g., Doty et al., 1973; Moscovitch, 1977]. Such a model of hemispheric competition during ontogeny would imply that in congenital absence of the corpus callosum, normally lateralized functions should develop redundantly in both hemispheres. This has in fact been suggested [e.g., Denenberg, 1981]. Jeeves [this volume] and others [e.g., Chiarello, 1980] have already reviewed the evidence that opposes such an assumption. Our own work on acallosal subjects also discredits the hypothesis of bilateral representation of functions in callosal agenesis [Lassonde et al., 1981, 1984]. Furthermore, a follow-up study of a child that underwent callosotomy at the age of six tends to show that hemispheric specialization continues to develop in the absence of callosal input [Lassonde et al., submitted].

An inhibitory role of the corpus callosum has also been suggested to account for the development of dominance of the contralateral over the ipsilateral pathway in the sensory and motor systems that appears to be essential for finely tuned sensation and motor control [Dennis, 1976; see also Jeeves, this volume]. On the clinical level, the callosum has sometimes been described as exerting an inhibitory influence on the build-up of epileptic discharges by keeping neural activity at subthreshold levels [Gastaut et al., 1980]. However, facilitatory influence of the callosal pathway has been more often invoked in the context of the pathogenesis of epilepsy [e.g., Bremer, 1967; Sperry et al., 1969; Geoffroy et al., this volume]. While both inhibitory and excitatory messages may be carried by this commissure, physiological evidence substantiating the inhibitory action of the callosum has been scarce. In fact, electrophysiological studies [Bremer, 1966, 1967], as well as observations of variations in cerebral blood flow or in electroencephalographic activity during performance of various cognitive tasks [for review, see Berlucchi, 1981, 1983] suggest that the primary function of the corpus callosum may be to equalize the activity of both hemispheres in order to maintain an adequate balance and to allow for optimal integration of cortical activity.

For the past ten years, our research team has concentrated on the study of acallosal subjects as well as children and adults who have undergone partial or total callosotomy for control of intractable epilepsy. The behavioral evidence we have gathered from these patients tends to confirm the notion of a facilitatory rather than an inhibitory role of the corpus callosum. Most of the experiments reported herein were originally designed to verify the applicability at the human level of results obtained from animal studies.

Three main themes were investigated: (a) the extent and limits of callosal plasticity, (b) the involvement of the corpus callosum in stereopsis, and (c) the organization of the visual field following callosal deprivation. The outcome of these three sets of studies was essentially similar in that intra- and interhemispheric deficits were observed. This suggests that the corpus callosum may not be solely involved in interhemispheric transfer but may also play an important role in the activation of each cerebral hemisphere.

EXTENT AND LIMITS OF CALLOSAL PLASTICITY

Most of the "split-brain" experiments conducted on human patients or on animals have emphasized the crucial role of the corpus callosum in interhemispheric transfer of sensory information. Typically, patients or animals having undergone section of all neocortical commissures or the corpus callosum alone are unable to compare sensory information separately channeled to the hemispheres [e.g., Sperry et al., 1969; Myers and Sperry, 1958]. This is particularly true for the visual and tactile modalities that are subserved by predominantly crossed pathways. On the other hand, interhemispheric communication does not seem to be disrupted when the callosum is congenitally absent. Thus, numerous studies of acallosal subjects [e.g., Ettlinger et al., 1972, 1974; Jeeves, 1965; Sauerwein et al., 1981; Saul and Sperry, 1968] have demonstrated that these patients are perfectly able to effect interhemispheric comparisons of visual and tactile information. The absence in these subjects of the typical disconnection deficits reported after surgical division of the hemispheres has often been attributed to the fact that the acallosal brain had the opportunity to start early in life to make use of neural plasticity in order to compensate for the agenesis of the principal commissure [Ettlinger et al., 1974; Milner and Jeeves, 1977]. The plasticity-hypothesis gains support from animal studies carried out in our laboratory that have shown that when tested in adulthood, split-brain kittens retain the ability to perform interhemispheric transfer of visual discrimination, provided that their callosum has been sectioned before its myelinization is completed [Ptito and Leporé, 1983]. However, the performance of these animals is limited compared to that of normal, non-operated animals with respect to speed of learning and transfer. In an attempt to verify whether such limitation is also present in our subjects born without the corpus callosum, we decided to compare their *inter*hemispheric performance to their *intra*hemispheric processing of a variety of simple visual discrimination tasks. This was done by monitoring both response accuracy and reaction times. In fact, we expected the latter measure to be more indicative of the efficiency of the intra- and interhemispheric pathways than the qualitative response.

Six patients with total callosal agenesis, as revealed by pneumo-encephalography and/or axial tomography, were compared to six control subjects of the same age and IQ. The subjects' ages varied between 13 and 24 and their IQ's ranged from 64 to 78. The task consisted of a same/different judgment of pairs of stimuli (letters, numbers, colors, or forms) that were presented tachistoscopically for 150 ms: (1) unilaterally, one on top of the other at 3° of eccentricity to the left or the right of a central fixation point (intrahemispheric condition) or (2) bilaterally, one to the left, the other to the right of the central point again with an eccentricity of 3° (interhemispheric condition). The presentation of the stimuli triggered a digital clock-counter, which, in turn, was stopped by the subject's oral response emitted into a microphone. A total of 160 trials were administered in each condition.

The results are depicted in Figure 1A,B. The two histograms represent the percentages of correct responses (Fig. 1A) and the reaction times (Fig. 1B) in the intra- and interhemispheric condition. It is apparent from this figure that acallosal subjects were able to effect interhemispheric comparisons at a rather high level of accuracy (Fig. 1A). In fact, their performance of the interhemispheric task did not differ from their intrahemispheric performance or, for that matter, from that of the control subjects. A different picture emerged when reaction times were compared (Fig. 1B). Here the acallosals required twice as much time to respond than the control group. This result was not particularly surprising, since the agenic subjects may be using a more indirect, slower route to accomplish these interhemispheric comparisons. However, contrary to our expectations, the same results were obtained in the intrahemispheric condition where visual input was channeled to the same hemisphere.

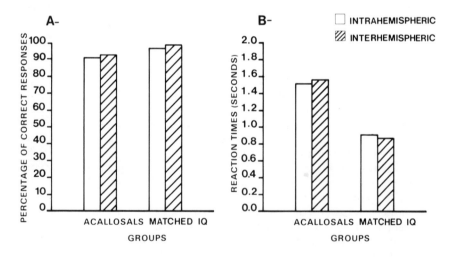

Fig. 1. Percentages of correct responses (A) and mean reaction times (B) obtained from acallosals and matched IQ subjects (n = 6) on an intra- and interhemispheric discrimination tasks.

The deficit observed in intrahemispheric comparisons of simple visual stimuli was not readily explainable on the basis of current knowledge. We first hypothesized that the absence of the callosum might result in a general decrease in the level of cortical responsiveness. The specific cellular changes that have been reported following callosal section [Glickstein and Whitteridge, 1976], or its congenital absence [Shoumura et al., 1975], could account for a certain decline in reactivity. However, reaction times to lateralized presentation of visual stimuli have usually been reported to be within normal range in acallosal subjects [Milner, 1982]. In fact, the reduced efficiency in intrahemispheric processing of visual information seen in the present study seems to be restricted to those situations in which visual discrimination is required. The same phenomenom has been occasionally observed in both acallosal [Ettlinger et al., 1972; Lassonde et al., 1984] and commissurotomized patients [Johnson, 1984; Kinsbourne, 1975]. Thus, it is entirely possible that the corpus callosum may participate in the bilateral activation of those regions specifically implicated in such specific visual activity. In the absence of this commissure, each hemisphere may be still able to carry out an adequate discriminative analysis as evidenced by the good qualitative performance observed in the intrahemispheric condition. However, deprived of the callosal input, neural activity in these regions may be somewhat reduced, resulting in delayed responsiveness. The results obtained from the second study tends to support this hypothesis.

The Involvement of the Corpus Callosum in Binocular Depth Perception

Stereopsis or binocular depth perception depends upon the integration by binocularly driven cells of retinal images falling on disparate positions in the two eyes [e.g., Bishop, 1981]. The anatomical substrate traditionally presumed to convey this information to binocular cells is the retinothalamic pathway, partially decussating at the optic chiasm. Section of the latter considerably reduces the number of cortical binocularly driven cells, while leaving unaffected a small proportion of units. These residual cells are thought to receive their binocular activation from the contralateral hemisphere via the corpus callosum. However, the callosal input to these binocular cells is limited to those units with large receptive fields that are situated close to the meridian vertical [Berlucchi and Rizzolatti, 1968]. At the behavioral level, the effects on stereopsis of lesions of either pathway have emphasized the predominant role of the optic chiasm. In cats, section of this structure has been shown to affect stereoacuity thresholds [Timney et al., in press] and the ability to perceive Julesz random-dot stereograms [Leporé et al., in press; see also Ptito et al., this volume], while the performance of these tasks is little, if at all, disrupted by callosal section in man and animal [Gazzaniga et al., 1962; Bridgman and Smith, 1945; Ettlinger et al., 1974; Timney et al., in press; Leporé et al., in press]. In fact, only one type of stereoscopic deficit has been reported after commissural section:

using a haploscope, impairments in midline coarse stereopsis were found in one commissurotomized patient [Mitchell and Blakemore, 1970] and in some agenic patients [Jeeves, 1979]. However, more recent evidence tends to indicate that midline stereopsis is only slightly impaired in the congenital absence of the callosal commissure [see Jeeves, this volume]. Furthermore, when Mitchell and Blakemore's study was replicated in callosotomized patients with the anterior commissure intact, no deficits in stereopsis were found [LeDoux et al., 1977]. In view of the rather discrepant results obtained from commissurotomized, callosotomized, and acallosal subjects, we decided to evaluate the role of the corpus callosum in stereopsis further by studying the performance of these three groups in a simple task requiring a judgment of distance (depth) between pairs of objects.

Four experimental groups composed of (1) six acallosal subjects; (2) five commissurotomized patients, (3) two callosotomized patients, and (4) two patients with section of the anterior part of the corpus callosum were compared to 15 control subjects matched on age, sex, and IQ with the experimental groups. The stereoscopic task consisted of judging the distance between pairs of familiar objects differing only in their color (yellow or green) and occasionally their size. The subjects were seated in a completely darkened room at a distance of 1.14 m from an illuminated diode that was placed in the center of a rectangular table. The table was covered with a black woolen sheet, and its height was adjusted so that it corresponded to the subjects' eye level when seated. The objects were presented on the table (a) one to the left, the other to the right of the fixation point with a distance of approximately 1° between each other (central condition); (b) at 4.5° both to the right or to the left of the fixation point (intraperiphery condition); and (c) at 4° of visual angle, one to the right, the other to the left of the central fixation point (interperiphery condition). The distance on a sagittal plane between each object and the fixation point was set to produce a retinal disparity of 0.5°. To prevent the occurrence of eye movements, the objects were illuminated for the brief period of 120 ms by a stroboscopic light mounted 3 m above the central fixation point. Each condition comprised 64 trials. The subject's task was to indicate verbally which of the two objects was closer, the yellow or the green.

The results are presented in Figure 2. It is quite clear from this figure that all experimental subjects, except those with anterior callosotomy, were significantly less apt to make depth judgments than their matched controls, regardless of the position of the stimuli. In fact, the performance of the group with anterior section of the corpus callosum and sparing of the posterior part was comparable to that of the control group. Only the absence of the posterior third of the callosum resulted in a deficit in binocular perception of depth. Once more, these results appeared to be rather surprising in several respects. First, the extent of the deficit was unexpected. Only in rare instances have acallosal subjects been reported to have problems in

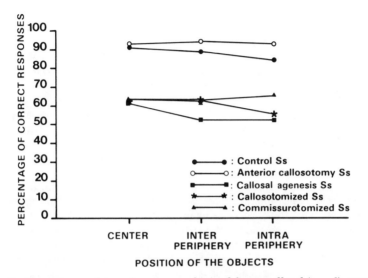

Fig. 2. Percentages of correct responses obtained from acallosal (n = 6), commissurotomized (n = 5), callosotomized (n = 2), anterior callosotomized (n = 2) patients, and control subjects (n = 15) in a task requiring a binocular evaluation of distance between two objects presented centrally (center), one to each hemisphere (interperiphery) or both to the same hemisphere (intraperiphery).

judging distances in normal, everyday life situations [Gazzaniga, 1970; Jeeves, this volume; Rohmer et al., 1959]. Actually, our acallosal subjects, as well as the commissurotomized and callosotomized patients in the present study, did not have any difficulties accomplishing our stereoscopic task during prolonged viewing. However, during tachistoscopic presentation, all patients with posterior callosal section performed the task at, or close to, chance level. Second, we had expected that absence or section of the corpus callosum would produce deficits only in those conditions requiring some kind of interhemispheric communication. Thus, it was not surprising to find impairment of perception of distance between objects presented centrally, since in this condition, the retinal images of each object were conveyed to different hemispheres. Similarly, the interperiphery condition was expected to present some difficulties for the experimental groups since it, too, required the evaluation of the distance between objects supposedly presented to different hemispheres. We were, however, surprised to find a deficit in the intraperiphery condition in which both objects should have been perceived by the same hemisphere. We soon rejected the verbal mode of response as a possible cause of failure. Although this response mode could have handicapped the commissurotomized and callosotomized patients when the objects were viewed by the right hemisphere, no differences were found between right and left visual field presentations in any of the subjects, including the split-brain patients. Furthermore, if the verbal aspect of the task would indeed be responsible for the deficits in the intrahemispheric condition, this should not have affected the performance of the agenic subjects, who are usually able to name stimuli presented to either hemifield [e.g., Sauerwein and Lassonde, 1983].

The finding of intra- as well as interhemispheric deficits led us to hypothesize that the role of the corpus callosum in stereopsis may not be restricted to relaying input from each eye to a small group of binocular neurons, a function which could only account for the impairments in the interhemispheric conditions. In order to explain the intrahemispheric deficit, we had to postulate along with others [e.g., Payne, this volume] that the corpus callosum would also exert a facilitatory influence on those binocular cells receiving their monocular input from both retinae through the thalamocortical pathway. This hypothesis gains further support from electrophysiological findings that have shown that callosal stimulation in cats facilitates the cortical response to stimuli arriving via the retinothalamic pathway [Bremer, 1967]. Such callosal activation should, in turn, become particularly important under liminal conditions, and we believed that the brevity of stimulus presentation used in our experiment might have created such a condition. A second stereoscopic study that we conducted with Patrick Cavanagh of the Université de Montréal confirmed the latter hypothesis [Lassonde et al., in preparation].

In this study, four agenic subjects were compared to four control subjects of the same age (17 to 24 years) and IQ (64 to 78). Their task was to determine whether the stimuli, two random-dot stereograms, appeared in front of, or in the same plane as, a central fixation point. The stereotargets consisted of two bars located on a vertical axis at a distance of 1.5 cm, one above, the other below the fixation point. The stimuli were generated by an Apple II computer and were presented on a color monitor at 0° or 5° to the right or the left of the central point. Three values of crossed disparities— 0.5°, 1.0°, and 1.5°—were used. The subjects, wearing red and blue filters, were seated 57 cm from the monitor screen. In order to familiarize them with the task, the stimuli were first presented at a duration of 4 s. When the performance had reached a level of 90% in a series of 40 trials, stimulus duration was progressively reduced to 200 ms, a period brief enough to prevent the occurrence of eye movements. The subjects were then submitted to a total of 200 trials. The results in terms of percentages of correct responses obtained at 0° and 5° of eccentricity are shown in Figure 3A,B, respectively.

At presentations of 200 ms, acallosal subjects performed above chance levels at all disparities and both eccentricities. However, their performance was inferior to that of the controls, regardless of whether the retinal images of the stimuli were conveyed to the same (eccentricity 5°) or different

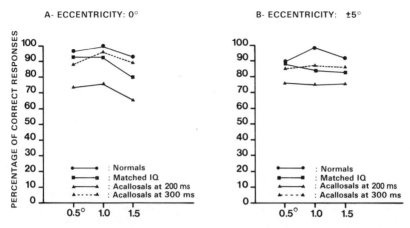

Fig. 3. Percentages of correct responses obtained from the various groups at a presentation of 200 ms. The results of the acallosal subjects (n = 4) with stimulus duration of 300 ms are also depicted. In A, the stimuli were presented centrally; in B, the stereotargets appeared at 5° to the left or the right of the central fixation point.

hemispheres (eccentricity 0°). This difference between acallosal and control subjects disappeared when the former were allowed to view the stereograms for a slightly longer period (300 ms).

The results of this experiment confirmed the presence of both intra- and interhemispheric deficits in stereopsis in the absence of the corpus callosum. They were also in agreement with our prediction that the facilitatory influence of the corpus callosum would be especially important around liminal conditions. On the basis of these results, we further postulated that in the absence of callosal facilitation and under specific limitating conditions, subtle bilateral deficits should be found. This hypothesis was partially confirmed by the results obtained in the following experiment.

VISUAL FIELD ORGANIZATION FOLLOWING CALLOSAL DEPRIVATION

The anatomical work of Innocenti and his colleagues carried out on cats has revealed that callosal connections are considerably more numerous at birth than in adulthood [see Innocenti, this volume]. Similarly, Elberger and her colleagues [see Elberger, this volume] have shown that callosal section in neonate cats may produce deficits that are often absent in animals operated in adulthood. For example, section of the posterior part of the callosum in neonate kittens was found to affect the organization of the visual field, producing a loss in visual responsiveness that included the field contralateral to the eye tested [Elberger, 1979; see also Elberger, this volume].

In order to test the applicability of these animal results to our human subjects, we compared the monocular and binocular visual fields of two agenic subjects, aged 17 and 24, to those of patients who had undergone at adulthood (a) a total callosotomy (n = 1), (b) a section of the posterior third of the corpus callosum (n = 1), or (c) an anterior callosotomy (n = 1). Four control subjects, matched on age and IQ with the agenic subjects, and four subjects with a normal IQ were also tested. The task consisted of pointing with either arm in the direction of a luminous square (2°) that appeared for 150 ms on one of two monitor screens. These monitors, located one in the left, the other in the right visual field, were mounted on pivots that could be silently rotated along a giant perimeter with a half-diameter of 1.14 m. On each trial, the monitors were positioned at different eccentricities (± 5°, 20°, 35°, 50°, 65°, 80°). The subjects were seated in a completely darkened room at a distance of 1.14 m from an illuminated diode located at eccentricity 0° on the table. The subject's eye level corresponded both to the height of this central diode and to that of the stimulus appearing on the screen. Once the subject had pointed to the luminous source, a curtain was closed to prevent him from seeing his responding hand, thus making the experimental situation an open-looped condition [e.g., Perenin and Vighetto, 1983]. A total of 480 trials were administered, consisting of 120 right and 120 left visual field presentations for each responding hand.

When tested under this paradigm, the results of the subjects were consistent with their neuroophthalmologic examination in that the monocular and binocular fields appeared normal. However, another type of difficulty was observed: when the percentages of correct pointing (i.e., within 10° of the target) were evaluated, it appeared that all patients deprived of their callosum, or its posterior part, were grossly inaccurate in their pointing. In fact, while control subjects and patients with anterior callosal section were able to make precise visually directed responses with either hand, acallosals, as well as callosotomized patients with total or posterior section, missed the targets often by more than 30°. This imprecision of gesture affected both hands and was to a certain degree apparent in both visual fields, although the responses with the right hand in the homolateral field were more often accurate (Fig. 4A,B). These difficulties in effecting visually directed hand movements, often referred to as optic ataxia, had, in fact, already been described in acallosal [Rohmer et al., 1959] and split-brain patients [Gazzaniga et al., 1965]. However, in these previous accounts, the specific disorder in visuomotor coordination had been reported only for the hand ipsilateral to the seeing hemisphere and had been attributed to a disconnection between the visual areas of the stimulated and the motor areas of the responding hemisphere [Rondot et al., 1977]. The deficit was thus interpreted as being part of the disconnection syndrome and had been labeled "bilateral crossed optic ataxia."

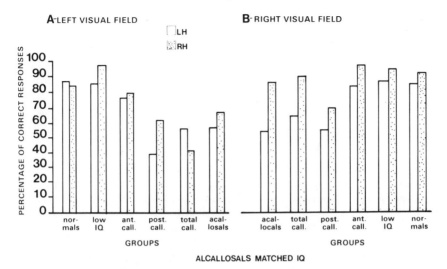

Fig. 4. Percentages of correct pointing responses for the various groups of subjects. RH = right hand; LH = left hand; normals = subjects with normal IQ (n = 4); low IQ = subjects with a mean IQ of 60 (n = 4); ant. call. = anterior callosotomy (n = 1); post. call. = posterior callosotomy (n = 1); total call. = total callosotomy (n = 1); acallosals = total agenesis of the corpus callosum (n = 2).

In contrast, our study revealed that the optic ataxia seen in agenic and callosotomized patients is not restricted to contralateral stimulus-response situations. In fact, there are other instances in which functional loss of the callosum seems to produce deficits in pointing that differ from the conventional crossed optic ataxia. For example, accurate pointing with the left hand to stimuli in the right visual field, but errors in indicating with the right hand the location of a stimulus in the contralateral visual field were observed by Levine and Calvanio [1980] in a patient with posterior section of the corpus callosum. Greater deficits in pointing with the contralateral hand to stimuli presented in the left visual field have also been observed in three callosal agenesis patients described by Rohmer et al. [1959]. In another case, the deficit was limited to pointing with the homolateral hand to visual stimuli presented to either half-field.

Although the cases reported here may vary in many respects, it appears nonetheless that optic ataxia following callosal deprivation cannot be solely explained by the disconnection syndrome. In fact, the pattern of our results closely resembles that reported in the case of a right superior parietal tumor [Levine et al., 1978]. Again, we were puzzled by this finding as well as by the observation that in all the cases cited above, the deficits disappeared with either prolonged practice or foveal presentation. At this point, it appeared to us that the absence of callosal influx resulted in a reduction in neural activity within each hemisphere which, under restricting conditions, mimicked the effects of uni– or bilateral lesions.

DISCUSSION

The results of our experiments suggest that the specific deficits in visual and visuomotor functions following section or congenital absence of the corpus callosum are not limited to *inter*hemispheric processing. The longer response latencies to unilateral input as welll as the difficulties in binocular perception of depth between objects presented to the same hemisphere rather indicate that *intra*hemispheric processing is also affected by the absence of callosal influx. These results lead us to postulate that in the intact cortex the corpus callosum exerts a facilitatory, or modulating influence on the neural activity in both hemispheres. In fact, Payne [this volume] has presented a model of how callosal input could operate as part of an "and" gate in the activation of cortical neurons.

The concept of a facilitatory action of the callosum may have some clinical relevance. Based on his electrophysiological studies, Bremer [1967] has proposed that the corpus callosum may play an important role in the pathogenesis of epilepsy by contributing through positive feedback to the activation of abnormal discharges in the lesioned part of the brain. Our own observations of callosotomized patients [see Geoffroy, this volume] suggest indeed that callosal section may not only abolish interhemispheric propagation of seizure discharges but may also reduce, or even arrest, abnormal activity in the initial focus. Moreover, numerous clinical reports lead us to believe that the corpus callosum, through its modulating action, may actively participate in the functional reorganization that takes place after brain injury. Already Goldstein [1948] had pointed out that the integrity of the corpus callosum was essential for recovery of language following left hemisphere damage. This observation was later confirmed by the postmortem studies of Russell and Espir [1961] and Russell [1963] of 255 patients that had been rendered aphasic by penetrating missile wounds. The authors noted that restitution of language functions had only occurred when the forebrain commissures had remained intact. By the same token, Campbell et al., [1981] have indicated that unilateral deficits seen in epileptic patients are more pronounced after surgical division of the neocortical commissures. These observations tend to affirm that the modulatory action of the corpus callosum may be an important means by which the intact hemisphere can help to compensate for loss or impairment of functions in the damaged hemisphere.

Conversely, the reciprocity of transcallosal facilitation would also imply that the lesioned hemisphere could interfere with normal activity in the intact hemisphere, thus compromising the functional efficiency of the latter. This view is supported by neuropsychological studies of hemispherectomized patients [Smith and Sugar, 1975], which have frequently revealed sensory and motor deficits in the residual, presumably intact, hemisphere. Finally, the absence of transcallosal enhancement of cortical activity could explain the appearance of uni- or bilateral symptoms following agenesis or section of the corpus callosum. We are referring here in particular to the difficulties experienced by our agenic and callosotomized patients in effecting precise visually directed movements that closely resemble optic ataxia observed after parietal lesions. In the same context, Milner and Kolb [see Milner, paper presented at conference] have reported bilateral impairments of complex arm and facial movements in commissurotomized patients. The extent of these deficits was found to be greater than that observed in patients with frontal or parietal lesions.

Clearly, the hypothesis of a predominantly excitatory action of the corpus callosum remains to be further investigated. The evidence put forth in this chapter is mostly behavioral, and more direct tests, including electrophysiological measurements, are still required. Furthermore, while the hypothesis of a facilitatory influence of the corpus callosum may best fit our results and a number of clinical findings, it is quite probable that the normal process of interhemispheric regulation requires a balance between both inhibitory and excitatory influences. Unfortunately, in the last two decades, much greater emphasis has been placed on the possible inhibitory role of the callosal pathway. Consequently, a dissociative view of the action of the two hemispheres has emerged, leaving little room for the development of an integrated model of brain functioning. Our conception of the corpus callosum as a modulator of cerebral activity predicts that each of the two functionally different hemispheres may achieve its full potential only in the presence of the other and thus offers a tentative response to the question addressed in this symposium: Two hemispheres, one brain?

ACKNOWLEDGMENTS

This research was supported by grants from the Ministère de L'Education du Québec, Fonds de la Recherche en Santé du Québec, and grants from the National Science and Engineering Council of Canada. I wish to thank Dr. Guy Geoffroy, Director of the Department of Neurology, Hôpital Sainte-Justine de Montréal; Dr. Jean-Marc Saint-Hilaire, Director of the Department of Neurology, Hôpital Notre-Dame, Montréal; and Dr. Joseph Bogen, Department of Neurological Surgery, University of Southern California for allowing access to their patients as well as for their help in the realization of these projects. I also want to express my gratitude to the graduate students, Nicole McCabe, Francois Paquette, Sylvain Bernier, Gilles Champoux, and Micheline Benoit, who participated in the testing of the patients. Finally, I am particularly indebted to Mrs. Hannelore Sauerwein for her continuing assistance in testing many of the subjects and for her kind revision of the text.

REFERENCES

Akelaitis AJ (1941): Psychobiological studies following section of the corpus callosum. Am J Psychiatry 97:1147–1158.

Berlucchi G (1981): Una ipotesi neurofisiologica sulle asimmetrie funzionali degli emisferi cerebrali dell'uomo. Ricerche di Psicologia 20:95–133.

Berlucchi G (1983): Two hemispheres but one brain. Behav Brain Sci 6:171–172.

Berlucchi G, Rizzolatti G (1968): Binocularly driven neurons in visual cortex of split-chiasm cats. Science 159:308–310.

Bishop PO (1981): Binocular vision. In Moses RA (ed): "Adler's Physiology of the Eye." St. Louis: Mosby, pp 575–649.

Bonhoeffer K (1914): Klinischer und anatomischer Befund zur Lehre von der Apraxie und der motorischen Sprachbahn, Monatsschr. Psychiatr Neurol 35:113–128.

Bremer F (1966): Le corps calleux dans la dynamique cérébrale. Experientia 22:201–208.

Bremer F (1967): La physiologie du corps calleux à la lumière de travaux récents. Laval Med 38:855–843.

Bridgman CS, Smith KU (1945): Bilateral neural integration in visual perception after section of the corpus callosum. J Comp Neurol 83:57–68.

Bryden MP (1982): "Laterality: Functional Asymmetry in the Intact Brain." New York: Academic Press.

Bykoff K (1925): Versuche an Hunden mit Durchschneiden des Corpus Callosum. Zentralbl Neurol Psychiat 39–40:199.

Campbell AI, Bogen JE, Smith A (1981): Disorganization and reorganization of cognitive and sensori-motor functions in cerebral commissurotomy. Compensatory roles of the forebrain commissures and cerebral hemispheres in man. Brain 104:493–511.

Chiarello C (1980): A house divided? Cognitive functioning with callosal agenesis. Brain Lang 11:128–158.

Déjerine J (1892): Des différentes variétés de cécité verbale. CR Man Soc Biol 44:61–90.

Denenberg VH (1981): Hemispheric laterality in animals and the effects of early experience. Behav Brain Sci 4:1–21.

Dennis M (1976): Impaired sensory and motor differentiation with corpus callosum agenesis: A lack of callosal inhibition during ontogeny? Neuropsychologia 14:455–469.

Doty RW, Negrão N, Yamaga K (1973): The unilateral engram. Acta Neurobiol Exp (Warsaw) 33:711–728.

Elberger AJ (1979): The role of the corpus callosum in the development of interocular eye alignment and the organization of the visual field in the cat. Exp Brain Res 36:71–85.

Elberger AJ (1986): The role of the corpus callosum in visual development. (This volume).

Ettlinger G, Blakemore CG, Milner AD, Wilson J (1972): Agenesis of the corpus callosum: A behavioral investigation. Brain 95:327–346.

Ettlinger G, Blakemore CG, Milner AD, Wilson J (1974): Agenesis of the corpus callosum: A further behavioral investigation. Brain 97:225–234.

Gastaut H, Regis H, Gastaut JC, Yermenos E, Low MD (1980): Lipomas of the corpus callosum and epilepsy. Neurology 30:132–138.

Gazzaniga MS (1970): "The Bisected Brain." New York: Appleton-Century Crofts.

Gazzaniga MS, Bogen J, Sperry RW (1962): Some functional effects of sectioning the cerebral commissures in man. Proc Natl Acad Sci USA 48:1765–1769.

Gazzaniga MS, Bogen JE, Sperry RW (1965): Observations on visual perception after disconnexion of the cerebral hemispheres in man. Brain 88:221–236.

Gazzaniga MS, Sperry RW (1967): Language after section of the cerebral commissures. Brain 90:131–148.

Geoffroy G, Lassonde M, Sauerwein H, Décarie M (1986): The effectiveness of corpus callosotomy for control of intractable epilepsy in children. (This volume).

Glickstein, M Whitteridge D (1976): Degeneration of layer III pyramidal cells in area 18 following destruction of callosal input. Brain Res 104:148–151.

Goldstein K (1948): "Language and Language Disturbances." New York: Grune and Stratton.

Innocenti GM (1986): What is so special about callosal connections? (This volume).

Jackson JH (1874): On the nature of the duality of the brain. Reprinted in Taylor J (ed): "Selective Writings of John Hughlings Jackson." New York: Basic Books, vol 2, 1958, pp 129–145.

Jeeves MA (1965): Psychological studies of three cases of congenital agenesis of the corpus callosum. In Ettlinger EG (ed): "Functions of the Corpus Callosum." London: Churchill, pp 73–94.

Jeeves MA (1979): Some limits to interhemispheric integration in cases of callosal agenesis and partial commissurotomy. In Russel IS, Van Hof MW, Berlucchi G (eds): "Structure and Functions of the Cerebral Commissures." London: McMillan, pp 449–474.

Jeeves MA (1986): Callosal agenesis: Neuronal and developmental adaptations. (This volume).

Johnson LE (1984): Vocal responses to left visual stimuli following forebrain commissurotomy. Neuropsychologia 22:153–166.

Kinsbourne M (1975): The mechanisms of hemispheric control of the lateral gradient of attention. In Rabbit PMA, Dormic S (eds): "Attention and Performance." New York: Academic Press, pp 81–97.

Lassonde M, Lortie J, Ptito M, Geoffroy G (1981): Hemispheric asymmetry in callosal agenesis as revealed by dichotic listening performance. Neuropsychologia 19:455–458.

Lassonde M, Paquette F, Cavanagh P (In preparation): Perception of Julesz random-dot stereograms in the absence of the corpus callosum.

Lassonde M, Ptito M, Laurencelle L (1984): Etude tachistoscopique de la spécialisation hémisphérique chez l'agénésique du corps calleux. Rev Can Psychol 38:527–536.

Lassonde M, Sauerwein H, Geoffroy G, Décarie M (Submitted): Effects of early and late transection of the corpus callosum in children: A study of tactual and tactuomotor integration.

LeDoux JE, Deutsch G, Wilson DH, Gazzaniga MS (1977): Binocular depth perception and the anterior commissure in man. The Physiologist 20:55.

Leporé F, Ptito M, Lassonde M (In press): Stereoperception in cats following section of the corpus callosum and/or the optic chiasm. Exp Brain Res.

Levine DN, Calvanio R (1980): Visual discrimination after lesion of the posterior corpus callosum. Neurology 30:21–30.

Levine DN, Kaufman KJ, Mohr JP (1978): Inaccurate reaching associated with a superior parietal lobe tumor. Neurology 28:556–561.

Levy J (1974): Cerebral asymmetries as manifested in split-brain man. In Kinsbourne M, Smith WL (eds): "Hemispheric Disconnection and Cerebral Function." Springfield, IL: Thomas, pp 165–183.

Liepmann H, Maas O (1907): Fall von Linksseitiger Agraphie und Apraxie bei rechtsseitiger Lähmung. J Psychol Neurol 10:214–227.

Maspes PE (1948): Le syndrome expérimental chez l'homme de la section du splénium calleux. Alexie visuelle pure hémianopsique. Rev Neurol 80:100–113.

Milner AD, Jeeves MA (1977): A review of behavioral studies of agenesis of the corpus callosum. In Russel IS, Van Hof MW, Berlucchi G (eds): "Structure and Function of Cerebral Commissures." Baltimore: University Park Press, pp 429–448.

Milner AD (1982): Simple reaction times to lateralized visual stimuli in a case of callosal agenesis. Neuropsychologia 20:411–419.

Milner B (1974): Hemispheric specialization: scope and limits. In Schmitt FO and Worden FG (eds): "The Neurosciences Third Study Program." Cambridge, MA: The MIT Press, pp 75–89.

Milner B (paper presented at conference): Specialization and integration of the hemispheres.

Mitchell DE, Blakemore C (1970): Binocular depth perception and the corpus callosum. Vision Res 10:49–54.

Moscovitch M (1977): Development of lateralization of language functions and its relations to cognitive and linguistic development: A review and some theoretical speculations. In Segalowitz SJ, Gruber FA (eds): "Language Development and Neurological Theory." New York: Academic Press, pp 193–211.

Myers RE, Sperry RW (1953): Interocular transfer of a visual form discrimination habit in cats after section of the optic chiasma and corpus callosum. Anat Rec 115:351–352.

Myers RE, Sperry RW (1958): Interhemispheric communication through the corpus callosum. Arch Neurol Psychiatry 80:298–303.

Payne BR (This volume): Role of callosal cells in the functional organization of cat striate cortex.

Perenin MT, Vighetto A (1983): Optic ataxia: A specific disorder in visuomotor coordination. In Hein A, Jeannerod M (eds): "Spatially-Oriented Behavior." New York: Springer Verlag, pp 305–326.

Ptito M, Leporé F (1983): Interocular transfer in cats with early callosal transection. Nature 301:513–515.

Ptito M, Leporé F, Lassonde M, Dion C, Miceli D (1986): Neural mechanisms for stereopsis in cats. (This volume).

Rohmer F, Wackenheim A, Vrousos C (1959): "Les agénésies du corps calleux." Paris: Masson.

Rondot P, De Recondo J, Ribadeau-Dumas JL (1977): Visuomotor ataxia. Brain 100:355–376.

Russell WR (1963): Some anatomical aspects of aphasia. Lancet 1:1173–1177.

Russell WR, Espir MIE (1961): "Traumatic Aphasia." London: Oxford University Press.

Sauerwein HC, Lassonde M (1983): Intra- and interhemispheric processing of visual information in callosal agenesis. Neuropsychologia 21:167–171.

Sauerwein HC, Lassonde M, Cardu B, Geoffroy G (1981): Interhemispheric integration of sensory and motor functions in agenesis of the corpus callosum. Neuropsychologia 19:445–454.

Saul RE, Sperry RW (1968): Absence of commissurotomy symptoms with agenesis of the corpus callosum. Neurology 18:307.

Shoumura K, Ando T, Kato K (1975): Structural organization of callosal OBg in human corpus callosum agenesis. Brain Res 93:241-252.

Smith A, Sugar O (1975): Development of above normal language and intelligence 21 years after left hemispherectomy. Neurology 25:813-818.

Sperry RW (1974): Lateral specialization in the surgically separated hemispheres. In Schmitt FO, Worden AG (eds): "The Neurosciences Third Study Program." Cambridge, MA: The MIT Press, pp 5-19.

Sperry RW, Gazzaniga MS (1967): Language following surgical disconnection of the hemispheres. In Millikan CH, Darley FI (eds): "Brain Mechanisms Underlying Speech and Language." New York: Grune and Stratton, pp 108-121.

Sperry RW, Gazzaniga MS, Bogen JE (1969): Interhemispheric relationships: The neocortical commissures, syndromes of hemisphere disconnection. In Vinken PJ, Bruyn GW (eds): "Handbook of Clinical Neurology." Amsterdam: North Holland Publishing Company, Vol 4, pp 273-290.

Thiébaut F (1955): Alexie et dominance hémisphérique. Rev Neurol 93:341-346.

Timney B, Elberger AJ, Vandewater ML (In press): Binocular depth perception in the cat following early corpus callosum section. Exp Brain Res.

Trescher JH, Ford FR (1937): Colloid cyst of the third ventricle. Report of a case; operation removal with section of the posterior half of corpus callosum. Arch Neurol Psychiatry 37:959-973.

Van Wagenen WP, Herren, RY (1940): Surgical division of commissural pathways in the corpus callosum. Arch Neurol Psychiatry 44:740-759.

Two Hemispheres—One Brain:
Functions of the Corpus Callosum, pages 403–421
© 1986 Alan R. Liss, Inc.

Callosal Agenesis: Neuronal and Developmental Adaptations

M.A. JEEVES

University of St. Andrews, St. Andrews, Fife KY16 9JU, Scotland

Presentations already given at this symposium have produced converging lines of evidence, anatomical, physiological, and behavioral, that confirm the key role of the neocortical commissures in the normal functioning of the brain. Thus, evidence has been presented from studies of the topography of the commissural pathways [Pandya, Innocenti], from electrophysiological studies of the commissures [Berlucchi], and from behavioral investigations using lesion techniques in animals [Doty, Alberger], which, taken together, amount to a formidable case for the importance of the commissures in the normal development and efficient, integrative activity of the brain. That being so, the enigma of people in whom the corpus callosum (and at times also the anterior commissure) are totally or partially absent at birth, remains as intriguing today as it was in 1910 when Levy-Valenci wrote, "the physiologist is no less embarrassed than the anatomist by these disconcerting cases" [Levy-Valenci, 1910]. The embarrassment felt by physiologists at the turn of the century is today shared by behavioral scientists in the light of the studies initiated by Sperry and his co-workers [e.g., Myers and Sperry, 1953].

In recent years, there has been a marked increase in the number of publications reporting studies of acallosal patients. These are well exemplified by the work of Lassonde and her colleagues just presented [Lassonde, this volume]. The relevance of such studies to this symposium may be focused by posing the following question: If it is the case that the normal development and functioning of the brain depends in some fundamental way upon the presence of the corpus callosum and anterior commissure, then what predictable consequences should follow if they are absent from birth? In so far as the predicted consequences do not occur, we are faced with the further question: What changes in brain organization might have occurred to compensate for functions normally carried out by the commissures? In order to address these questions more directly, we shall select two supposedly essential functions attributed to neocortical commissures, namely, inhibition and integration, and ask whether the findings from studies of acallosals give support to such essential roles or not.

AN INHIBITORY ROLE

At the end of the 1961 John Hopkins' conference on "Interhemispheric Relations and Cerebral Dominance," Richard Jung [Jung, 1962], speaking as a neurophysiologist, said "For a neurophysiologist, it seems evident that interhemispheric co-ordination and all the functions which have been discussed at the conference, including transfer of training, can only occur *with a considerable amount of inhibition*" [my italics]. This theme has been taken up at regular intervals in the last decade. Thus, Doty and his colleagues [Doty et al, 1973] suggested that unilateralization of language may depend upon callosal inhibition. Dennis [1976] spelled out why callosal inhibition of uncrossed sensory and motor pathways was necessary for the development of topographic sensation and precise motor control. Galin [1977] argued that the development of normal hemispheric specialization depends upon the crucial role played by the corpus callosum. Moscovitch [1977] argued that the corpus callosum is necessary to suppress linguistic development in the right hemisphere. Corballis and Morgan [1978] put forward a theory of cerebral lateralization that implicated an inhibitory role of the callosum in maintaining a left/right gradient in the development of cerebral dominance. Most recently, Denenberg [1981], developing the view put forward by Davidson [1978], argued for a key role for the neocortical commissures in order to guarantee the normal development of hemispheric specialization. Running through these miscellaneous views of an inhibitory role for the neocortical commissures are two recurring themes. First, an inhibitory role in the course of normal development such that the callosum prevents the unnecessary duplication of specialized functions; this is seen particularly clearly in the well-documented left-hemisphere specialization for language and right hemisphere specialization for visuospatial processes. Second, a role in the inhibition of ipsilateral sensory and motor pathways.

Assuming these claims for an inhibitory role for the neocortical commissures are correct, we may go on to ask what predictable consequences follow if the commissures fail to develop either totally or partially. Two have been canvassed that are open to empirical investigation in acallosals. First, functions that normally are lateralized might be bilaterally represented. In this regard, most attention has focused on language lateralization [Sperry, 1968b]. Second, in the absence of the hypothesized normal inhibition of ipsilateral sensory and motor pathways, there might be deficits on tasks of sensory discrimination and motor performance. In examining the evidence from studies of acallosals relevant to these two issues, we must remember that when the commissures fail to develop normally, there are other identifiable structural changes evident in acallosal brains.

As yet, there is no adequate account of the insult that prevents the normal development of the corpus callosum [Loeser and Alvord, 1968; Rakic and Yakovlev, 1968]. It is clear, however, that the time of fetal life when the insult occurs determines the extent of the absence of the callosum. If the insult occurs before the tenth embryonic week of life, it will prevent the development of all the forebrain commissures. An insult in the tenth or eleventh week will spare only the anterior commissure. At a slightly later stage, a defect will not affect the anterior and nascent hippocampal commissures but will result in callosal agenesis. If the insult occurs later in embryonic life, varying degrees of partial agenesis will occur. There is some evidence [Geschwind, 1974] that when the corpus callosum has failed to develop, certain functioning "callosal" fibers still cross via the anterior commissure.

Rakic and Yakovlev [1968] argue that callosal agenesis is not a failure of fibers to grow but a misdirection of their growth. The most noteworthy structural abnormality of acallosal brains is the presence of the Probst bundle [Stefanko and Schenk, 1979]. This is a massive longitudinal bundle lying above the fornix and running fronto-occipitally in the medial wall of each hemisphere. In recent years, several studies have indicated otherwise normal cyto-architecture in some acallosal brains [Bossy, 1970; Stefanko and Schenk, 1979]. Doubtless there are other undetected cerebral anomalies, although in the past perhaps too much stress has been placed on these and not sufficient recognition given to the equal or greater likelihood of similar anomalies in the brains of commissurotomized patients, most of whom have a long history of epilepsy. Nevertheless, it would be prudent not to place too much weight upon reported behavioral and/or cognitive changes in acallosals unless either they have been reported on a number of cases, preferably by different investigators working in different laboratories, or are substantiated by careful, systematic, and controlled laboratory studies and not simply by clinical observation.

An Inhibitory Role in the Development of Lateralized Functions

Is there evidence of abnormal cerebral lateralizations of functions in acallosals? Is there evidence for bilateral representation of language? In answering these questions, five lines of evidence will be reviewed and data from recent studies of the programming and execution of bimanual motor coordination will be presented in some detail.

The results of amytal testing.

Gazzaniga [1970] reported that a patient had been tested by B. Milner using this technique and that normal lateralization of language was present. Gott and Saul [1978] used the technique on two acallosals; one showed lateralization, the other, a nonfamilial left-hander, produced evidence of bilateral representation of speech. Before too much weight is placed on this latter finding, it is worth remembering that 15% of all nonfamilial left-handers also show bilateral representation for speech.

Lateralized visual/verbal input.

Studies using visual input typically present words or letters tachistoscopically to the left or right visual field and measure accuracy and latency of responding. When such tasks are given to acallosals, it is found that they are able to read the words whether presented in the right or the left visual field. Such differences as there are between the two visual fields are within the range found with normals; that is, there is a slight right visual field advantage, though in some acallosals seemingly less than in some normals [Martin, 1981]. There is one clear exception to this general finding. Donoso and Santander [1982] described an acallosal who was unable to read words in the right half of the visual field. They argued that this was evidence for the absence, not only of the corpus callosum, but also of the anterior commissure. We shall comment further on this case later.

Studies using dichotic listening show no consistent pattern of results to justify the conclusion that acallosals have speech and language bilaterally represented. While some have reported an absence of the normal right-ear advantage [Geffen, 1981] there is reason to believe that this may have been due to a ceiling effect [Jeeves, 1979]. Others [Bryden and Zurif, 1970; Lassonde et al., 1981] have shown clear symmetries, though at times with the left ear showing superior performance. This author's own studies with acallosals [Jeeves, 1979] have consistently revealed a clear right-ear advantage using Geffen's tapes. The asymmetry found both in terms of accuracy and speed is, in fact, more robust on retest than occurs with some normals [Jeeves and Silver, in preparation].

Vocal responses to unstructured light stimuli.

Milner and Lines [1982] required normal subjects to make a vocal response to a light stimulus presented in the right or left visual field. They found that in normals the response to the stimuli in the right visual field was consistently and systematically faster than to those in the left visual field. This, they believed, was evidence of the normal lateralization of language and speech in the left hemisphere. Applying the same technique to an acallosal patient, Milner [1982] found that the asymmetry was again evident but to a more marked degree.

Handedness.

Chiarello [1980] reviewed the evidence from the behavioral testing of 29 acallosals and pointed out that of the 29, 21 were right-handed and 8 left-handed. In other words, they are usually right-handed [Milner and Jeeves, 1979; Chiarello, 1980], not left-handed as has sometimes been suggested. This is further evidence of asymmetry of motor control in acallosals. Presumably, if there was no dominance for motor control, one might expect a substantial number of acallosals to be reported as ambidextrous. There is no evidence that this is the case. Since the proportion of left-handers is generally greater in neurological patients than in normals, it would be difficult to argue from Chiarello's data that the overall proportion of right-

and left-handers is markedly different in acallosals owing to the absence of the callosum.

Cerebral dominance for motor activity.

Left-hemisphere dominance for motor control has been argued by, for example, Kimura and Archibald [1974], Heilman [1979], and B. Milner [paper presented at conference]. Evidence consistent with this view was reported by Preilowski [1972, 1975] in his studies of commissurotomy patients. Preilowski [1972] used tasks (see Fig. 1) that required the bimanual motor control of a pen in which a subject had to execute simultaneous mutually adjusted rotary movements of both upper limbs, such that in the movement of each limb, the action of the contralateral limb had to be continuously taken into account. The movement of the pen vertically depended upon the activity of the left hand only, while the movement of the pen horizontally depended upon the activity of the right hand only. In order to trace a line at 112.5° (see Fig. 2), the left hand must turn more than twice as fast as the right, whereas at 157.5°, the right hand must turn more than twice as fast as the left. The subject's task was to trace a line within parallel guidelines and to do so as quickly and accurately as possible. Preilowski confirmed the findings of earlier studies of bimanual activity that had shown that bimanual coordination can be maintained by using visual and proprioceptive feedback as long as performance is slow. However, for perfor-

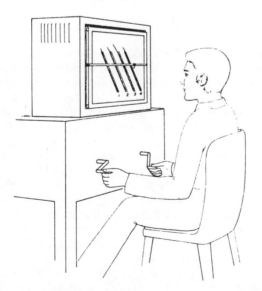

Fig. 1. Task used by Preilowski to study bimanual motor coordination [Preilowski, 1972].

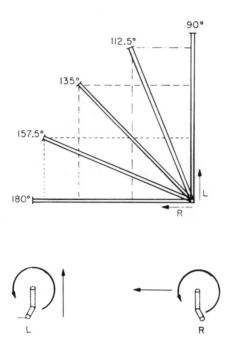

Fig. 2. Directions of lines drawn by subjects in Preilowski's task [Preilowski, 1972].

mance to remain efficient at high speeds, a faster, more direct, and finer bimanual control is necessary, such as would be provided by the interhemispheric exchange of corollary or feed-forward discharges arising directly from the motor outflow. Such motor corollary discharges have been proposed by Sperry [1950], von Holst and Mittelstaedt [1950], and Teuber [1964]. Preilowski found significantly lower quality and speed of performance in surgical "partial split" patients in whom the anterior part of the callosum had been sectioned. These patients also showed a persistent asymmetry such that performance was worse when the left hand had to contribute a greater output than the right hand. (On Preilowski's task this was when patients were required to draw lines at 112.5°.) Preilowski explained his results by referring to the normal left cerebral dominance for motor control. He argued that, if the left hemisphere is dominant, then the major flow of inhibitory impulses through the intact commissures is from the right to the left hemisphere, since, to maintain a state of balance between the hemispheres, the dominant left hemisphere, because it is "dominant," requires greater inhibition from the right hemisphere to maintain equality of activity. Applying this reasoning to the bimanual coordinated activity called for on Preilowski's task, we see that when required to move the pen along a line at 112.5°, the left hemisphere controlling the right arm has to be inhibited in order to extend its lesser output, while the greater output of the left hand controlled by the right hemisphere is taking place. It is argued that the patients with anterior commissurotomies lack the necessary inhibitory transcallosal control and that the result is the disturbance observed in both quality and speed of performance. As the proportion of the right limb output to the left limb output increases in favor of the right extremity, the lack of callosal inhibition becomes less detrimental and results in a relatively better performance at 157.5°. Consistent with this view, Preilowski found that in the absence of visual feedback, there was a trend toward a greater output with the right hand even though overall there was a general tendency toward equality of output by the two hands. Thus, when visual feedback was withdrawn halfway through a trial, the deviation at 112.5° was greater than at 157.5°. As is shown in Figures 3–5, the same effect is found in the performances of the two acallosals tested on the same task. This asymmetry also applies to the speed of performance (Fig. 6). At 112.5°, where the right limb—that is, the left hemisphere—must be inhibited most, we see the greater disturbance in terms of reduced speed, while at 157.5°, when the right hand, the left hemisphere, is inhibited less, we observe better coordination and faster performance. All of this is consistent with the view that in the acallosals studied, left hemisphere dominance for motor control is present. When two acallosals were tested systematically over nine sessions (540 trials), it became evident that the quality and speed of their performance, as compared with normals, was similar to that of Preilowski's anterior commissurotomy patients. Moreover, their performance when visual feedback was withdrawn could be interpreted as indicating normal left hemisphere dominance for motor control.

The Inhibition of Ipsilateral Sensory and Motor Pathways

It is interesting to consider further some aspects of the performance of the acallosals on this task in the framework of Dennis's [1976] hypothesis about the elaboration of ipsilateral sensory and motor pathways in acallosals. Dennis had argued that normally the callosum performs an inhibitory role in the suppression of ipsilateral sensory and motor pathways that otherwise compete with the crossed pathways. In her view, in the absence of the callosum, the ipsilateral outputs compete with the contralateral outputs and result in generally lower performance levels as measured by speed of performance. A general deficit of acallosals in carrying out bimanual perceptuomotor tasks under speed stress has been confirmed many times since our initial report [Jeeves and Rajalakshmi, 1964; Sauerwein et al., 1980]. The generally lower level of performance of acallosals on the X-Y plotter task (Fig. 6) when measured in terms of time taken to complete a trial on the task supports Dennis's view.

Dennis believed that the same argument could explain poor coding of stimulus topography in acallosals, which is characteristic of the represen-

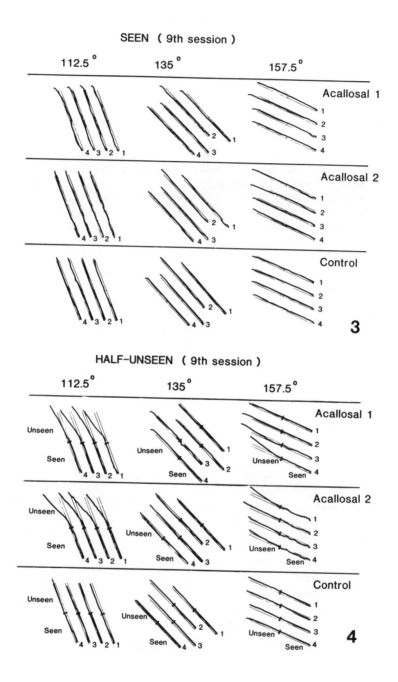

SEEN (9th session)

112.5° 135° 157.5°

HALF-UNSEEN (9th session)

112.5° 135° 157.5°

tation of sensory information by uncrossed and extralemniscal pathways. Dennis [1976] found that topognosis was impaired in acallosals both within hand and between hands. In further support of her view, she reported that unintentional movements within and between hands occurred more often in acallosals than in normals. Her argument was that if voluntary movement of the distal extremities is as much under the control of the contralateral hemisphere in acallosals as in normals, then there should be no difference between the two groups in carrying out independent finger movements. To the extent that motor output is mediated by uninhibited ipsilateral projections, unintended associated movements will occur. Acallosals, in fact, made significantly more unintended movements with both hands [Dennis, 1976]. To sum up, the evidence from our study of bimanual coordination can be interpreted as (1) showing asymmetry of motor control in acallosals and, in that sense, *not* supporting a necessary inhibitory role of the callosum in the development of this aspect of cerebral asymmetry, and (2) lending support to the view that there *is* an inhibitory role for the callosum in the normal efficient control of bimanual motor output. The latter view is, moreover, consistent with a similar inhibitory role for the callosum in suppressing ipsilateral sensory inputs as argued by Dennis [1976].

AN INTEGRATIVE ROLE

Several lines of evidence support the view that when the callosum is absent from birth, there is a reduced level of integration of the activity of the two cerebral hemispheres.

Tactile

On tasks using tactile discrimination and localization, the reports of Dennis [1976] and this author [Jeeves, 1979] consistently identify small but reliable deficits in cross-tactile localization. These, it seems, are not entirely attributable to the ipsilateral difficulties reported by Dennis [1976]. In a recent study by Nilsson [1983], it is evident that the performance in the crossed condition is markedly less efficient than in the uncrossed condition in the acallosals as compared with the normals. There is a suggestion from Nilsson's data that the extent of the deficit in the crossed condition is, if anything, greater in the younger than in the older acallosals (see Fig. 7).

Fig. 3. Performance levels achieved by two acallosals and a typical normal control on a task of bimanual motor coordination with visual feedback after extended practice.

Fig. 4. Performances of two acallosals and a normal control after extended practice on a task of bimanual motor coordination when visual feedback is withdrawn halfway through a trial.

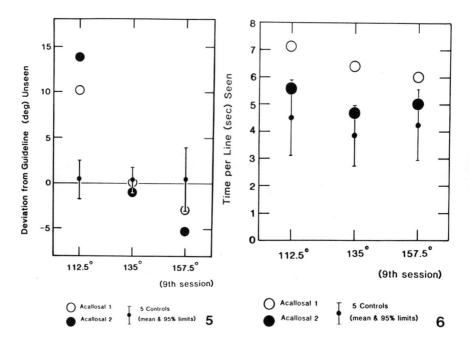

Fig. 5. Deviation in performance when visual feedback is withdrawn on a task of bimanual motor coordination. A comparison of two acallosals and five controls.

Fig. 6. Speed of performance of two acallosals on a task of bimanual motor coordination compared with five controls.

Visual

Acallosals give no evidence of any difficulties in cross-matching drawings of simple shapes or letters or pictures of objects. Gott and Saul [1978], however, reported a deficit when subjects were required to compare *complex* figures such as Chinese characters. Their result confirms an earlier report of Ettlinger et al. [1972], who found a deficit in matching dot patterns in the two visual fields. In the study by Donoso and Santander [1982] mentioned above, the investigators reported that when their patient was required to make complex visual comparisons between the two visual fields, he behaved like patients in whom the anterior commissure and corpus callosum had been surgically sectioned, and made many errors. When the patient was required to name colored patches presented in the right or left visual field, he showed a clear right visual field (RVF) superiority, indicating an inability to effectively integrate the left visual field (LVF, i.e., right

ACALLOSALS ONE FINGER STIMULATED

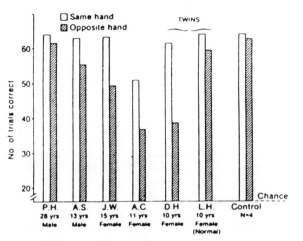

Fig. 7. Crossed and uncrossed responding on a task of tactile topography in acallosals and normals [Nilsson, 1983].

hemisphere) visual input with the presumed left hemisphere competence for language. Likewise, in the naming of pictures of objects, there was a right visual field superiority, as in the naming of syllables. This inability to integrate LVF information with left hemisphere language contrasted with the patient's ability to grasp objects with the left hand, drawings of which had been projected to the left visual field. The authors conclude that the most notable defect of their case was this inability to *name* stimuli presented in the left visual field. They comment further that the existence of a visual path providing significant ipsilateral representation is very improbable, as is shown from studies of patients with hemispherectomies. They believe that in patients lacking only the corpus callosum visual integration could normally occur via the anterior commissure, and they believe, therefore, that in their patient, both the corpus callosum *and* the anterior commissure are absent. If this is so, then it means that visual integration via subcortical pathways is of severely limited capacity.

Several contributors to this symposium have already drawn attention to the role that the neocortical commissures play in integrating the activity in the two visual half-fields [Berlucchi, Marzi, Lassonde]. They have pointed out that efficient cross-connections through the splenium of the corpus callosum and, to a lesser extent, the anterior commissure exist that permit interhemispheric integration between all known cortical areas concerned with visual processing, starting with the primary projection area, VI (or area 17 [Berlucchi, 1972; Zeki, 1970]) and extending into the temporal lobe

[Zeki, 1973]. An earlier study of the patient K.C. [Reynolds and Jeeves, 1974] by Dunn [1977], in which chimeric faces were presented tachistoscopically, reported preliminary findings suggesting that this acallosal patient failed to detect that the pictures were chimeric [Levy et al., 1972]. Findings largely in accordance with these earlier results were subsequently reported by this author [Jeeves, 1979] in studies of three more acallosals on the same task: there seemed to be a failure to detect the difference between the constituted half-faces that form a chimeric face (the join falling along the vertical midline of the visual field). Repeated testing, however, found the deficit disappearing and the question therefore arose of whether the acallosals had developed behavioral strategies to circumvent the task demands. However, acallosal subjects do not fail to see the incompleteness of partial pictures or words cut off at the visual midline [Dunn, 1977; Trevarthen, 1974b] and therefore never experience total perceptual completion as split-brain subjects sometimes do [Trevarthen, 1974a,b].

Earlier in this symposium, Lassonde [this volume] presented evidence showing quite specific deficits in binocular depth perception in acallosals. This author [Jeeves, 1965] had reported that a 9-year-old acallosal boy, P.H., had difficulty in judging distance and that his stereoscopic vision was defective when tested on a coordinascope. An adult acallosal tested at the same time, however, showed no such abnormalities. Mackay [1976], working with Rogers, tested the clinically asymptomatic patient K.C. on a midline stereoscopic task using conditions similar to those of Mitchell and Blakemore [1970] and found a similar deficit, i.e., significantly poorer midline but relatively unimpaired peripheral performance. This result was replicated by this author [Jeeves, 1979].

However, subsequent studies by students working with Rogers on a number of other acallosal patients [Rogers and Cooper, in preparation] have indicated that midline stereopsis is only slightly poorer than peripheral ($> 3°$ eccentricity) stereopsis when appropriate forced-choice procedures are used to record the responses. A possible resolution between the earlier results of Mitchell and Blakemore and the later findings of other workers may be found in the necessary distinction between "fine" stereopsis and "coarse" stereopsis [Bishop and Henry, 1971]. As Cowey [1984, in press] pointed out, it is perhaps a pity that in the Mitchell and Blakemore study much smaller disparities were not tested, because the nasotemporal overlap along the vertical retinal meridian may well be able to handle disparities smaller than $0.5°$. It may also be, as hinted at by Cowey, that patients tested over several sessions on these tasks, as is the case with the studies carried out by Rogers and colleagues, are able, whether thinkingly or unthinkingly, to develop strategies to cope with the particular way this task is presented. Thus, for example, eccentric fixation by the patient may have allowed information about disparity to reach the same hemisphere directly. However, in a subsequent experiment on K.C. that required the patient to report the near-threshold luminance changes of the fixation point (to ensure good fixation), Rogers and Cooper [in preparation] found only a marginally poorer performance for midline stimuli with 0.5–2° disparity. Clearly, further studies are called for in which eye movement is monitored very carefully before any firm conclusions can be drawn on these intriguing data.

Olfactory

None of the studies that have investigated naming of the odors of familiar substances such as peppermint or tobacco have reported deficits either in naming stimuli correctly in either nostril or in correctly cross-matching stimuli presented to both nostrils. It has been presumed that the anterior commissure is responsible for such error-free performance. Unfortunately, Donoso and Santander [1982] did not carry out olfactory testing on their patient, in whom it is presumed that the anterior commissure is also absent.

MOTOR INTEGRATION

One of the first clear deficits reported on acallosals [Jeeves and Rajalakshmi, 1964; Jeeves, 1965] was on simple tasks requiring bilateral motor coordination under speed stress. This deficit, moreover, does not disappear with growth to maturity [Jeeves, 1979,1984]. Patients followed up over a period of more than 20 years continue to show deficits on these tasks. One possible reason for this may be the reduced speed of interhemispheric transmission. This author's earlier [Jeeves, 1969] estimates of an interhemispheric transmission time of 2 msecs in normals has been confirmed in subsequent reports [Berlucchi et al., 1971; Jeeves, 1979; Bashore, 1981; Milner, 1982]. In acallosals our own and others estimates of interhemispheric transmission times range from 10 to 20 msecs. Milner [1982] has produced evidence that he interprets as showing that while the interhemispheric transmission time is measuring a motor transmission pathway in normals [Berlucchi, 1971; Milner, 1982], in acallosals it is a sensory pathway that is being measured. Milner demonstrated that if the intensity of the light stimulus to which the motor response is made is reduced, there is a lengthening of the interhemispheric transmission time. This does not occur in normals [Milner et al., 1985].

A third line of evidence that could be interpreted as being consistent with less efficient interhemispheric information transfer in acallosals comes from the study of bimanual coordination reported above. Here it is argued that the hypothesised motor corollary outflow necessary for fast, accurate performance is occurring with reduced efficiency in acallosals, hence their overall lower speed of performance. Another possibility is that the slower performance is due to the competing crossed and uncrossed outputs. The large deviation in performance when visual feedback is withdrawn could certainly be interpreted as failure of motor corollary outflow in acallosals to cross the midline at all.

COMPENSATORY MECHANISMS IN ACALLOSALS

Since some of the expected consequences of callosal agenesis do not occur (e.g., normal lateralization is present) or, if they do occur, are present in an attenuated form, we may ask what kinds of changes, neural or behavioral, may have taken place by way of compensation. Four possibilities separately or in combination have been proposed [Jeeves, 1965; Sperry, 1968; Dennis, 1972; Milner and Jeeves, 1979; Chiarello, 1980; Jeeves, 1984]. The extent to which they occur in any individual will doubtless depend upon whether there is total or partial absence of the callosum and upon whether or not the anterior commissure is present [cf. Donoso and Santander, 1982].

Behavioral Strategies

Commissurotomized patients have been reported as developing subtle behavioral strategies to circumvent the task demands [Sperry, 1968; Gazzaniga, 1970]. Occasionally acallosals develop such behavioral strategies within a long testing session. One patient being tested on touch localization made *gross* movements of the finger touched on one hand [Jeeves, 1979]. Presumably such gross movements would involve proximal musculature, and thus give a clue to prime the hemisphere making a distal response with the other hand. Generally speaking, however, this seems to be an unlikely type of compensatory mechanism in acallosals since some of the deficits observed in childhood at age 6, such as in bimanual coordination, are still evident 20 years later [Jeeves, 1984]. If adequate behavioral compensations could have occurred, then over a 20-year interval they should have appeared but did not.

Bilateral Representation of Functions That Are Normally Lateralized

In view of the evidence reviewed above, we believe that while such a possibility cannot be completely ruled out, it seems unlikely. Certainly language dominance and motor dominance are evident in at least some of the acallosal cases. As long as there are some such cases with normal dominance, then the argument cannot be sustained that the callosum is *essential* for normal lateralization.

Elaboration of Ipsilateral Pathways

Dennis [1976] has argued for this possibility most cogently. It recognizes that sensory input has access to both hemispheres via the simultaneous use of crossed and uncrossed projections. It then assumes that normally the callosum serves as a pathway for the suppression of ipsilateral input and hence prevents competition between crossed and uncrossed inputs. Dennis believes that the dissociation shown by acallosal patients between tasks of tactile discrimination and localization supports her hypothesis. Certainly sensory input via uncrossed and extralemniscal pathways are known to give poor coding of stimulus topography. Dennis [1981] has extended the hypothesis about failure to suppress ipsilateral input to explain one of the difficulties encountered by an acallosal patient in a linguistic acoustic task. In applying some of Dennis's [1981] tasks to three further acallosals, we [Jeeves and Temple, in preparation] found no consistent picture of language deficits and thus urge caution in applying an argument about lack of suppression of ipsilateral auditory input to explain the language deficits observed in Dennis's patient. The evidence presented above on the X—Y plotter task showing generally lower performance levels by acallosals could be interpreted as being in part due to competition between the crossed and uncrossed motor outputs that are normally suppressed by the callosum. Evidence from animal work [Brinkman and Kuypers, 1973] would support this.

Subcortical and Anterior Commissural Pathways

The possibility of an increased role for the anterior commissure as a multimodal sensory system is argued by Risse et al. [1978]. A subsequent report by McKeever et al. [1981] led to different conclusions. The importance of the anterior commissure is certainly highlighted by the results reported by Donoso and Santander [1982] cited above and supported by the animal studies of Doty and Negrao [1973].

In addition, Jeeves [1965], Ettlinger et al. [1972], and Sperry [1968b] have argued for an increased role for the commissures of the midbrain visual system and recent work by Ptito and Lepore [1983] can be interpreted as supporting this view.

CONCLUSIONS

Careful study of patients born without the corpus callosum and/or the anterior commissure provides another way of evaluating claims that are made for the supposedly *essential* functions of the neocortical commissures in the normal development of the brain. In the light of the evidence currently available, it has been argued that the assertion that the corpus callosum performs an essential inhibitory role in normal development in order to ensure cerebral lateralization of specialized functions such as language, is not supported. However, available evidence is consistent with the view that the callosum may play an important inhibitory part in preventing unnecessary competition between crossed and uncrossed sensory and motor pathways. The claim that the corpus callosum plays an indispensable role in interhemispheric integration is weakened by studies of acallosals, but at the same time, there do appear to be certain residual integrative processes that are never fully compensated for in acallosals either neurally or behaviorally.

REFERENCES

Bashore TR (1981): Vocal and manual reaction time estimates of interhemispheric transmission time. Psychol Bull 89:352–368.

Berlucchi G (1972): Anatomical and physiological aspects of visual functions of corpus callosum. Brain Res 37:371–392.

Berlucchi G, Heron W, Hyman R, Rizzolatti G, Umilta C (1971): Simple reaction times of ipsilateral and contralateral hand to a lateralized visual stimulus. Brain 94:419–430.

Bishop PO, Henry GH (1971): Spatial vision. Ann Rev Psychol 22:119–160.

Bossy JG (1970): Morphological study of a case of complete, isolated and asymptomatic agenesis of the corpus callosum. Arch Anat (Strasb) 53:289–340.

Brinkman J, Kuypers HGJM (1973): Cerebral control of contralateral and ipsilateral arm, hand and finger movement in the split-brain rhesus monkey. Brain 96:653–674.

Bryden MP, Zurif EB (1970): Dichotic listening performance in a case of agenesis of the corpus callosum. Neuropsychologia 8:371–377.

Chiarello C (1980): A house divided? Cognitive functioning with callosal agenesis. Brain Lang 11:128–158.

Corballis MC, Morgan MJ (1978): On the biological basis of human laterality. I. Evidence for a maturational left right gradient. Behav Brain Sci 1:261–269.

Cowey A (1985): Disturbances of stereopsis by brain damage. In Ingle D, Jeannerod M, Lee D (eds): "Brain Mechanisms and Spatial Vision." Nijhof: Martinus, pp 259–278.

Davidson RJ (1978): Lateral specialisation in the human brain: Speculations concerning its origins and development. Behav Brain Sci 1:291–299.

Denenberg VH (1981): Hemispheric laterality in animals and the effects of early experience. Behav Brain Sci 4:1–21.

Dennis M (1976): Impaired sensory and motor differentiation with corpus callosum agenesis: A lack of callosal inhibition during ontogeny? Neuropsychologia 14:455–469.

Dennis M (1981): Language in a congenitally acallosal brain. Brain Lang 12:33–53.

Donoso AD and Santander M (1982): Hemialexia y afasia hemianoptica en agenesia del cuerpo calloso. Rev Chil Neuropsiquiat 20:137–144.

Doty RW, Negrao N (1973): Forebrain commissures and vision. In Jung R (ed): " Handbook of Sensory Physiology." Berlin: Springer-Verlag, Vol VII/3B, pp 543–582.

Doty RW, Negrao N, Yamaga K (1973): The unilateral engram. Acta Neurobiol Exp (Warsaw) 33:711–728.

Dunne JJ (1977): The role of the corpus callosum in midline perception. MA dissertation (unpublished). University of St. Andrews, Fife, Scotland.

Ettlinger G, Blakemore CB, Milner AD, Wilson J (1972): Agenesis of the corpus callosum. A behavioral investigation. Brain 95:327–346.

Galin D (1977): Lateral specialization and psychiatric issues: speculations on development and the evolution of consciousness. Ann NY Acad Sci 299:397–411.

Gazzaniga MS (1970): "The Bisected Brain." New York: Appleton-Century Crofts.

Geffen G, Caudrey D (1981): Reliability and validity of the dichotic monitoring test for language laterality. Neuropsychologia 19:413–424.

Geschwind N (1974): Late changes in the nervous system: An overview. In Stein DG, Rosen JJ, Butters N (eds): "Plasticity and Recovery of Function in the Central Nervous System." New York: Academic Press, pp 467–508.

Gott PS, Saul Re (1978): Agenesis of the corpus callosum: Limits of functional compensation. Neurology 28:1272–1279.

Heilman KM (1979): Apraxia. In Heilman KM, Valenstein E (eds): "Clinical Neuropsychology." New York: Oxford University Press, pp 159–185.

Holst E von, Mittlenstaedt H: Das Reafferenzprinzip (Wechselwirkung zwischen Zentralnervensystern und Peripherie). Die Naturwissenschaften 37:464–476.

Jeeves MA (1965): Psychological studies of three cases of congenital atresia of the corpus callosum. In Ettlinger EG (ed): "Functions of the Corpus Callosum." London: Churchill, pp 77–94.

Jeeves MA (1969): A comparison of interhemispheric transmission time in acallosals and normals. Psychonam Sci 16:245–246.

Jeeves MA (1979): Some limits to interhemispheric integration in cases of callosal agenesis and partial commissurotomy. In Russell IS, Van Hof, MW, Berlucchi G (eds); "Structure and Function of the Cerebral Commissures." London: Macmillan, pp 449–474.

Jeeves MA (1984): Functional and neuronal plasticity—The evidence from callosal agenesis. In Almli CR, Finger S (eds): "Early Brain Damage, Research Orientation and Clinical Observations." Vol 1. New York: Academic Press, pp 233–252.

Jeeves MA, Rajalakshmi R (1964): Psychological studies of a case of congenital agenesis of the corpus callosum. Neuropsychologia 2:247–252.

Jeeves MA, Silver PH (in preparation): Dichotic listening in callosal agenesis.

Jeeves MA, Temple CM (in preparation): A further study of language function in callosal agenesis.

Jung R (1962): In Mountcastle VB (ed): "Interhemispheric Relations and Cerebral Dominance." Baltimore: Johns Hopkins Press, pp 274–275.

Kimura D, Archibald Y (1974): Motor functions of the left hemisphere. Brain 97:337–350.

Lassonde MC, Lortie J, Ptito M, Geoffroy G (1981): Hemispheric asymmetry in callosal agenesis as revealed by dichotic listening performance. Neuropsychologia 19:455–458.

Levy J, Trevarthen C, Sperry RW (1972): Perception of bilateral chimeric figures following hemispheric deconnexion. Brain 95:61–78.

Levy-Valensi J (1910): "Le Corps Calleuz." Paris Theses 448. Paris: Steinheil.

Loeser JD, Alvord EC (1968): Agenesis of the corpus callosum. Brain 91:553–570.

Mackay B (1976): An investigation into two perceptual impairments with agenesis of the corpus callosum; depth perception and the completion of one visual halffield for a chimeric stimulus. Unpublished MA thesis, University of St. Andrews, Fife, Scotland.

McKeever WF, Sullivan KF, Ferguson SM, Rayport M (1981): Typical cerbral hemisphere disconnection deficits following corpus callosum section despite sparing of the anterior commissure. Neuropsychologia 19:745–755.

Martin A (1981): Visual processing in the acallosal brain: A clue to the different functions of the anterior commissure and the splenium. Paper presented at the 9th Annual Meeting of the International Neuropsychological Society.

Milner AD (1982): Simple reaction times to lateralized visual stimuli in a case of callosal agenesis. Neuropsychologia 20:411–419.

Milner AD, Jeeves MA (1979): A review of behavioral studies of agenesis of the corpus callosum. In Russell IS, van Hof MW, Berlucchi G (eds): "Structure and Function of the Cerebral Commissures." London: MacMillan, pp 428–448.

Milner AD, Lines CR (1982): Interhemispheric pathways in simple reaction time to lateralized light flash. Neuropsychologia 20:171–179.

Milner AD, Jeeves MA, Silver PH, Lines CR, Wilson J (1985): Reaction time to laterlised visual stimuli in hemisphere agenesis: stimulus and response factors. Neuropsychologia 23:323–332.

Mitchell DE, Blakemore C (1970): Binocular depth perception and the corpus callosum. Vision Res 10:49–54.

Moscovitch M (1977): Development of lateralization of language functions and its relations to cognitive and linguistic development: A review and some theoretical speculations. In Segalowitz SJ, Gruber FA (eds): "Language Development and Neurological Theory." New York: Academic Press, pp 193–211.

Myers RE, Sperry RW (1953): Interocular transfer of a visual form discrimination habit in cats after section of the optic chiasma and corpus callosum. Anat Rec 175:351–352.

Nilsson J (1983): The effects of corpus callosum lesions and hemispheric specialization on tactile perception. Unpublished PhD thesis. Flinders University, South Australia.

Preilowski BFB (1972): Possible contribution of the anterior forebrain commissures to bilateral motor co-ordination. Neuropsychologia 10:267–277.

Preilowski BFB (1975): Bilateral motor interaction: Perceptual motor performance of partial and complete "split-brain" patients. In Zulch KT, Creutzfeld O, Galbraith GC (eds): "Cerebral Localization." Berlin: Springer, pp 116–131.

Ptito M, Lepore F (1983): Interocular transfer in cats with early callosal transection. Nature 301:513–515.

Rakic P, Yakovlev PI (1968): Development of the corpus callosum and cavum septi in man. J Comp Neurol 132:14–72.

Reynolds DM, Jeeves MA (1974): Further studies of crossed and uncrossed pathways responding in callosal agenesis—reply to Kinsbourne and Fisher. Neuropsychologia 12:287–290.

Risse GL, Le Doux J, Springer SP, Wilson DH, Gazzaniga MS (1978): The anterior commissure in man: functional variation in a multisensory system. Neuropsychologia 16:23–31.

Rogers BJ, Cooper A (in preparation): Midline stereopsis in normal and acallosal subjects.

Sauerwein HC, Lassonde MC, Cardu B, Geoffroy G (1981): Interhemispheric integration of sensory and motor functions in agenesis of the corpus callosum. Neuropsychologia 19:445–454.

Sperry RW (1950): Neural basis of the spontaneous optokinetic response produced by visual inversion. J Comp Physiol Psychol 43:482–489.

Sperry RW (1968a): Mental unity following surgical disconnection of the cerbral hemispheres. Harvey Lecture 6:293–323.

Sperry RW (1968b): Plasticity of neural maturation. Dev Biol, Suppl 2:306–327.

Stefanko SZ, Schenk VWD (1979): Anatomical aspects of the agenesis of the corpus callosum in man. In Russell IS, Berlucchi G (eds): "Structure and Function of the Cerebral Commissures." London: Macmillan, pp 479–483.

Teuber HL: The riddle of frontal lobe function in man. In Warren JM, Akert R (eds): "The Frontal Granular Cortex and Behavior." New York: McGraw Hill, pp 410–444.

Trevarthen C (1974a): Analysis of cerebral activities that generate and regulate consciousness in commissurotomy patients. In Dimond SJ, Beaumont JG (eds): "Hemisphere Function in the Human Brain." London: Elek, pp 235–263.

Trevarthen C (1974b): Cerebral embryology and the split brain. In Kinsbourne M, Smith WL (eds): "Hemisphere Disconnection and Visual Function." Springfield, IL: Thomas, pp 208–236.

Zeki SM (1970): Interhemispheric connections of prestriate cortex in monkey. Brain Res 19:63–75.

Zeki SM (1973): Comparison of the cortical degeneration in the visual regions of the temporal lobe of the monkey following section of the anterior commissure and the splenium. J Comp Neurol 143:167–175.

Two Hemispheres—One Brain:
Functions of the Corpus Callosum, pages 423–433
© 1986 Alan R. Liss, Inc.

Effects of Partial and Complete Corpus Callosotomy on Central Auditory Function

FRANK E. MUSIEK AND ALEXANDER REEVES

Sections of Otolaryngology, Audiology and Neurology, Dartmouth-Hitchcock Medical Center, Hanover, New Hampshire 03756

The purpose of this report is to review our auditory research findings on patients with complete and anterior half sections of the corpus callosum. Our data on audiological correlates of complete corpus callosotomy will be briefly overviewed, but the emphasis of this report will be on auditory results obtained from patients who have had the anterior half of the corpus callosum surgically divided.

There are relatively few studies investigating the auditory system of patients who have undergone complete callosotomy [Sparks and Geschwind, 1968; Milner et al., 1968; Gazzaniga et al., 1975; Springer et al., 1978; Musiek et al., 1979, 1980, in press; Musiek and Wilson, 1979]. Most of the reports on auditory performance in (complete) split-brain subjects involve a single type of dichotic listening task. However, a few studies have employed a broader spectrum of auditory tests from which additional information has been gained [Sparks and Geschwind, 1968; Springer et al., 1978; Musiek et al., 1979, 1984].

Although there has been great variability in procedures, stimuli, and subject characteristics, dichotic speech tests results have consistently revealed a left ear deficit, usually of a marked degree. More recent reports indicate that complete split-brain subjects may have difficulty in verbally reporting various patterns of tonal sequences, regardless of which ear receives these monaural patterns [Musiek et al., 1980; Musiek and Kibbe, 1985].

This brief review on audition and partial callosotomy will be limited to reports in which the anterior half of the corpus callosum, or some portion thereof, has been sectioned. Springer and Gazzaniga [1975] reported dichotic consonant-vowel (CV) results for a patient with only part of the splenium left intact and another with only the anterior third of the corpus callosum sectioned. The first subject revealed a greater left ear deficit than the second. Nevertheless, the second subject demonstrated a moderate left ear deficit (i.e., RE = 67%, LE = 37%). By selectively attending to the left ear stimulus, this subject improved his left ear score by 30%; however, in this same test condition, the first subject showed no left ear improvement. The first subject was also tested dichotically using animal names rather than CVs, and his scores were similar for each ear [Gazzaniga et al., 1975]. Geffen [1980] reported on one subject who had a 30-mm section of the callosal trunk sectioned. This subject demonstrated a marked left ear deficit for the recognition of preselected "target words" presented in a dichotic paradigm. Interestingly, this subject performed normally on phonological fusion tasks (see example below).

Stimulus	Correctly fused response
Left ear: back	black
Right ear: lack	

Considering the relative paucity of auditory data on complete and partial callosotomy patients, especially in regard to preoperative and postoperative comparisons, presentation of our current research findings seems timely.

METHODS AND PROCEDURES
Subjects

All ten subjects had either partial or complete surgical section of the corpus callosum for intractable seizures. Four individuals had a complete section of the corpus callosum with the anterior commissure left intact. Six patients had only the anterior half of the corpus callosum divided with the anterior commissure left intact. The subjects were tested 10 days to 2 weeks after surgery. Usually multiple test sessions were required to complete the assessment. All were right-handed and ranged in age from 17 to 42 years. Peripheral hearing for the four subjects with complete callosotomy was within the normal range bilaterally, both preoperatively and postoperatively. This meant that pure tone thresholds were 25 dB HL or better for frequencies 500 through 4,000 Hz; speech discrimination ability, as measured by the Northwestern University Test Number Six, was 90% or better bilaterally. (Peripheral hearing measures for the subjects with anterior section of the corpus callosum are discussed in the Results section.)

All subjects were tested in a sound-treated room. Pure tone and speech discrimination tests were performed using conventional audiologic methods. Central test stimuli were recorded on high-fidelity tape and were played back on a reel-to-reel tape recorder at 7.5 i.p.s. These stimuli were passed through the speech circuitry of a diagnostic audiometer and presented to the subjects through TDH-49 earphones. Responses were by verbal report, and all subjects were encouraged to guess if they were unsure of a response.

Central Auditory Test Procedures

The following section describes the central auditory tests done preoperatively and postoperatively with the patients in this study.

Low-pass-filtered speech (LPFS).

A low-pass-filtered speech test was administered to three of the four subjects with complete callosotomy preoperatively and postoperatively. Test items consisted of CNC (monosyllables) words passed through a 500-Hz low-pass filter with an 18-dB/octave roll-off. Fifty words were presented at a 50-dB sensation level (SL) re: SRT (speech reception threshold, i.e., the lowest intensity level of two-part words that can be accurately repeated 50% of the time). Right and left ear scores (percent correct) were recorded.

Dichotic Tests

Three dichotic tests were administered. These included the staggered spondaic word (SSW) test [Katz, 1962], the competing sentence test [Willeford, 1977], and a dichotic digits test [Musiek and Wilson, 1979; Musiek, 1983a,b].

Competing sentence test.

This test requires presenting a different sentence to each ear simultaneously. The "target" sentence is presented at 35 dB SL (re: SRT), while the "competing" sentence is presented to the opposite ear at 50 dB SL (re: SRT). The patient is asked to repeat the target sentence and ignore the competing sentence.

For example:

Left ear: I think we'll have rain today (target).
Right ear: There was frost on the ground (competing).

The sentence pairs are presented, and a percentage score for correct repetition of the target sentences is reported for each ear. For detailed scoring information on this test, see Musiek [1983b].

Staggered spondaic word test.

The staggered spondaic word (SSW) test [Katz, 1962] consists of 40 pairs of spondees or bisyllabic words that are presented so they overlap in time as shown in the following example:

Right ear: race   horse
Left ear: streetcar

In the example, *race* is presented to the right ear in a noncompeting condition, followed by *horse* and *street*, which are presented simultaneously in a competing or dichotic condition to the right and left ears. *Car* is then presented to the left ear in a noncompeting condition. The test is designed to alternate the lead word between ears. Test items were presented at 50 dB SL (re: SRT), and the listener was asked to repeat all words heard. Only right and left ear scores of percentage correct for the competing condition are reported.

Dichotic digits tests.

Our dichotic digits test [Musiek, 1983a,b] involves the presentation of paired digits to each ear simultaneously as shown in the below example:

Right ear: 2,6
Left ear: 5,1

The listener's task is to repeat all four digits verbally. The digits are presented at 50 dB SL (re: SRT). There are a total of 40 digits (20 pairs) presented to each ear. Percentage correct scores are reported for each ear.

Frequency Patterns (Monaural)

This auditory task was developed by Pinheiro and Ptacek in 1971. Three tones are presented, one differing in frequency from the other two by being higher or lower. The tone that is different is placed in any one of the three temporal positions generating the following six patterns: high-low-high; low-high-low; low-low-high; high-low-low; low-high-high; and high-high-low. The tone bursts are 150 msec long (10-msec rise-fall time) with a 200-msec interstimulus interval. The frequencies used are 880 and 1,220 Hz presented at 50 dB SL. Thirty patterns are presented to each ear with a percentage correct score reported for each ear.

RESULTS
Before and After Complete Callosotomy

There was essentially no change in pure tone hearing or speech discrimination ability for either ear after surgery. The mean central auditory test scores were grossly within normal limits prior to complete callosotomy (Fig. 1A,B). However, after surgery, all of the dichotic speech tests (competing sentences,[1] SSW, dichotic digits) revealed marked left ear deficits. Frequency pattern scores were dramatically reduced bilaterally after surgery. The mean LPFS[2] scores were not affected by the surgery.

---

[1]Test administered to only two patients

[2]Test administered to only three patients

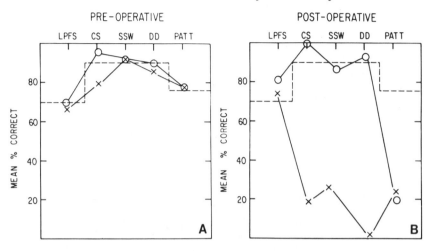

Fig. 1. A. Preoperative right (○) and left (X) ear mean scores for low-pass-filtered speech (LPFS), competing sentences (CS), staggered spondaic words (SSW), dichotic digits (DD), and frequency patterns (PATT). B. Results on these tests after complete corpus callosotomy. The dashed lines indicate lowest limits of normal performance for adults on these tasks.

Before and After Anterior Corpus Callosotomy

The preoperative mean pure tone and speech discrimination scores were grossly within the normal range. At 4,000 Hz, two of the patients did show a mild sensorineural hearing loss. Mean postoperative pure tone thresholds and speech discrimination ability showed little change from preoperative scores bilaterally (Fig. 2A,B).

The mean preoperative scores from five central auditory tests indicated slightly better function for the right ear (Fig. 3A,B). This trend was maintained after surgery. Overall, the mean score comparison preoperatively and postoperatively showed little change in either ear for the five tests (Fig. 4). The competing sentences test results were most affected by surgery, but this was due primarily to a rather dramatic effect in only one subject. It is important to note the considerable variability in both preoperative and postoperative scores bilaterally for all subjects (Table 1). The left ear showed slightly more deficit after surgery than the right ear.

DISCUSSION
Complete Callosotomy

It is clear from the data on the four subjects with complete callosotomy that there are certain central auditory trends. These trends have been discussed before, and thus, they will be only briefly reviewed here [Sparks and Geschwind, 1968; Musiek et al., 1979, 1980, 1984]. Essentially, there is

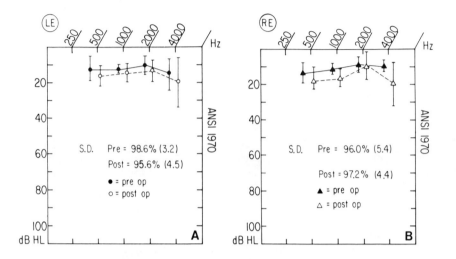

Fig. 2. Mean pure tone speech discrimination (S.D.) scores before and after anterior callosotomy. A. Left ear. B. Right ear.

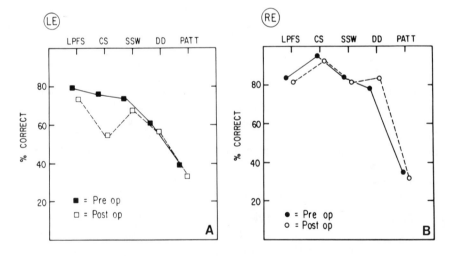

Fig. 3. Mean central auditory test scores before and after anterior callosotomy. (Test abbreviations same as for Fig. 1.) A. Left ear. B. Right ear.

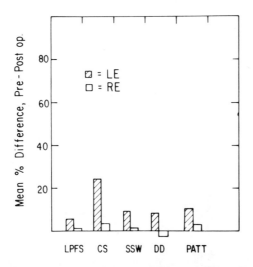

Fig. 4. Mean difference in scores before and after anterior callosotomy for the five central auditory tests. This graph reflects the mean percentage decrease in scores postoperatively with the exception of dichotic digits (DD) for the right ear, which showed an improvement after surgery.

no effect of complete callosotomy on low-pass-filtered speech; however, the dichotic tests show a marked left ear deficit. This deficit is related to the brain's inability to transfer the left ear/right hemisphere auditory information to the left hemisphere for a speech output. The right ear has a direct route to the left hemisphere; hence, speech processing is readily available. This left ear deficit is readily noted for the dichotic speech tasks, because in this situation the ipsilateral auditory routes to the cortex are suppressed, leaving the dominant contralateral pathways to supply acoustic information to each cortex [Kimura, 1961].

The bilateral deficit for auditory frequency patterns has been shown and discussed in two recent reports [Musiek et al., 1980, 1984]. Both hemispheres of the brain must interact to report the patterns verbally. Lesions in either auditory hemisphere or the auditory portion of the corpus callosum result in deficits in both ears [Pinheiro, 1976]. It is theorized [Musiek et al., 1980] that the right hemisphere must recognize the "pattern contour" and then this information must be transferred to the left hemisphere for linguistic labeling and speech output. A breakdown in any of these three processing areas of the brain disallows proper decoding and verbal report of a pattern, regardless of which ear receives the patterns.

Anterior Section of the Corpus Callosum

The central auditory test results before and after division of the anterior half of the corpus callosum reveal high variability in performance; however,

TABLE 1. Scores on Five Central Auditory Tests for Six Patients Who Had Undergone Anterior Callosotomy[1]

	LPFS		Completing sentences		SSW		Dichotic digits		Frequency patterns	
	LE	RE	LE	RE	LE	RE	LE	RE	LE	RE
Preoperatively	78.7 ± 5.9	80.8 ± 9.5	78.3 ± 19.1	97.2 ± 4.9	76.7 ± 23.8	83.0 ± 6.3	63.6 ± 28.6	80.6 ± 9.3	39.3 ± 32.8	35.5 ± 37.4
Postoperatively	74.2 ± 10.3	79.7 ± 12.7	55.8 ± 42.7	93.7 ± 6.8	70.3 ± 28.4	82.3 ± 10.3	58.2 ± 27.1	84.3 ± 16.3	31.0 ± 22.3	33.2 ± 26.3

[1]Values expressed as mean ± one standard deviation. LE = left ear; RE = right ear.

these results, though variable, obviously differ for those obtained for patients with complete callosotomy.

Preoperatively, the "anterior" group demonstrated lower mean scores, especially for the left ear, than the complete commissurotomized group. This finding probably reflects the fact that two of the patients had more right than left hemisphere damage. The remaining patients appeared to have more symmetrical involvement. Greater right hemisphere damage or involvement should yield a greater deficit for the left ear on central auditory testing.

The recognition of the presence of auditory deficits prior to surgery is clearly a critical factor in testing callosotomized patients. Despite this rather obvious consideration, few auditory studies on complete, and fewer on partial, callosotomy subjects report preoperative data. Patients undergo surgical division of the brain usually because of intractable seizures; therefore, brain damage must exist. In these patients, the areas of brain damage may or may not affect the auditory areas. Without preoperative testing, one cannot be sure if the postoperative deficits are truly related to sectioning the corpus callosum or to previous brain damage.

In general, the anterior group revealed considerably less deficits on all central tests than the group with a complete callosotomy, with the exception of LPFS. The LPFS test is a monotic test that is probably less dependent on interhemispheric interaction than the other central tests administered [Musiek et al., 1984].

The lack of auditory effect in the "anterior" sectioned compared to the "complete" sectioned group appears to have an anatomical correlate. Pandya and associates [Pandya, et al., 1971; Pandya, 1982, 1984] have shown that in the monkey, the fibers in the corpus callosum that connect the auditory portions of the two hemispheres are located in the posterior half of this commissure (Fig. 5). If the human corpus callosum anatomy is similar to that of the monkey, then one would not expect an auditory disconnection deficit with division of the anterior half of the corpus callosum.

There was considerable variability among patients' test scores in the anterior callosotomy group. This may be attributable to several factors. There could be individual variances in this structure of the corpus callosum. The auditory area of the corpus callosum borders on the most posterior aspect of the surgical division of the anterior half of this structure in the subjects with anterior commissurotomy. Perhaps, in individual cases, the auditory fibers are located more anteriorly than conceptualized from Pandya's data. There also could be some variation in the surgical measurement reference points, which could have resulted in slight differences in the amount of callosal tissue sectioned. Finally, auditory measurements, especially psychophysical ones, can vary greatly for individuals with central nervous system involvement. The attention level, comfort, and motivation, as well as many other facets of behavior, may be highly variable in a patient with a CNS disorder and these, in turn, can affect test results.

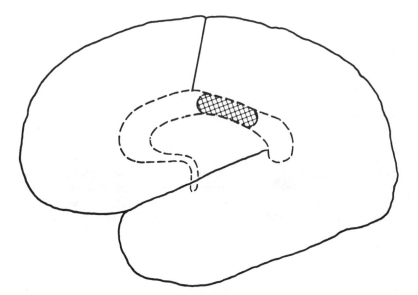

Fig. 5. Author's interpretation of Pandya's [1971] data, which localizes the auditory area (cross-hatched) of the corpus callosum.

SUMMARY

Preoperative and postoperative audiological results are reported for four patients with complete corpus callosotomy and for six patients with only the anterior half of the corpus callosum sectioned. Audiological measures included peripheral tests of pure tone thresholds and speech discrimination ability and central tests of low-pass-filtered speech (LPFS), competing sentences (CS), staggered spondaic words (SSW), dichotic digits (DD), and frequency patterns (PATT).

Complete callosotomy resulted in decreased left ear scores for all the dichotic tests (CS, SSW, DD) and bilateral deficits for frequency patterns. Peripheral tests and LPFS were unaffected by this surgical procedure. Anterior callosotomy patients yielded considerable variability on the audiological tests; however, mean scores from these tests were similar to preoperative scores. The differences in the effect of complete versus anterior corpus callosotomy appear to have an anatomical basis. Animal studies have indicated that the "auditory" area of the corpus callosum is located in its posterior half. Therefore, one may expect a greater "auditory effect" from complete callosotomy than from sectioning the anterior half.

REFERENCES

Gazzaniga M, Risse G, Springer S, Clark E, Wilson D (1975): Psychological and neurological consequences of partial and complete commissurotomy. Neurology 25:10–15.

Geffen G (1980) Phonological fusion after partial section of the corpus callosum. Neuropsychologia 18:613–619.

Katz J (1962): The use of staggered spondaic words for assessing the integrity of the central auditory system. J Aud Res 2:327–337.

Kimura D (1961): Some effects of temporal lobe damage on auditory perception. Can J Psychol 15:157–165.

Milner B, Taylor S, Sperry R (1968): Lateralized suppression of dichotically presented digits after commissural section in man. Science 161:184–185.

Musiek F, Wilson D, Pinheiro M (1979): Audiological manifestations in split-brain patients. J Am Aud Soc 5:25–29.

Musiek F, Wilson D (1979): SSW and dichotic digit results pre- and post-commissurotomy: a case report. J Speech Hear Disord 44:528–533.

Musiek F, Pinheiro M, Wilson D (1980): Auditory pattern perception in split-brain patients. Arch Otolaryngol 106:610–612.

Musiek F (1983a): Assessment of central auditory dysfunction: The dichotic digit test revisited. Ear Hear 4:79–83.

Musiek F (1983b): The results of three dichotic speech tests on subjects with intracranial lesions. Ear Hear 4:318–323.

Musiek F, Kibbe K (1985): An overview of audiological test results in patients with commissurotomy. In Reeves A (ed): "Epilepsy and the Corpus Callosum." New York: Plenum Press, pp 393–399.

Musiek F, Kibbe K, Baran J (1984): Neuroaudiological results from split-brain patients. Seminars in Hearing 5:219–229.

Pandya D, Karol E, Heilbornn D (1971): The topographical distribution of interhemispheric projections in the corpus callosum of the rhesus monkey. Brain Res 32:31–43.

Pandya D (1982): Some observations on the trajectories and topography of commissural fibers. Presented at the Conference on Epilepsy and the Corpus Callosum. Hanover, NH, July 13.

Pandya D (1984): Topography of commissural fibers. Presented at the Symposium on Two Hemispheres, One Brain. Montreal, Canada, May 16.

Pinheiro M, Ptacek P (1971): Reversals in the perception of noise and tone patterns. J Acoust Soc Am 49:1778–1782.

Pinheiro M (1976): Auditory pattern perception in patients with right and left hemisphere lesions. Ohio J Speech Hear 12:9–20.

Sparks R, Geschwind N (1968): Dichotic listening in man after section of neocortical commissures. Cortex 4:3–16.

Springer S, Gazzaniga M (1975): Dichotic testing of partial and complete split-brain patients. Neuropsychologia 13:341–346.

Springer S, Sidtis J, Wilson D, Gazzaniga M (1978): Left ear performance in dichotic listening following commissurotomy. Neuropsychologia 16:305–312.

Willeford J (1977): Assessing central auditory behavior in children: A test battery approach. In Keith R (ed): "Central Auditory Dysfunction." New York: Grune and Stratton, pp 43–73.

Two Hemispheres—One Brain:
Functions of the Corpus Callosum, pages 435–459
© 1986 Alan R. Liss, Inc.

Callosal Dynamics and Right Hemisphere Language

ERAN ZAIDEL

Department of Psychology, University of California, Los Angeles, California 90024

INTRODUCTION

From Function to Structure

Breakthroughs in modern biology, unlike modern physics, have been characterized by highly concrete rather than abstract discoveries. Typically, such discoveries consist of identifying localized anatomical, molecular structures or physiological processes that correspond to well-demarcated functions and conform to our everyday temporal-spatial intuitions. To some extent this state of affairs reflects a science that is predominantly empirical and as yet largely atheoretical. However, such structural empiricism can have a constructive, moderating effect on unconstrained theory. It is in that role that the structure of brain contributes to the functional analysis of mind. Today neuroscience meets cognitive psychology on the ground of experimental neuropsychology. Our goal is to constrain theoretical cognitive models by neurobiologic data and principles.

The recent history of research on hemispheric specialization critically involved a connectionist, anatomic, structural interpretation of complex psychological functions. Animal experiments emphasized the connecting function of the corpus callosum rather than the functional independence of the two hemispheres. What was originally an investigation of the corpus callosum, a well-defined anatomical structure, turned out eventually to bear upon much wider and more complex problems of cognitive function and mind.

The late 19th-century diagram makers in the tradition of Carl Wernicke and Jules Dejerine, believed in left hemisphere (LH) dominance for language; and Hugo Liepmann extended this to LH dominance for motor programing or praxis, of which speech was an important special case. It followed that when the left hand executed a complex motor sequence, the motor cortex in the RH had to be controlled by "praxis centers" in the LH, and that such control was mediated by the corpus callosum. Consequently, callosal disconnection owing to a lesion could result in a unilateral left-hand apraxia. Thus, the concept of hemispheric specialization led to the concept of interhemispheric callosal mediation.

The Akelaitis-Van Wagenen series of commissurotomy surgeries for epilepsy [1944] severely challenged this connectionist view by failing to demonstrate any disconnection syndrome. But systematic animal work starting with Sperry and Meyers [1953] demonstrated in cats and monkeys that interhemispheric disconnection results in interruption of the flow of information between the two hemispheres. The subsequent study of the Bogen-Sperry series of commissurotomy patients as well as Geschwind and Kaplan's study of patients with natural callosal lesions were inspired and guided by these animal experiments and demonstrated dramatically the classic disconnection syndrome. The corpus callosum "regained" its original function and was no longer relegated to the support of the two hemispheres from falling into each other (Lashley), or to the propagation of electrical seizures between the two hemispheres (McCulloch). As the concept of functional hemispheric independence and complementarity developed in the wake of human split-brain research, the theoretical role of the corpus callosum became increasingly important as a channel of communication between the two cerebral hemispheres.

The Corpus Callosum as Channels of Communication

Today, an attractive view is that the corpus callosum houses a set of communication channels, each represented in a different anatomical part and integrating different cortical regions, and each transmitting modality- or function-specific messages in different codes or languages. The transmission in each channel has a definite rate, capacity, and measurable information loss. On this view interhemispheric interaction requires translation to and from a callosal code and messages that can not be so coded must remain locked in one hemisphere, even in the intact brain.

It is possible to regard the communication channels along the corpus callosum from posterior to anterior poles as ordered along a set of increasingly complex or abstract cognitive functions. As sensory visual information, for example, is subjected to progressive stages of analysis and becomes more elaborate, its interhemispheric transfer is said to be mediated by more anterior parts of the corpus callosum [Hamilton, 1982]. Thus, middle and posterior callosal sections should result in sensory-motor disconnection, whereas anterior section could result in disruption of traffic of concept formations and plans across the neocortical commissures as long as such concepts could not be recoded in terms of sensory information. So far, these predictions received only slight and mixed support. While it is generally acknowledged that the splenium and anterior commissure mediate visual transfer, it is also true that a splenial section does not always result in complete visual disconnection. Partial callosal lesions, whether natural or surgical, suggest that auditory functions are mediated through the posterior part of the callosum just anterior to the splenium [Michel, personal communication; cf. Pandya, Imig, this volume], but this again is not universally true. Of particular theoretical interest would be a case of selective disconnection of conceptual but not sensory interhemispheric communicaton with anterior callosal section leaving the splenium intact. Such cases are yet to be reported. They presuppose independent and specialized processing by one hemisphere that can not be communicated to the other by sensory information alone.

It would seem that the corpus callosum is a complex dynamic channel of both facilitatory and inhibitory codes such that partial section can result in a redistribution of channels, leading to compensatory shifts and even apparent paradoxical increases in connectivity.

Alternative Conceptualizations

Brown [1977] regards symptoms seen after callosal section, such as left-hand anomia, as the result of partial or early bilateral processing that has not reached the level of verbal awareness, rather than as a result of independent hemispheric processing or lack of transfer. According to this analysis, the hemispheres act linguistically as one up to a certain cognitive stage that will vary according to the degree of lateralization in the individual. Beyond this level, asymmetric structures carry cognition further in the left hemisphere only. On this hierarchical, microgenetic model, the inability to name objects with the left hand reflects an early level of processing (semantic but not phonological) dictated by RH cognition and language. (Brown believes that degree of lateralization and of RH language varies across individuals.) This interpretation is consistent with the presence of some semantic transfer from the disconnected RH to the LH in the absence of correct verbalization. However, Brown's model fails to account for the discrepancy between the cognitive level of RH and LH perception in the disconnected hemispheres. Why can the right hand not retrieve the same object retrieved by the left hand? It is easy to demonstrate complex nonverbal awareness of a stimulus in the disconnected RH that is simply not available to the LH.

Kinsbourne [1984], too, deemphasizes the role of the corpus callosum as a channel of communication for symbolic information and interprets the disconnection syndrome as a failure of the unstimulated and unactivated hemisphere to assume readiness to perform. Here the corpus callosum is conceptualized as a means for equilibrating interhemispheric activation as well as, or rather than, for transmitting information. Callosal section reduces the resources available to any lateralized cognitive task, resulting, according to Kinsbourne, in a general reduction of level of performance in mental testing. The problem with this account is, first, that it fails to distinguish presence of hemispheric activation from absence of interhemispheric exchange. Suppose that when information is presented to one hemisphere the other hemisphere fails to act upon it. On the one hand, no amount of simultaneous stimulation of the inactive hemisphere will make it able to act on the information locked in the other side. Indeed, no amount of directed attention or set effect will abolish some disconnection symptoms, such as unilateral anomia or a massive right-ear advantage (REA) in dichotic listening to nonsense stop-consonant vowel syllables. On the other hand, by prior training it would be easy to initiate some independent complex activity in the inactive hemisphere simultaneously with the presentation of information to the other side. This would show that the inactive hemisphere is not unready to perform, only ignorant of the relevant stimulus information.

The sharp contrast between the structural-anatomic and attentional models of callosal function serves to highlight the theoretical assumptions and empirical support for each. Although the structural model is probably ultimately too mechanistic, it seems heuristically most useful for a breakthrough in the field in its current preliminary state.

CONVERGING MODELS OF BEHAVIORAL LATERIALTY EFFECTS
Models

Three main classes of models are available to account for behavioral laterality effects in normal subjects. The first two are anatomically motivated, whereas the third one is more psychologically motivated. The anatomical models assume that information transfer through the corpus callosum results in measurable losses of time and stimulus quality. The first, *direct-access*, model assumes that the hemisphere that receives the sensory information first will process it, for better or worse. Laterality differences here are due to relative differences in the perceptual-cognitive competencies of the two hemispheres. The second, *callosal-relay* model, assumes that only one hemisphere can process the information, so that if sensory information reaches the other hemisphere first, the information will have to shuttle across the corpus callosum to the specialized hemisphere prior to processing [cf. Moscovitch, 1973; Rizzolatti, 1979; Bashore, 1981; Zaidel, 1983; but see Swanson et al., 1978]. A third class of models of laterality effects in normal subjects, first proposed by Kinsbourne [e.g., 1975], involves a *dynamic shift* of hemispheric control. Hemispheric activation is said to depend on psychological set effects and thus on a host of task parameters. In this view dual-task priming can increase hemispheric activation, but overloading can eventually shift control to the other hemisphere [Hellige et al., 1979; Moscovitch and Klein, 1980; Friedman et al., 1982; Kinsbourne and Hiscock, 1983; Hellige, 1984]. Dynamic-shift models utilze both the direct-access assumption of bilateral competence and the callosal-relay emphasis on cross-callosal transfer.

Direct-access models are often suggested by split-brain as well as lesion studies showing different performance styles in the two hemispheres for certain cognitive tasks. Callosal-relay models for various functions are suggested by selective cognitive deficits following hemispheric lesions. Individual differences in laterality effects (behavioral specialization effects in laterality experiments) in a callosal-relay task can be due in part to individual differences in callosal connectivity. On the other hand, individual differences in laterality effects in direct-access tasks must reflect differences in relative hemispheric specialization exclusively. In principle, therefore, it is possible to factor out individual differences in laterality effects into a hemispheric specialization component and a callosal connectivity component. A crucial question that remains unanswered in our formulation of a direct-access task concerns the nature of interhemispheric transfer when input is restricted to one hemisphere. Does the sensory information transfer to the other hemisphere? If so, does parallel processing proceed in that other hemisphere and then how is it inhibited from response? To answer these questions, we need to develop experimental paradigms for tapping "on-the-fly" different stages of processing in each hemisphere.

A direct-access task should show small and comparable behavioral laterality effects in the split and normal brains since no callosal transfer is involved. Examples of this are certain versions of the dot localization task (Gordon and Zaidel, unpublished data) and a lateralized matching-to-sample task of nonsense Vanderplass shapes of intermediate complexity [Hellige et al., 1979; Letai, 1981]. A callosal-relay task, on the contrary, will show a massive laterality effect in the split brain but a relatively small, even if significant, laterality effect in the normal brain. In our lab the direct-access pattern was found for lexical decision of concrete lateralized words [Zaidel, 1983], and a callosal-relay pattern was observed for dichotic listening to nonsense stop consonant-vowel syllables [Zaidel, 1976, 1983].

What are the behavioral criteria for interpreting laterality data in normal subjects as reflecting a direct-access or a callosal-relay task? In terms of experimental design, we would characterize the direct-access model by a response hand × stimulus visual half-field interaction; the callosal-relay model would be characterized by main effects both of hand and of visual field [Zaidel, 1983] (Fig. 1). Conversely, conditions for refuting this model analysis include a main-hand effect without a visual-hemifield effect, or a main-hand effect opposite to the hemifield effect. In fact, of the scarce experiments in the literature that report enough data, few conclusively satisfy or refute either model. When central processing and manual response programming interfere with each other, we may get a contralateral hand-field advantage instead of the ipsilateral one shown in Fig. 1. In both cases, however, a significant hand × field interaction indicates direct-access. When a task combines a sequence of direct-access and callosal-relay components, the net hand × field pattern is callosal-relay, with the visual field advantage determined by the first callosal-relay component, and the hand advantage determined by the last callosal-relay component.

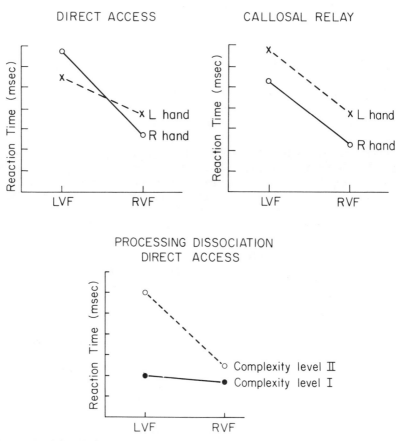

Fig. 1. Models of behavioral laterality effects. Top left: interaction of response hand with hemifield of presentation, signifying direct access. Top right: main effect of hand together with main effect of ipsilateral hemifield, signifying callosal relay. Bottom: processing dissociation signifying direct access.

Are there alternative behavioral criteria for model fitting? A commonly used solution is the "processing dissociation" criterion for direct access, where there occurs a significant interaction between visual hemifield of stimulus and degree of stimulus complexity (Fig. 1). For example, consider a lexical decision task with the word stimuli consisting of English nouns. Suppose we observe a significant interaction between the concreteness of the nouns and visual hemifield of presentation such that the left visual field (LVF) has a selective deficit in recognizing the abstract nouns. Then we may conclude that this task is direct access on the assumption that concrete and abstract nouns of similar visual complexity would relay across the corpus callosum at the same rate. It could be argued that concrete and abstract nouns use different callosal channels and are relayed at different rates. However, we believe that it is much more likely that different callosal channels are distinguished by more general features of modality and cognitive class (e.g., words vs. pictures) rather than by specific semantic class or dimension. Systematic model fitting and parameter estimation can be undertaken by comparing results with split-brain patients and normal subjects on compatible laterality tests. Furthermore, without separate hand-field analyses for each stimulus dimension, we can not conclude that both are processed through direct-access.

Another way to determine whether a lateralized task is direct access or callosal relay is to pair it with a secondary task of known lateralization in a dual-task interference paradigm. Suppose the secondary task is exclusively specialized to the LH. Assume also that if the primary task is direct access then it shares no resources with the unstimulated hemisphere. We say that the primary task interferes with the secondary task if the decrement in performance of the secondary task is sensitive to the complexity of the primary task [Navon and Gopher, 1980]. Table 1 shows the possible combinations of interference patterns and their interpretations. Pattern 3 is indeterminate since either the primary task is callosal relay and specialized in the LH without sharing any resources with the secondary task in the same hemisphere, or else the primary task is direct access and still shares no resources with the secondary task when processed in the LH. Patterns 1 and 2 distinguish callosal relay from direct-access tasks. The interpretations can be confirmed by pairing the primary task with a secondary one that is callosal relay, specialized in the RH.

As already mentioned, the distinction between callosal-relay and direct-access tasks is theoretically crucial because it separates laterality effects owing to degrees of hemispheric specialization from those owing to degrees of callosal connectivity, which presupposes a certain degree of hemispheric independence. The two factors may contribute independently and unequally

TABLE 1. Patterns of Interference Between a Callosal-Relay Secondary Task Specialized in the LH, and a Primary One Presented in the RVF (I = Interference That is Sensitive to Difficulty of Primary Task)

Condition	RVF	LVF	Interpretation
1	I	I	Primary task is callosal relay, specialized in the LH
2	I	No I	Primary task is direct access
3	No I	No I	? (Differentiated resources within the hemispheres)
4	No I	I	Impossible

to individual differences in laterality effects. In a given individual, different regions of the corpus callosum may vary in their relative connectivities, and the growth of connectivity of specific regions during ontogenesis may control the development of hemispheric specialization. It is possible, therefore, that individuals differ in their regional patterns of callosal connectivity. Thus women and left-handers may show weaker behavioral laterality effects than men and right-handers, respectively, not only because they have a more bilateral representation of the function tested and thus a smaller relative hemispheric specialization for the task, but also bacause they have better callosal connectivity. Individual differences in callosal connectivity are detectable with callosal relay but not with direct-access tasks. On the other hand, individual differences in relative hemispheric specialization should be detected with either direct-access or callosal-relay tasks. For example, we have observed sex differences in laterality effects not only in dichotic listening to nonsense syllables—a callosal-relay task with exclusive LH specialization—but also in lexical decision of concrete nouns, a direct-access task [Zaidel, 1983]. Such results suggest that women have weaker relative specialization in addition to any possible advantage in callosal connectivity.

Interhemispheric Transfer Time

Different callosal-relay delays occur in different tasks. Simple motor reaction-time experiments yield callosal transmission time estimates of 3 msec and have the clearest anatomical interpretation [Poffenberger, 1912; Rizzolatti, 1979; Bashore, 1981]. Here the estimate is plausibly due to the presence of an extra synapse and a long fiber, assuming that the largest callosal fibers mediate the behavioral response. In contrast, estimates of callosal transmission time obtained from choice reaction-time experiments are on the order of 30 msec. Although this estimate, too, is consistent with callosal transmission through many smaller myelinated and unmyelinated fibers, the estimate is probably a reflection of psychologic (i.e., dynamic) as well as fixed, structural anatomic effects. A population of unmyelinated fibers can take as long as 300 msec to code and relay information across the corpus callosum [Doty, personal communication].

As Rizzolatti [1979] points out, in choice reaction-time experiments, a transfer of information cannot occur at the level of the primary visual cortical areas, where hemispheric differences in analyzing stimuli are unlikely, because these areas are not, as far as we know, connected with each other across the callosum except along the vertical meridian. Thus, transfer time much more likely depends on the association areas where the stimulus is processed, and on the part of the corpus callosum that unites these areas. In this way interhemispheric transfer time may well be a function of the complexity of the stimuli. This is especially true if transfer occurs following a preliminary level or stage of psychological processing by the stimulus-receiving hemisphere in the callosal-relay situation. In that case, some recoding may be necessary with some attendant latency and accuracy cost. At the present time we have a weak anatomical basis for variations in callosal connectivity as a function of psychological variables. One way to start the search for underlying anatomical models would focus, say, on modality callosal effects, where some specificity of callosal connections is already established [cf. Pandya, this volume].

As mentioned, since Poffenberger [1912], parametric analyses of simple manual reaction time to lateralized unpatterned visual stimuli routinely disclose a hemifield by response-hand interaction, supporting direct-access and providing consistent estimates of interhemispheric transfer times (about 3 msec). These estimates do not appear to vary as a function of handedness or sex and are not sensitive to spatial compatibility effects [see review in Bashore, 1981]. By minimizing both cognitive and response demands, a reasonably pure measure of input and output operations can be derived [Bashore, 1981]. The simple tasks can be executed relatively quickly and with smaller variance so that the brief interhemispheric transfer time can be measured reliably.

Bashore [1981] points out that within certain small limits there is an apparent inverse relation between RT and interhemispheric transfer time. Thus slower RTs owing to eccentric stimuli or crossed hands tend to produce shorter estimates of callosal transfer. As task demands increase in complexity, e.g., when stimulus detection or response decisions are required, longer and more variable RTs are obtained as well as longer estimates of callosal transfer time. Thus, estimates of interhemispheric transfer time that derive from two-choice RT experiments are not only generally longer than are those from simple RT and stimulus detection studies, but also much more sensitive to spatial compatibility effects. Practice is said to reduce the stimulus-response compatibility effect for the dominant hand in the crossed and uncrossed response conditions, whereas this effect is said to persist in the nondominant hand [Brebner, 1973, cited in Bashore, 1981]. This suggests that spatial compatibility is a consequence of hemispheric specialization rather than the general cause of laterality effects or a factor independent of hemispheric specialization.

Bashore [1981] speculates that fast callosal transfer in simple RT tasks is mediated by larger-diameter, myelinated axons, which account for 10% of callosal fibers, whereas slower callosal transfer in choice RT tasks is mediated by the 60% of smaller and slower fibers. The question occurs whether the spatial distribution of different types of fibers in the corpus callosum can be associated with differences in type and modality of the conveyed information.

As tasks increase in complexity, they would intuitively seem less likely to fit either the direct-access or callosal-relay model and should be more likely to invoke interhemispheric interactions and involve considerably longer response times than callosal-relay, let alone direct-access, tasks. Yet, paradoxically, this is not always the case. Dahlia W. Zaidel [1982] administered a hemifield tachistoscopic test of category membership with stimuli consisting of pictorial exemplars to normal subjects and found a significant interaction between visual half-field of presentation and degree of typicality of category instances. Furthermore, she obtained a massive and highly significant overall left visual field advantage (LVFA) of about 400 msec. Thus, this complex task that taps long-term semantic memory and requires rather long RTs (a mean of 1,400 msec for positive responses by male subjects) still satisfies the processing dissociation criterion of direct access. Direct access or hemispheric independence can be observed even in tasks that require final responses by one hemisphere exclusively [Levy et al., 1983].

An interesting example of an anatomically inspired interpretation of laterality effects in normal subjects was discussed by Berlucchi and his associates [1971]. Consider simple reaction times to lateralized visual stimuli and the difference between responses with the ipsilateral and contralateral hand. The authors suggest that if this difference changes as a function of degree of eccentricity of the visual stimuli, then interhemispheric transfer occurs at the level of the visual, rather than, say, motor cortex. This is because presumably only the cortical areas related to the vertical meridian of the visual field give origin to and receive commissural fibers. More eccentric stimuli that do not have direct commissural connections would then require longer cross callosal transfer time and result in a bigger difference between crossed and uncrossed (visual field-hand) responses (the former require visual callosal transfer, the latter do not). Failure of an eccentricity effect to occur would remain ambiguous. It could be due to exclusively more anterior callosal transfer of more processed or abstract information which is consistent with a callosal relay model. In fact the data of Berlucchi et al. did not show an eccentricity effect (on the difference between crossed and uncrossed responses) and did show a visual field × hand interaction, which fits a direct-access model with a motor transfer.

Several assumptions of the callosal-relay model remain problematic. One paradox is the failure of some plausible consequences of callosal relay to be supported by seemingly relevant experiments. Thus, callosal relay is said to result in a measurable temporal delay and signal degradation. Yet temporally advancing the stimulus to the inferior ear in a dichotic listening paradigm does not decrease the observed perceptual asymmetry [Berlin, 1977]. (However, this manipulation may preclude real dichotic listening and require a new analysis.) Similar failures were observed in visual tests with bilateral hemifield presentations [McKeever and Huling, 1971]. Correspondingly, increasing the intensity of the left-ear signal in a consonant-vowel dichotic listening test does not erase the right-ear advantage [Studdert-Kennedy and Shankweiler, 1970]. The intensity manipulation also failed to erase the right-ear advantage in the commissurotomy patients [Cullen, 1975; Efron et al., 1977].

The reasons for these counterintuitive results have not been explored. It is not clear, for example, whether the temporal offset in the lag manipulation should be in the range of 3 msec (callosal transfer of a motor command in a simple RT task), in the range of 30 msec (callosal transfer in a choice RT task), or in some other range. In fact, the lag condition may introduce an independent backward masking effect that washes out the change in ear advantage (Bertelson, personal communication).

Another apparent paradox is the absence of disconnection effects in some patients with partial callosal lesions, natural or surgical. Splenial sections result in hemialexia [Trescher and Ford, 1937; Maspes, 1948; Gazzaniga and Freeman, 1973; Sugishita et al., 1984], and yet section of the anterior commissure and corpus callosum sparing the splenium results in no disconnection symptoms [Gordon et al., 1971]. Middle callosal sections sometimes do and sometimes do not result in auditory disconnection [Geffen et al., 1980], but this may reflect the extent to which the posterior callosum anterior to the splenium is involved.

There exist callosal-relay and direct-access tasks.

It now appears quite likely that there exist direct-access and callosal-relay tasks that are specialized in the left hemisphere and in the right hemisphere, both verbal and nonverbal, auditory and visual. Even if no real task of interest were to fit the models, they could still have theoretical value in explicating the microstructure of cross-callosal communication during strategic points in the information-processing sequence. But as a matter of fact there seem to exist a variety of tasks instantiating both models. I will illustrate both models with linguistic tasks—one auditory, the other visual. This will provide an opportunity to discuss the paradigms of dichotic listening and hemifield tachistoscopy, with special reference to the contribution of the commissurotomy syndrome to our understanding of the mechanisms involved.

Dichotic listening to nonsense syllables.

Consider a dichotic tape with linguistic stimuli. More accurate perception of right-ear stimuli is commonly thought to reflect LH specialization for language. Three independent assumptions are made in this interpretation. First, it is assumed that the LH is specialized for processing the input [Kimura, 1961]. Second, it is supposed that the ipsilateral signal from the left ear to the LH is suppressed, perhaps at a subcortical level [Kimura, 1967]. Berlin [1977] suggests that ipsilateral suppression occurs at the medial geniculate bodies. Third, stimuli presented to the left ear will first reach the RH, then cross the corpus callosum to be processed in the LH. This left-ear signal then competes or interferes with, but does not dominate, the direct contralateral right-ear signal, resulting in the observed right-ear advantage (REA) [Milner et al., 1968; Sparks and Geschwind, 1968]. The split brain offers a unique opportunity for testing the three assumptions.

In 1974, I verified the three hypotheses on a task with natural tokens of the dichotic stop consonant-vowel nonsense syllables ba, da, ga, pa, ta, and ka prepared at Haskins Lab in New Haven [Zaidel, 1976]. The stop-consonant syllables were chosen because they are highly coded phonetically. The LH is said to be specialized for phonetic analysis, whereas both hemispheres may be able to do acoustic analysis [Studdert-Kennedy and Shankweiler, 1970]. Perception of the dichotic pairs was assessed separately by verbal report and by lateralized visual probes. In the visual probe condition each dichotic pair was followed immediately by a triplet of letters (from the set B, D, G, P, T, K, corresponding to the six dichotic syllables) representing the left-ear syllable, the right-ear syllable, and a syllable differing from both in one or two phonetic features (voicing and place of articulation) in order to allow for error analysis. The subject was required to point to the letter representing the sound she/he was most sure of having heard in either ear. These tests were administered to normal subjects, hemispherectomy patients, and commissurotomy patients.

The results showed the usual small but quite reliable REA with normal subjects both using verbal report and with visual probes in either visual half-field. This was true in more than 90% of right-handed males. Commissurotomy patients showed a massive REA but not as complete as that shown by a case of right hemispherectomy. Monotic presentation resulted in good and equal verbal report (LH) from either ear. When the answers were presented only to the RH, there was no competence for responding to stimuli perceived in either ear in both the dichotic and monotic condition. Thus all three assumptions are verified. In particular, given the verification of exclusive LH specialization and of ipsilateral left ear suppression, the large difference between the REA in normals and in split-brain patients verifies the assumption of callosal interference and shows that this is a callosal-relay task. The exclusive specialization of the LH for perceiving stop consonant-vowel nonsense syllables probably reflects LH specialization for detecting fast formant transitions in the linguistic material.

Lexical Decision of Concrete Nouns

As an example of the direct-access model, consider a lexical decision task with concrete, imageable targets and pronounceable nonwords, that can be performed by each disconnected hemisphere. I will argue that the decision task fits the direct-access model. The behavioral criteria cited in evidence consist of (1) the observation of a relatively small and comparable visual-field advantage in the split and in the normal brain, and (2) a pattern of results with normal subjects satisfying the "processing dissociation" criterion for direct access in lexical decision with semantic facilitation (assuming that if lexical decision is "direct access" with semantic facilitation, it remains so when unaccompanied by primes). Thus, although the disconnected RH is seen to be inferior to the normal RH in semantic facilitation, the two are similar in competence for lexical decision itself.

The test stimuli were prepared by Allen Radant, then an honors senior at UCLA [1981]. They included 128 letter strings. Half of the stimuli were highly imageable, concrete, and frequent words, the other half were orthographically regular pronounceable nonwords. Stimuli were presented randomly and briefly to one visual hemifield or the other, and the subject was required to press a button as fast as possible if the stimulus was a word. In the case of commissurotomy patients the hand ipsilateral to the stimulated field responded. Normal subjects responded with their right hand. Of six commissurotomy patients (two partials) tested, five could lexically decide targets in both hemifields. Most patients showed more accurate LH decisions (Fig. 2), but of those patients whose accuracy was above chance bilaterally, most were equally fast with both hemispheres. Normal subjects also showed a small but significant LH superiority on this task.

Radant also paired each of 128 target letter strings with a frequent, concrete, and imageable lateralized prime word that preceded the targets. Half of the word targets were highly associated with their primes and half were not. Associated target word pairs (8), unassociated target word pairs

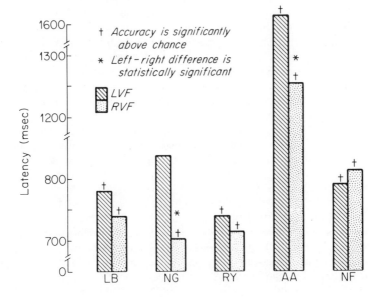

LEXICAL DECISION IN THE SPLIT BRAIN

Fig. 2. Lexical decision by commissurotomy patients.

(8), and the target nonword pairs (16) were assigned to each of four presentation conditions: (i) prime in the LVF and target in the LVF (LL); (ii) prime in the RVF and target in the LVF (RL); (iii) prime in the left and target in the right (LR); and (iv) prime in the right and target in the right (RR). Again, a go/no-go paradigm was used, requiring speeded right-hand presses to word targets. All subjects saw the lateralized primes for 100 msec, and after an interstimulus interval of 500 msec, they saw the lateralized targets for 50 msec. We can compare reaction time on a prime-target pair to reaction time on the target alone. Then faster RT on associated pairs would reflect semantic facilitation or priming; the slower RT to unassociated pairs would reflect inhibition relative to targets alone. Unexpectedly, the results showed a significant facilitation and a significant inhibition only in the RVF. This satisfies the "processing dissociation" criterion of direct access and verifies that lexical decision can be done by either hemisphere, whether disconnected or normal.

DYNAMICS OF INTERHEMISPHERIC CONTROL
Cross-Callosal Inhibition

We have already discussed above the hypothesis that individual differences in callosal connectivity may partly underlie sex and handedness effects in behavioral laterality measures in the normal brain. More generally, such individual differences in relative hemispheric independence, in degree of interhemispheric integration or in callosal flexibility, may explain individual differences in cognitive repertoires and styles. Some problems may require facile interhemispheric integration, while others may call for a unique hemispheric processing style and may actually be inhibited by the other hemisphere. Thus, performance on the latter may actually improve under conditions of decrease in callosal traffic. There is now evidence that the amount of callosal traffic may depend not only on genetic factors, such as sex or handedness, but also on environmental conditions, such as anxiety, sleep, or hypnosis, that can be controlled experimentally.

An example of a perceptual ability that improves with callosal disconnection may be Thurstone's second visual closure factor, the ability to perceive details in more complex gestalts, also known as Witkin's cognitive style of "field independence," measured by performance on his Embedded Figures Test. There is evidence from both hemispheric damage and the disconnected brain that the LH is specialized for field independence [Zaidel, 1979]. Furthermore, Cohen et al. [1973] showed that left-sided electroconvulsive shock decreases a person's field independence (in this case performance on Witkin's Rod and Frame Test), whereas right-sided treatment improves the score above normal. This would suggest that the normal RH partly inhibits the normal LH in its performance on field dependence measures, and that removal of that inhibition either by temporary paralysis of the RH or through functional callosal section results in improved field independence in the LH. Complementary Russian data reported by Jakobson and Santelli [1979] suggest that verbal fluency and syntactic complexity may increase after right-sided electroconvulsive therapy (ECT), whereas musical ability is said to increase after left-sided ECT.

There is evidence for even more dramatic pathologic inhibition through the corpus callosum in unilateral lesion states. The data come from a comparison between the cognitive deficits of patients with left- and right-hemisphere lesions, on the one hand, and the cognitive competence of the disconnected hemispheres in the split brain or the isolated hemispheres following hemispherectomy, on the other. Both disconnected hemispheres are dramatically free of many of the severe perceptual-cognitive deficits that often follow hemispheric damage. Thus, the disconnected LH does not have a facial recognition deficit nor does it exhibit a unilateral neglect of the left half of space or a visuospatial agnosia. Similarly, the disconnected RH is not globally aphasic, nor, for example, does it have the severe deficit on the Raven Progressive Matrices that some posterior aphasics exhibit.

Therefore, the behavior of hemisphere-damaged patients must signal the net effect of residual LH processing, of some RH compensation, and of some pathologic inhibition of the healthy RH by diseased tissue in the LH, through the neocortical commissures. The unilateral lesion impairs performance of the whole brain, giving rise to a "negative dominance" effect even though the undamaged hemisphere does have competence for the task [Zaidel, 1983]. For example, a smaller area of representation in the healthy hemisphere may be inhibited by a lesion in a much larger area of representation in the diseased side. In that case, inhibition in the opposite direction will not reveal detectable deficits, however, because it will suppress only a small part of a redundant system. Alternatively, although negative dominance effects reflect a net result of asymmetric inhibition, they may nonetheless originate from a failure in the balance of interhemispheric influences owing, say, to loss of normal facilitation in the other direction.

Cross-callosal pathologic inhibition as a result of a unilateral lesion may indeed reflect a disability of a central control mechanism or process that regulates interhemispheric interaction. Impairment of the process may result in a failure to release control to the intact, usually secondary, hemisphere. In the normal brain, the same process would inhibit callosal transfer when independent hemispheric processing leads to conflicting information on each side. On other occasions, when interhemispheric integration is required, the process would facilitate callosal transfer in one or the other direction. It is plausible that within each function-specific callosal region, different pathways mediate facilitatory and inhibitory effects.

Landis, Regard, and associates describe several examples of the modulation of cross-callosal inhibition of RH reading by LH lesions. The first example consists of reduced stimulus exposure beyond the range of LH "competence" in a letter-by-letter reader with pure alexia owing to a LH gliobastoma (Landis et al. [1980] and see below Alexia Without Agraphia). The second example is the preponderance of positively emotional words in the semantic paralexias of unselected aphasics. This pattern correlated better with the LVF than with the RVF error pattern of normal subjects [Graves et al., 1981]. The occurrence of paralexias was also correlated with the size of LH lesion and the crucial area seemed to be the left angular gyrus. The third example is the occurrence of a seizure in a patient with partial complex epilepsy owing to a left limbic lesion. Depth electrode recording showed that a massive RVF advantage prior to the seizure on a bilateral hemifield lexical decision task with function words switched to a comparable LVFA soon after the seizure and back to the usual RVFA a short time later (Landis and Regard, personal commmuncation). This lexical decision task shows a RVFA in normals as well. By contrast, no comparable shift in VFA was observed in this patient on a facial recognition task that shows a LVFA in normal subjects. Thus, greater speed of stimulus presentation, greater size of aphasiogenic lesion, and increased seizure activity all seem to release RH reading from pathologic LH inhibition.

Callosal Mediation of Right-Hemisphere Contribution to Reading in Aphasia

The comparison between semantic facilitation of lexical decision in disconnected and normal RHs discloses greater lexical semantic competence in the normal RH than in the RH of the split brain. [Zaidel, 1983]. It would thus seem that normal LH contribution to RH language increases the linguistic competence of the RH from what is found in the commissurotomized or hemispherectomized brain. Therefore, the linguistic profile of the disconnected RH may well underestimate the linguistic competence of the normal RH. This would mean that the partitioning and allocation of some language functions into direct access RH components is a function of the cognitive resources available to it and may be different for the normal and the split brains. Consequently, a laterality effect reflecting a direct-access task in the disconnected RH may not be the same as that in the normal LVF for the same task. In any case, there remains the paradox of complete breakdowns of specific linguistic functions in aphasic patients with lesions restricted to the LH and leaving the RH intact. I argue that such cases of aphasia reflect either inadequate testing or pathological inhibition of RH competence. Below, I will demonstrate experimental conditions for the release of such competence.

Alexia without agraphia.

The classic disconnection account of pure alexia is credited to Dejerine [1982], although according to Albert [1979], it was only Quensel who stressed in 1931 the necessity of the callosal lesion. This account was revived by Geschwind in 1965. A lesion in the left visual area that does not encroach on reading centers in the angular gyrus interrupts visual information entering the LH from reaching these centers. At the same time, visual stimuli entering the intact RH are interrupted by a splenial lesion in the corpus callosum. The lesions need not result in right homonymous hemianopsia or in a splenial lesion per se. The left angular gyrus can be simply undercut and isolated from visual information from both left and right visual cortices. Thus this model is consistent with the view of the corpus callosum as a set of selective channels of communication and denies any role in reading to the RH.

Frequently, pure alexics can name some objects, letters, or digits; and, as mentioned, the right-half-field blindness is not a necessary feature of the syndrome. In order to explain such selective preserved naming in the face of visual disconnection, Geschwind invoked the "channels of communication" view of the corpus callosum. He suggested [1965] that some visual stimuli can evoke nonvisual sensory associations in the RH and that these new representations may cross the corpus callosum through the more anterior, uninterrupted regions. Colors, lacking tactile associations, would not be transferred and would not be named.

Coltheart [1984] extended this view to the hypothesis that in the case of reading the splenium of the corpus callosum carries abstracted phonological or semantic information, whereas more anterior parts of the callosum mediate the transfer of raw sensory and ideographic information. Then deep dyslexia (see below) would involve a more anterior callosal lesion, whereas pure alexia or letter-by-letter reading would involve a splenial lesion with semantic disconnection. This suggestion is conceptually appealing but it is not supported by the anatomic data nor by the failure to find visual disconnection in partial commissurotomy patients with only the spleniums intact [Schweiger et al., 1985].

Could RH reading be revealed in pure alexia with assessment techniques that do not involve speech or action, such as reading comprehension with pointing to multiple choice pictures? Patterson and Kay [1982], Warrington and Shallice [1980], and F. Michel (personal communication) all failed to show such reading comprehension by pure alexic patients. However, Landis et al. [1980] tested a patient with pure alexia caused by a tumor. They found that he could correctly point to objects in response to brief tachistoscopic words at speeds that did not allow him to name individual letters and led him to deny that he had seen anything. Furthermore, the patient subsequently lost this ability when he improved enough to be able to name individual letters of the flashed words.

It is plausible that by using tachistoscopic presentations Landis et al. may have succeeded in releasing RH reading from LH inhibition. For example, this could be achieved by making the task too difficult for the LH but not for the RH. Or, it could be due to RH priming or activation resulting in decreased callosal traffic and reduced LH inhibition from left to right. In turn, failure of the central regulating process to release control to RH when letter-by-letter reading is present may reflect a deficit state owing to misleading input from the language area in the LH, or owing to a disorder in the regulating process itself. Another example of a dynamic shift in hemispheric control of reading as a function of task parameters can be demonstrated in acquired aphasia with deep dyslexia.

Deep dyslexia.

Patients with deep dyslexia characteristically make semantic errors in reading aloud, read concrete nouns better than abstract function words, and cannot translate orthography to sound, thus failing to read nonsense words. (Many authors distinguish the concrete-abstract effect from the part-of-speech effect, but both effects may be due to a common underlying dimension in lexical semantic reference.) Some deep dyslexics maintain these symptoms not only in reading aloud but also during reading comprehension. In the case of reading comprehension semantic errors consists of pointing to pictures of words related in meaning to the stimulus. Similarly, speech-free assessment of the ability to translate orthography to sound consists of failure to match written words for rhyming. It turns out that reading in the disconnected RH also satisfies the same criteria when tested with speech-free comprehension tests [Zaidel and Peters, 1981; Menn and Zaidel, unpublished data]. Consequently, Coltheart [1980] formulated a "right-hemisphere hypothesis" for deep dyslexia, according to which the deep dyslexic uses his intact RH for lexical semantic access, and this is the source of the semantic errors [see also Zaidel and Peters, 1981]. On this view, the RH would provide the semantic address of a written word, but phonological interpretation and articulation would be completed in the damaged LH following R to L semantic transfer through the corpus callosum.

Recently, Avraham Schweiger in my lab has been studying a 39-year-old deep dyslexic (and deep dysgraphic) woman, R.W., with no visual field defect. RW showed the deep dyslexic symptoms on the same reading comprehension tests that were administered to the disconnected RHs of two complete commissurotomy patients, although her overall reading ability is superior to that of the disconnected RH. We administered R.W. the same lexical decision task that had shown bilateral competence with LH superiority in both the disconnected and normal brains (see above). She had equal accuracy (about 80%) in both visual fields but significantly faster RTs and a significantly smaller standard deviation in the LVF [Schweiger et al., 1985]. By contrast, she had no visual field differences in either accuracy or RT on a control task using the same stimuli and requiring her to press the button if the target was more than four letters long (regardless of whether it was a word or not). The same task showed no visual field advantage in normal subjects. This result suggests that unlike the normal RH and her own premorbid state (assuming she had been a typical right hander), R.W. has shifted control to the intact RH in lexical decision [cf. also Saffran et al., 1980].

The second experiment demonstrated that R.W.'s RH does not assume control over all reading functions, nor of any single reading function all of the time. In this task she was asked to read aloud another list of 64 words presented to each hemifield in two sessions, in a counterbalanced manner. The words were flashed for 90 msec in order to reduce the LH's ability to read them, thus increasing the chances that the RH would take over lexical semantic access, resulting in more semantic errors. The patient had 22 semantic errors in reading aloud, with a majority of 16 (73%) occurring in the LVF. In sharp contrast, of a total of 51 words read correctly, a majority of 28 (55%) occurred in the RVF. This pattern is consistent with the conclusion that the LH still controls reading aloud, but that semantic errors are due to occasional RH takeover when LH reading fails. Here the corpus callosum is presumed to mediate both release of control to the RH (perhaps through removal of LH inhibition) as well as the transfer of accessed semantic information from the right to the left hemisphere.

Shifts in Callosal Connectivity?

Are there any examples of systematic changes in callosal connectivity such that their cognitive consequences can be evaluated? There is some anatomical, electrophysiological, and behavioral evidence that callosal connectivity increases with age. The corpus callosum is completely formed at birth and matures very slowly. It is one of the last systems to myelinate, beginning at the end of the first year of life, being substantially advanced by age 4, and continuing to increase to age 10 and beyond [Lecours, 1975]. Somatosensory evoked-response studies of contralateral and ipsilateral manual stimulation also show a relative increase of ipsilateral responses with age, reflecting better callosal conduction of the cross-callosal signal between the two sensory cortices [Salamy, 1978]. Moreover, Galin et al. [1979] showed a significant increase in manual cross-retrieval of simple texture discrimination from ages 3 to 5, and Geffen [1985] showed a developmental increase between ages 5 and 7 in children's ability to achieve cross-finger localization.

On the other hand, auditory tests do not support the hypothesis of increased functional cross-callosal connectivity with age. If true, the hypothesis would predict that young children should approximate the disconnection syndrome, and should show a massive right-ear advantage in verbal report during dichotic listening to nonsense stop consonant-vowel syllables, comparable to the disconnected LH. No such findings have been reported. Berlin et al. [1973] showed early (as young as age 5) and fairly constant LH specialization superimposed on a gradual increase in performance. Bryden and Allard [1978] found a later and gradual development of ear asymmetry, reaching significance only at age 12, in direct opposition to the prediction of the hypothesis. Similarly, using a disconnection battery of visual, auditory, and kinesthetic tests with children as young as 5 years old, we failed to show any disconnection effect [White, Zaidel, and Schweiger, unpublished data]. The same tests showed failure of interhemispheric sensory transfer in the split brain. Thus, even if anatomical and physiological callosal connectivity does increase with age, the functional significance of this remains unclear.

A curious recent study by Gott et al. [1984] reports on a woman who can selectively activate her LH or RH at will. One measure of hemispheric activation was the degree of interhemispheric transfer of somatosensory signals recorded by vibrotactile somatosensory evoked potentials. Hemispheric activation is said to be associated with decreased connectivity into the active hemisphere relative to connectivity out of it [Inoyue et al., 1981]. In fact, relative hemispheric activation may be modulated by callosal signals in the normal brain. This would mean that callosal connectivity is not independent of hemispheric activation. Consequently, if we are to separate the effects of callosal connectivity from relative hemispheric specialization (not activation) in the etiology of behavioral laterality effects in the normal brain (callosal relay vs. direct access tasks), then we need to use bilateral tasks that activate both hemispheres simultaneously. Nonetheless, it may still be true that the development of callosal connectivity can mediate the development of hemispheric specialization [cf. Jeeves, this volume; Denenberg, 1981]. In fact, callosal connectivity may develop at different rates in different regions, thereby mediating the specialization of different hemispheric functions.

There is also preliminary evidence that state anxiety [Spielberger et al., 1970] is associated with decreased callosal connectivity from the LH to the RH, perhaps owing to increased RH activation [Radant, 1981]. Conversely, a possible interpretation of reduced laterality effects (REA) in dichotic listening to phonetic stimuli under hypnosis [Frumkin et al., 1978] is that connectivity from the RH to the LH is selectively inhibited [cf. Zaidel, 1976, 1983; McKeever et al., 1981].

CONCLUSIONS AND PROSPECTS

Complete commissurotomy patients are paradoxically free of any apparent gross behavioral deficits, with the possible exception of some kinds of memory dysfunction [Zaidel and Sperry, 1974]. Since neither disconnected hemisphere shows the many kinds of severe perceptual or cognitive deficits that often accompany unilateral damage [Zaidel, 1973; Plourde and Sperry, 1984], it would seem that the corpus callosum mediates functionally inhibitory influences from the lesioned to the intact hemisphere. One could argue that since the absence of the neocortical commissures has no apparent clincial consequence, it would also seem that these pathways have little use in normal everyday life. However, the unified behavior of commissurotomy patients can be explained by several factors, both normal and compensatory, following disconnection. Unified behavior is supported by visual and manual exploration of space, conjugate eye movements, some bilateral representation of sensory information, shared autonomic system functions, and perhaps midbrain control of attention [Sperry, 1974]. Furthermore, there is increased functional use of ipsilateral sensory and motor projections in the long term in those patients, especially on the left side [Zaidel, 1978]. There is even evidence for noncallosal semantic transfer from the RH to the LH, presumably mediated by the spread of affect through shared brainstem structures [Zaidel, 1978; Sperry et al., 1979].

But it is also likely that more subtle perceptual, cognitive, and construtual tasks will reveal long-term deficits in complete commissurotomy patients attributable to lack of normal interhemispheric integration. For example, these patients have a persistent inability to focus attention on complex tasks for long periods of time and bring them to successful completion. They may well exhibit subtle cognitive deficits such as loss of lexical richness and nuance, inability to execute speeded scanning, etc., because the disconnected LH does not benefit from RH contribution to reading. Indeed, these patients are generally neither productive nor creative [Bogen and Bogen, 1969].

I argued that some simple experimental tasks require callosal relay, and some do not (direct access). Most everyday tasks probably require complex interhemispheric interaction, although we know little or nothing about the rate and extent of such communication. It probably varies with requisite function and with mediating callosal region. Thus increased hemispheric activation may increase the flow of relevant incoming stimuli and decrease the flow of irrelevant, competing, or functionally incompatible stimuli. Therefore, strictly speaking, callosal connectivity is dependent on hemispheric activation and thus also on individually wired-in limits of relative hemispheric specialization.

Conceptualizing the corpus callosum as a set of channels of communication may ultimately prove too mechanistic and simpleminded. But this conceptualization is appropriate for the current Zeitegeist in neuropsychological theorizing, which is dominated by block-diagram information-processing models. Within such models, the information-theoretic function of the corpus callosum seems heuristically productive: it focuses attention on modes of interhemispheric interaction and hints at exciting prospects for experimental shifts in hemispheric activation and competence through modulation of callosal transfer.

ACKNOWLEDGMENTS

Thanks to Doreen Aghajanian for assistance, to Diane Brodahl for word processing, and to C.R. Hamilton and J.E. Bogen for comments on the manuscript. This work was supported by NIH grant NS 20187 and NIMH RSDA MH00179 to E. Zaidel.

REFERENCES

Akelaitis AJ (1944): A study of gnosis, praxis and language following section of the corpus collosum and anterior commissure. J Neurosurg 1:94–102.

Albert ML (1979): Alexia. In Heilman KM, Valenstein E (eds): "Clinical Neuropsychology." New York: Oxford, pp 59–91.

Bashore TR (1981): Vocal and manual reaction time estimates of interhemispheric transmission time. Psychol Bull 89:352–368.

Berlin CI (1977): Hemispheric asymmetry in auditory tasks. In Harnad S, Dody RW, Goldstein I, Jaynes J, Krauthamer G (eds): "Lateralization in the Nervous System." New York: Academic Press, pp 303–323.

Berlin CI, Hughes LF, Lowe-Bell SS, Berlin HL (1973): Dichotic ear advantage in children 5 to 13. Cortex 9:393–401.

Berlucchi G, Heron W, Hyman R, Rizzolatti G, Umilta C (1971): Simple reaction times of ipsilateral and contralateral hand to lateralized visual stimuli. Brain 94:419–430.

Bogen JE, Bogen GM (1969): The other side of the brain III: The corpus callosum and creativity. Bull Los Angeles Neurol Soc 34:191–220.

Brown J (1977): "Mind, Brain and Consciousness: The Neuropsychology of Cognition." New York: Academic Press.

Bryden MP, Allard F (1978): Dichotic listening and the development of linguistic processes. In Kinsbourne M (ed): "Hemispheric Asymmetry of Function." Cambridge: The University Press.

Cohen BD, Berent S, Silverman AJ (1973): Field-dependence and lateralization of function in the human brain. Arch Gen Psychiatr 28:165–167.

Coltheart M (1980): Deep dyslexia: A right hemisphere hypothesis. In Coltheart M, Patterson K, Marshall JC (eds): "Deep Dyslexia." London: Routledge and Kegan Paul, pp 326–380.

Coltheart M (1984): The right function and disorders of reading. In Young AW (ed): "Functions of the Right Cerebral Hemisphere." London: Academic Press, pp 171–201.

Cullen JK, Jr. (1975): Tests of a model for speech information flow (doctoral dissertation, Louisiana State University). Dissertations Abstracts International, 36, 1167A (Unversity Microfilms No. 75-19, 262).

Dejerine J (1892): Contribution a l'etude anatomo-pathologique et clinique des differentes varietes de cecite verbale. Mem Soc Biol 4:61–90.

Denenberg VH (1981): Hemispheric laterality in animals and the effects of early experience. Behav Brain Sci 4:1–49.

Efron R, Yund FW, Bogen JE (1977): Perception of dichotic chords by normal and commissurotomized human subjects. Cortex 13:137–149.

Friedman A, Polson MC, Dafoe CE, Gaskill SJ (1982): Divided attention within and between hemispheres: Testing a multiple resources approach to limited-capacity information processing. J Exp Psychol HP&P 8:625–650.

Frumkin LR, Ripley HS, Cox GB (1978): Changes in cerebral hemispheric lateralization with hypnosis. Biol Psychiatr 13:741–749.

Galin D, Johnstone J, Nakell S, Herron J (1979): Development of the capacity for tactile information transfer between hemispheres in normal children. Science 204:1330–1332.

Gazzaniga MS, Freeman H (1973): Observations on visual processes after posterior callosal section. Neurology 23:1126–1130.

Geffen G, Nillson J, Quinn K (1985): Interhemispheric transfer of tactile information in the developing and corpus callosum lesioned human brain. Poster presented at the Thirteenth Annual INS Meeting, San Diego, CA, February 8.

Geffen G, Walsh W, Simpson D, Jeeves M (1980): Comparison of the effects of transcortical and transcallosal removal of intraventricular tumors. Brain 103:773–778.

Geschwind N (1965): Disconnexion syndromes in animals and man. Brain 88:237–294, 585–644.

Gordon HW, Bogen JE, Sperry RW (1971): Absence of disconnection syndrome in two patients with partial section of the neocommissures. Brain 94:327–336.

Gott PS, Hughes EC, Whipple K (1984): Voluntary control of two lateralized conscious states: Validation by electrical and behavioral studies. Neuropsychologia 22:65–72.

Graves R, Landis T, Goodglass H (1981): Laterality and sex differences for visual recognition of emotional and non-emotional words. Neuropsychologia 19:95–102.

Hamilton CR (1982): Mechanisms of interocular equivalence. In Ingle DJ, Goodale MA, Mansfield RJW (eds): "Analysis of Visual Behavior." Cambridge: MIT Press, pp 693–717.

Hellige JB, Cox JP, Litvac L (1979): Information processing in the hemispheres: Selective hemisphere activation and capacity limitations. J Exp Psychol Gen 108:251–279.

Hellige JB, Sergent J (1985): Role of task factors in visual field asymmetries. Brain and Cognition (in press).

Inouye T, Yagasaki A, Takahashi H, Shinosaki K (1981): The dominant direction of interhemispheric EEG changes in the linguistic process. Electroenceph Clin Neurophysiol 51:265–275.

Jakobson R, Santelli K (1979): "Brain and Language: Cerebral Hemispheres and Linguistic Structure in Mutual Light." Columbus: Slavica.

Kimura D (1961): Cerebral dominance and the perception of verbal stimuli. Can J Psychol 15:166–171.

Kimura D (1967): Functional asymmetry of the brain in dichotic listening. Cortex 3:166–178.

Kinsbourne, M. (1975): The mechanisms of hemispheric control of the lateral gradient of attention. In Rabbitt PMA, Dornic S (eds): "Attention and Performance V." London: Academic Press, pp 81–97.

Kinsbourne M (1984): The material basis of mind. Unpublished manuscript.

Kinsbourne M, Hiscock M (1983): Asymmetries of dual-task performance. In Hellige JB (ed): "Cerebral Hemisphere Asymmetry: Method, Theory and Application." New York: Praeger, pp 255–334.

Landis T, Regard M, Serrat A (1980): Iconic reading in a case of alexia without agraphia caused by brain tumor: A tachistoscopic study. Brain Lang 11:45–53.

Lecours AR (1975): Myelogenetic correlates of the development of speech and language. In Lenneberg EH, Lenneberg E (eds): "Foundations of Language Development, V.I." New York: Academic Press, pp 121–135.

Letai AD (1981): Performance on lateralized visual and auditory single and dual tasks. Unpublished manuscript, Department of Psychology, UCLA.

Levy J, Heller W, Banich MT, Burton LA (1983): Are variations among right-handed individuals in perceptual asymmetries caused by characteristic arousal differences between hemispheres? J Exp Psychol HP&P 9:329-359.

Maspes PE (1948): Le syndrome experimental chez l'homme de la section du splenium du corps calleux. Alexie visuelle pure hemianopsique. Rev Neurol 80:100-113.

McKeever WF, Huling MD (1971): A note on Filby and Gazzaniga's "Splitting the brain with reaction time." Psychonom Sci 22:222.

McKeever WF, Larrabee GJ, Sullivan KF, Johnson HJ, Ferguson S, Rayport M (1981): Unimanual tactile anomia consequent to corpus callosotomy: Reduction of anomic deficit under hypnosis. Neuropsychologia." 19:179-190.

Milner B, Taylor L, Sperry RW (1968): Lateralized suppression of dichotically presented digits after commissural section in man. Science 161:184-186.

Moscovitch M (1973): Language and the cerebral hemispheres: Reaction time studies and their implications for models of cerebral dominance. In Plimer P, Alloway T, Krames L (eds): "Communication and Affect: Language and Thought." New York: Academic Press, pp 89-126.

Moscovitch M, Klein D (1980): Material-specific perceptual interference for visuals, words and faces: Implications for models of capacity limitations, attention and laterality. J Exp Psychol HP&P 6:590-604.

Navon D, Gopher D (1980): Task difficulty, resources, and dual-task performance. In Nickerson RS (ed): "Attention and Performance VIII." Hillsdale, NJ: Erlbaum, pp 297-315.

Patterson KE, Kay J (1982): Letter-by-letter reading: Psychological descriptions of a neurological syndrome. Qu J ExpPsychol 34A:311-442.

Plourde G, Sperry RW (1984): Left hemisphere involvement in left spatial neglect from right-sided lesions: A commissurotomy study. Brain, 107, 95-106.

Poffenberger AT (1912): Reaction time in retinal stimulation with special reference to time lost in conduction through nerve centers. Arch Psychol 27:17-25.

Radant A (1981): Facilitation in a lexical decision task: Effects of visual field and anxiety. Honors undergraduate thesis, Department of Psychology, The Unversity of California, Los Angeles.

Rizzolatti G (1979): Interfield differences in reaction times to lateralized visual stimuli in normal subjects. In Russell IS, Van Hof MW, Berlucchi G (eds): "Structure and Function of Cerebral Commissures." Baltimore: University Park Press, pp 390-399.

Saffran EM, Bogyo LC, Schwartz MF, Marin OSM (1980): Does deep dyslexia reflect right hemisphere reading? In Coltheart M, Patterson K, Marshall JC (eds): "Deep Dyslexia." London: Routledge and Kegan Paul, pp 381-406.

Salamy A (1978): Commissural transmission: Maturational changes in humans. Science 200:1409-1411.

Schweiger A, Zaidel E, Field T, Dobkin B (1985): Intermittent right hemisphere dominance for reading in an aphasic with deep dyslexia. (Submitted.)

Sparks R, Geschwind N (1968): Dichotic listening in man after section of neocortical commissures. Cortex 4:3-16.

Sperry RW (1974): Lateral specialization in the surgically separated hemispheres. In Schmitt FO, Worden FG (eds): "The Neurosciences: Third Study Program." Cambridge: MIT Press, pp 5–19.

Sperry RW, Myers RE (1953): Interocular transfer of a visual discrimination habit in cats after section of the optic chiasm and corpus callosum. Anat Rec 115:351–352.

Sperry RW, Zaidel E, Zaidel D (1979): Self-recognition and social awareness in the disconnected minor hemisphere. Neuropsychologia 17:153–166.

Spielberger CD, Gorsuch RL, Lushene RE (1970): "STAI Manual." Palo Alto, California, Consulting Psychologists Press.

Studdert-Kennedy M, Shankweiler D (1970): Hemispheric specialization for speech perception. J Acoust Soc Am 48:579–594.

Sugishita M, Shinohara A, Shimoji T, Ogawa T (1985): A remaining problem in hemialexia: Tachistoscopic hemineglect and hemialexia. In Reeves J (ed): "Epilepsy and the Corpus Callosum." New York: Plenum 417–434.

Swanson J, Ledlow A, Kinsbourne M (1978): Lateral asymmetries revealed by simple reaction time. In Kinsbourne M (ed): "Asymmetrical Function of the Brain." New York: Cambridge University Press, pp 274–292.

Trescher HH, Ford FR (1937): Colloid cyst of the third ventricle. Report of a case; operative removal with section of posterior half of corpus callosum. Arch Neurol Psychiatr 37:959–973.

Warrington EK, Shallice T (1980): Word form dyslexia. Brain 103:99–112.

Zaidel D, Sperry RW (1974): Memory impairment after commissurotomy in man. Brain 97:263–272.

Zaidel DW (1982): Long-term memory and hemispheric specialization: Semantic organization for pictures (Doctoral dissertation, University of California at Los Angeles). Dissertation Abstracts International, 42 (University Microfilms No. 82-06,093).

Zaidel E (1973): Linguistic competence and related functions in the right cerebral hemisphere of man following commissurotomy and hemispherectomy. (Doctoral dissertation, California Institute of Technology.) Dissertation Abstracts International, 34, 2350B (University Microfilms No. 73-26,481).

Zaidel E (1976): Language, dichotic listening and the disconnected hemispheres. In Walter DO, Rogers L, Finzi-Fried JM (eds): "Conference on Human Brain Function." Brain Information Service/BRI Publications Office, UCLA, 103–110.

Zaidel E (1978): Concepts of cerebral dominance in the split brain. In Buser P, Rougeul-Buser A (eds): "Cerebral Correlates of Conscious Experience." Amsterdam: Elsevier, pp 263–284.

Zaidel E (1979): Performance on the ITPA following cerebral commissurotomy and hemispherectomy. Neuropsychologia 17:259–280.

Zaidel E (1983): Disconnection syndrome as a model for laterality effects in the normal brain. In Hellige J (ed): "Cerebral Hemisphere Asymmetry: Method, Theory and Application." New York: Praeger, pp 95–151.

Zaidel E, Peters AM (1981): Phonological encoding and ideographic reading by the disconnected right hemisphere: Two case studies. Brain Lang 14:205–234.

SECTION VI
HUMAN NEUROPSYCHOLOGY II

Two Hemispheres—One Brain:
Functions of the Corpus Callosum, pages 463–469
© 1986 Alan R. Liss, Inc.

The Nature of Complementary Specialization

M. P. BRYDEN

Department of Psychology, University of Waterloo, Waterloo, Ontario Canada N2L 3G1

In the contemporary view of brain function, the two cerebral hemispheres are seen as acting in different but complementary fashion. It is common, for instance, to hear of the left hemisphere described as being verbal, analytic, or a sequential processor, while the right hemisphere is often depicted as being concerned with global or Gestalt attributes, or as being a simultaneous processor [e.g., Semmes, 1968; Cohen, 1973; Bradshaw and Nettleton, 1981]. In many eyes, this view implies that one hemisphere takes on a certain set of functions *because* the other hemisphere is involved in opposing operations. Thus, Bradshaw and Nettleton [1981] argue that the right hemisphere acquires its capacities only in response to the development of other capacities in the left hemisphere. Similarly, Corballis [1983] states that "... left-hemispheric specialization is essentially superimposed on a brain that would otherwise be bilaterally symmetric. Right hemisphere specialization is therefore achieved by default." A similar position is taken by LeDoux et al. [1977], who states that "... the superior performance of split-brain patients on a variety of manipulospatial tasks may not reflect the overall cognitive style and evolutionary specialization but may instead represent local processing in the left-parietotemporal junction due to the presence of language."

For the sake of our discussion, I should like to call this position that of *causal complementarity*. The argument is that the specialization of the left hemisphere for language causes the right hemisphere to become apparently specialized for a variety of nonlinguistic processes, since the left hemisphere is at least in part otherwise occupied. Such a view implies that any normal individual who develops right-hemisphere language will show a *left*-hemisphere superiority for those processes commonly associated with the right hemisphere.

An alternative view is what I shall term *statistical complementarity*. By this argument, certain factors lead the brain to develop in such a way as to bias the left hemisphere for subserving language functions in the majority of people, and other factors lead to a preponderance of right-hemisphere control over visuospatial and musical processes in the majority of people.

However, these factors may well be quite independent of one another, with the result that the cerebral lateralization of language is statistically independent of the lateralization of visuospatial processes or of musical processes. By this view, complementarity, in the sense that the two cerebral hemispheres have different functions, is the modal state of affairs, but for statistical reasons rather than causal ones. Most people have left hemisphere language *and* right hemisphere visuospatial functions simply because the likelihood that language will be left-hemispheric is about 95%, and the likelihood that visuospatial functions will be right hemispheric is about 80%, with the result that the joint probability will be the product of these two, or about 76%.

Virtually all of my own research has dealt with laterality effects in normal subjects, and my interest in this issue arose because of the repeated observation that laterality effects obtained on such tasks as dichotic listening and tachistoscopic recognition did not show the expected pattern of interrelations. For example, the argument of causal complementarity would predict that there should be a negative correlation between laterality effects for verbal and nonverbal tasks, yet it is often reported that the same hemisphere is superior for both verbal and nonverbal processes [cf. Bryden, 1973; McGlone and Davidson, 1973]. Similarly, my recent studies of the right-hemispheric superiority for the perception of emotional intonation and expression have shown no correlation between the left-hemisphere superiority for verbal tasks and the right-hemisphere superiority for affective tasks [Ley and Bryden, 1982; Saxby and Bryden, 1984].

In addition, we have recognized for a long time that the incidence of right-hemisphere language representation is much higher in left-handers than it is in right-handers [e.g., Rasmussen and Milner, 1977; Segalowitz and Bryden, 1983]. However, visuospatial deficits following unilateral right-hemisphere damage seem to be similar in left-handers and in right-handers [e.g., Hécaen and Sauguet, 1971; De Renzi, 1982; Masure and Benton, 1983]. If the value of handedness as a predictor of the effects of unilateral brain damage is different for language and for visuospatial ability, then it becomes more unlikely that functional complementarity is causal in nature.

In the present paper, I should like to provide two bits of evidence that complementarity is in fact statistical rather than causal, and then suggest some alternative ways of thinking about why the human cerebral cortex is organized as it is.

The first bit of evidence comes from a large-scale study of the effects of unilateral brain damage carried out by Henri Hécaen and his colleagues in Paris [Hécaen et al., 1981]. Before his death, Professor Hécaen was kind enough to send me his data on 270 cases of unilateral brain damage, and I carried out a further analysis of these data, which was published in 1983 [Bryden et al., 1983]. The population consisted of 140 left-handers and 130 right-handers with unilateral brain damage, classified as to the presence or absence of aphasia and as to the presence or absence of visuospatial disorders.

If complementary specialization were causal, in the sense I have described above, then one should expect a *negative* association between the occurrence of aphasia and the occurrence of visuospatial disorder; that is, individuals would be expected to manifest one symptom but not both. This is not what we observed. Among right-handers, there was simply no association between aphasia and visuospatial disorder following either left hemisphere lesions or right hemisphere lesions (Table 1).

In the left-handers, the only significant association between aphasia and visuospatial disorder appeared in those with left-hemisphere damage, but it was positive rather than negative in direction (Table 2). That is, those subjects who were aphasic were more likely to manifest a visuospatial disorder than those who were not aphasic. This is the opposite of what would be predicted by a theory of causal complementarity. As we suggested in our paper, such data are best explained by assuming that a reasonable percentage of left-handers have bilateral representation of language, visuospatial abilities, or both [cf. Rasmussen and Milner, 1977; Satz, 1980; Segalowitz and Bryden, 1983]. If such is the case, unilateral damage to either hemisphere would disrupt the functions that are bilaterally represented, and the likelihood that both language and visuospatial functions will be disturbed would be higher than in individuals in whom both functions are unilaterally represented.

The second source of data I want to discuss is from normal adult subjects. We have recently completed a study of dichotic listening performance in a large sample of university undergraduates [Bryden, 1984]. In this study, 60 left-handers and 60 right-handers, equally divided among the two sexes, were given two different dichotic listening tasks. One involved the recogni-

TABLE 1. Association Between Aphasia and Spatial Dysfunction in 130 Right-Handed Patients With Unilateral Brain Damage[1]

Lesion side	Spatial dysfunction	No spatial dysfunction	
Left			
Aphasic	9	27	36
Not aphasic	7	27	34
	16	54	$\chi^2 = 0.19$[2]
Right			
Aphasic	3	2	5
Not aphasic	28	27	55
	31	29	$\chi^2 = 0.15$[2]

[1]Data from Bryden et al. [1983].
[2]Not significant.

TABLE 2. Association Between Aphasia and Spatial Dysfunction in 140 Left-Handed Patients With Unilateral Brain Damage[1]

Lesion side	Spatial dysfunction	No spatial dysfunction	
Left			
Aphasic	34	32	66
Not aphasic	5	16	21
	39	48	$\chi^2 = 4.94$*
Right			
Aphasic	12	5	17
Not aphasic	17	19	36
	29	24	$\chi^2 = 2.54$[2]

[1]Data from Bryden et al. [1983].
[2]Not significant.
*p < .05.

TABLE 3. Association Between Verbal and Musical Dichotic Ear Effects in 120 Normal Subjects[1]

Verbal	Music		
	Left ear better	No difference	Right ear better
Left ear better	4	14	5
No difference	9	11	7
Right ear better	18	29	23

[1]χ^2 (4) = 3.68, NS. Data from Bryden [1984].

tion of consonant-vowel (CV) syllables and normally leads to a right-ear superiority in right-handers. The other involved the recognition of the melodic line in musical passages, and usually produces a left-ear effect in right-handers. If complementary specialization were a causal matter, one should expect to find opposite asymmetries for the two tasks. Yet, as Table 3 shows, there was virtually no association between the laterality effects observed in the two tasks. Although the data in this table have been combined across both sex and handedness groups, no association between the two laterality measures is found in any of the subgroups.

This is not an isolated finding, for we have noticed similar effects in other studies [e.g., Bryden, 1973], and other people have also failed to find strong associations between putatively verbal and nonverbal laterality tasks. Such observations suggest that complementarity is not a causal matter, but that the lateralization of verbal functions is determined by one set of factors, while the lateralization of nonverbal processes is determined by a quite different set of factors.

There is support for such notions from other areas. Recent neuroanatomical data suggest that verbal dichotic performance is correlated with the size of the temporal plane [Strauss et al., 1985]. One might therefore postulate that visuospatial and musical laterality effects would correlate with the anatomical size of different areas in the right, rather than the left, hemisphere. In a similar vein, Howard Gardner, in his excellent book *Frames of Mind* [1983], has argued for the modularity of different intelligences, suggesting that verbal skills, musical skills, kinesthetic skills, and visuospatial skills are independent intelligences, with different brain localizations and different origins.

To pursue this argument, I might note that it is common to place considerable emphasis on the association between handedness and left-hemisphere language lateralization, and we are all taught that the general rules do not apply to left-handers. In fact, Kimura's [1979] model is based on a direct link between language and gesture. However, in a statistical sense, the correlation between handedness and language lateralization is really rather poor, on the order of magnitude of .05, since the majority of left-handers are also left-hemispheric for language. While I am sure that the search for a better predictor of right-hemisphere language will go on, the weak correlation suggests that Gardner may be right in viewing language and motor skill as separable abilities, both biased to the left hemisphere, but not causally connected.

In another recent paper consistent with the view I am espousing, Graves [1983] has argued that lateralization in verbal tachistoscopic tasks, in verbal dichotic tasks, and in the asymmetry of mouth expression all index different aspects of language lateralization, and that the various aspects of language are not necessarily lateralized in the same way. The recent electrostimulation work of George Ojemann and his colleagues [Ojemann and Mateer, 1979; Fried et al., 1982] are also consistent with this view. Thus, it may be necessary to postulate not merely a few separable components to brain organization, but a great many.

If complementary specialization is statistical rather than causal, what implications does this have for our research? First, and perhaps most obvious, it suggests that we should not *assume* that visuospatial and other nonverbal functions are lateralized to the right hemisphere simply because we have lateralized language to the left hemisphere. This in turn has implications for those who would argue that artistic or musical training will somehow improve the functioning of the right hemisphere and make us more creative.

Second, I believe that it suggests that we—and by we I especially mean those of us who do research with normal subjects—should concentrate more on the exceptional patterns of brain organization than on the modal pattern. That is to say, we should stop focusing on right-handers and begin to pay more attention to left-handers. It is clear that at least some left-handers are different, but it is not yet established which left-handers are the different ones, nor why. Many suggestions, from familial sinistrality [Hécaen and Sauguet, 1971] to handwriting posture [Levy and Reid, 1978], from patterns of arm crossing [Sakano, 1982] to sex [McGlone, 1980], have been offered, but none have yet provided a clear differentiation between various groups of left-handers. Even if handedness is not causally linked to language lateralization or to visuospatial ability, left-handers do represent a group that is neurologically more variable than right-handers, and we need such variability to help us understand the underlying mechanisms. If we work only with right-handers, we may be misled into believing that variables are causally associated when they are not. There is a significant problem here, and one that deserves our attention.

ACKNOWLEDGMENTS

Preparation of this paper was aided in part by a grant from the Natural Sciences and Engineering Research Council of Canada.

REFERENCES

Bradshaw JL, Nettleton NC (1981): The nature of hemispheric specialization in man. Behav Brain Sci 4:51–91.

Bryden MP (1973): Perceptual asymmetry in vision: Relation to handedness, eyedness, and speech lateralization. Cortex 9:418–435.

Bryden MP (1984): Dichotic listening and cognitive abilities in left-handers. Paper presented at annual meeting of Canadian Psychological Association, Ottawa, June.

Bryden MP, Hécaen H, DeAgostini M (1983): Patterns of cerebral organization. Brain Language 20:249–262.

Cohen G (1973): Hemispheric differences in serial vs. parallel processing. J Exp Psychol 97:349–356.

Corballis MC (1983): "Human Laterality." New York: Academic Press.

DeRenzi E (1982): "Disorders of Space Exploration and Cognition." Chichester, England: John Wiley.

Fried I, Mateer C, Ojemann G, Wohns R, Fedio P (1982): Organization of visuospatial functions in human cortex: Evidence from electrical stimulation. Brain 105:349–371.

Gardner H (1983): "Frames of Mind." New York: Basic Books.

Graves R (1983): Mouth asymmetry, dichotic ear advantage, and tachistoscopic visual field advantage as measures of language lateralization. Neuropsychologia 21:641–649.

Hécaen H, DeAgostini M, Monzon-Montes A (1981): Cerebral organization in left handers. Brain Lang 12:261–284.

Hécaen H, Sauguet J (1971): Cerebral dominance in left-handed subjects. Cortex 7:19–48.

Kimura D (1979): Neuromotor mechanisms in the evolution of human communication. In Steklis HD, Raleigh MJ (eds): "Neurobiology of Social Communication in Primates." New York: Academic Press.

LeDoux J, Wilson DH, Gazzaniga M (1977): Manipulo-spatial aspects of cerebral lateralization: Clues to the origin of lateralization. Neuropsychologia 15:743–749.

Levy J, Reid M (1978): Variations in cerebral organization as a function of handedness, hand posture in writing, and sex. J Exp Psychol [Gen] 107:119–144.

Ley RG, Bryden MP (1982): A dissociation of right and left hemispheric effects for recognizing emotional tone and verbal content. Brain Cognition 1:3–9.

Masure MC, Benton AL (1983): Visuospatial performance in left-handed patients with unilateral brain lesions. Neuropsychologia 21:179–181.

McGlone J (1980): Sex differences in human brain asymmetry: A critical review. Behav Brain Sci 3:215–263.

McGlone J, Davidson W (1973): The relation between cerebral speech lateralization and spatial ability with special reference to sex and hand preference. Neuropsychologia 11:105–113.

Ojemann G, Mateer C (1979): Human language cortex: Localization of memory, syntax, and sequential motor-phoneme identification systems. Science 205:1401–1403.

Rasmussen T, Milner B (1977): The role of early left-brain injury in determining lateralization. Ann NY Acad Sci 299:355–369.

Sakano N (1982): "Latent Left-Handedness: Its Relation to Hemispheric and Psychological Functions." Jena: VEB Gustav Fischer Verlag.

Satz P (1980): Incidence of aphasia in left-handers: A test of some hypothetical models of cerebral speech organization. In Herron J (ed): "The Neuropsychology of Left-Handedness." New York: Academic Press.

Saxby LN, Bryden MP (1984): Left-ear superiority in children for processing auditory emotional material. Dev Psychol 20:72–80.

Segalowitz SJ, Bryden MP (1983): Individual differences in hemispheric representation of language. In Segalowitz SJ (ed): "Language Functions and Brain Organization." New York: Academic Press.

Semmes J (1968): Hemispheric specialization: A possible clue to mechanism. Neuropsychologia 6:11–26.

Strauss E, Lapointe JS, Wada JH, Gaddes W, Kosaka B (1985): Language dominance: Correlation of radiological and functional data. Neuropsychologia (in press).

Two Hemispheres—One Brain:
Functions of the Corpus Callosum, pages 471–481
© 1986 Alan R. Liss, Inc.

Speech Functions Related to Local Changes of Cerebral Blood Flow and Metabolism

DAVID H. INGVAR

Department of Clinical Neurophysiology, University Hospital, S-221 85 Lund, Sweden

INTRODUCTION

It is pertinent at this symposium to include a review of studies that have been made in recent years on how speech production and speech perception alter the blood flow of the cerebral cortex and also the regional cerebral metabolism. In this paper the main emphasis will be given to measurements of regional cerebral blood flow (rCBF) by means of intra-arterial or intravenous administration of Xenon 133. These methods have a two-dimensional character; i.e., they measure changes in the rCBF from the side of the head, on one or both sides. Such measurements record mainly changes of the blood flow in the cerebral cortex. Measurements of regional cerebral metabolic rate (rCMR) are made with positron-emission tomography (PET) of the regional glucose uptake or the regional oxygen consumption. Very few PET studies related to speech have, however, been made.

The techniques mentioned have opened up a new chapter in speech physiology. For the first time, it is possible to record how the brain works when it perceives speech or when it produces speech. It is evident that speech engages much wider regions of the brain than has hitherto been known, and also that most speech patterns show important symmetrical features in the two hemispheres. Certain side differences can, however, be demonstrated and they will be emphasized below. One important feature of all speech patterns recorded is that the prefrontal cortex is highly involved, possibly owing to the role that this part of the cortex plays in the temporal organization of behavior and perception. The new results obtained with the blood flow and metabolic measurements appear to necessitate a reevaluation of how the classical speech centers of Broca, Wernicke, and Penfield participate in the production and perception of speech. A more extensive review of the present topic has been published recently by this author [Ingvar, 1983].

METHODOLOGICAL CONSIDERATIONS

The Xenon 133 clearance techniques imply in principle that the gamma-emitting isotope Xenon 133, which has a half-life of about 6 days, is dissolved in a small amount of saline. The solution is administered either into the intracarotid artery, or intravenously. In both cases the arrival of the isotope and its subsequent clearance is recorded by an array of detectors that look at the side of the head [Lassen and Ingvar, 1961; Lassen et al., 1963; Lassen and Ingvar, 1972]. In this manner mainly superficial parts, i.e., the cerebral cortex, of the hemisphere are recorded. With the intra-arterial technique only one hemisphere is injected, and hence only unilateral measurements are possible. Bilateral measurements can be made with the intravenous technique [Nilsson et al., 1982]. It is also possible to administer Xenon 133 by means of inhalation [Risberg, 1980]. Only a few speech studies have, however, been made with this variant. It is pertinent to mention that the Xenon 133 technique has recently been supplemented with the so-called SPECT technique (single photon-emission computerized tomography), which also enables recording of the cerebral blood flow in deep structures of the brain [Stokeley et al., 1980]. No speech studies with SPECT have, however, been reported so far.

Measurements of the regional cerebral metabolic rate (rCMR) of glucose or oxygen are made by positron-emission tomography (PET) [Reivich et al., 1979; Phelps et al., 1982; Alavi et al., 1982; cf. Greitz et al., 1985]. Positron-emitting isotopes ($^{15}O_2$ or ^{18}F) are administered either in pure form or incorporated into metabolically relevant molecules. During the short existence of the positron-emitting isotope in the brain, its distribution is measured by means of rotating detectors in a so-called positron camera. Only a few rCMR studies related to speech have been carried out so far. Details concerning the character of the tests used for speech production and speech perception, as well as for technical details concerning the rCBF and rCMR methods, are given in the original papers referred to below.

RESULTS

In the present context, findings in patients without major neurological disturbances and with normal speech, normal skull x-ray, CT-scan, cerebrospinal fluid, etc., will be mainly considered. They will be briefly related to observations in patients with aphasia and psychotic language.

Automatic Speech

The initial rCBF studies with the intra-arterial rCBF Xenon 133 method were made with automatic speech, i.e., during naming of the weekdays over and over again, a simple speech test with low semantic content that can be performed automatically with only slight cognitive effort [Ingvar and Schwartz, 1974; Ingvar, 1975]. Automatic speech gives an extensive activation in both hemispheres of the upper premotor-prefrontal region, corresponding to the supplementary motor area (the upper speech cortex of Penfield) and regions prefrontal to it. A marked peak was also found in the lower rolandic region corresponding to the mouth-tongue-larynx area. A moderate increase of rCBF was also recorded in the superior temporal region, possibly caused by auditory feedback. During reading of a simple text a clear-cut activation of occipital (visual and paravisual) areas was recorded in addition in the same study.

The main rCBF level of the hemispheres did not change significantly, indicating that automatic speech mainly gave a redistribution of the flow (function) in the hemisphere. It was somewhat unexpected that the test did not give rise to a clear-cut augmentation of rCBF in the Broca field. In regions pertaining to the Wernicke area a very moderate augmentation was recorded. This observation, as well as the Z-like activation pattern on both sides, was confirmed in a subsequent intra-arterial rCBF study, also with automatic speech, by Larsen et al. [1978] with an instrument with high spatial resolution.

Silent speech, automatic speech without vocalization of well-known word series, e.g., counting silently from 1 to 100, have in a few observations been found to give a selective activation of upper prefrontal regions [Lassen et al., 1978; Lassen and Larsen, 1980] (Fig. 1).

Word perception (in pretrained subjects) of short expressions like "bang," "crack," etc., augmented the mean hemisphere flow about 10% on both sides [Nishisawa et al., 1982]. Focal increases were seen bilaterally in (1) the superior temporal regions along the sylvian fissure, (2) the prefrontal area anterior to area 6, (3) in frontal eye fields, and (4) in the lower prefrontal cortex anterior to Broca's field. The activation in the superior temporal region was more widespread and of greater intensity on the left side. Related observations have been made by Maximilian [1982] in rCBF studies with the inhalation technique.

rCMR measurements with positron-emission tomography using 18-F-deoxyglucose show that the perception of verbal messages augments the regional metabolism in lower frontal regions of the left side and also in the left thalamic region as well as in the caudate nucleus [Reivich et al., 1983; Mazziotta et al., 1982, 1983; Metter et al., 1982].

In contrast, *auditory discrimination* of temporally highly structured tonal patterns gave a more dominant right-sided temporal activation in addition to bilateral activation of premotor and prefrontal areas [Roland et al., 1981]. rCMR augmentations dominating the temporal region on the right side have also been recorded during perception of music [Mazziotta et al., 1982, 1983].

Reading

During silent reading the following fields are activated: (1) the frontal eye fields, (2) the lower frontal regions including Broca's area, (3) the

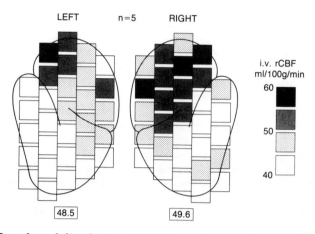

Fig. 1. Hyperfrontal distribution of rCBF in resting consciousness. Superimposed bilateral intravenous (IV) rCBF determinations in five healthy young men (aged 27–34 years). rCBF values are denoted in accordance with scale to the right. Mean values for each hemisphere are given in boxes below hemisphere outlines (48.5 and 49.6 ml/100 g/min, respectively. Normal mean value for both hemispheres was 49.1 SD ± 5.2 ml/100 g/min). Note higher values in regions anterior to the rolandic and sylvian fissures. Note also slight asymmetry between hemispheres. Replotted from color TV display [Ryding et al., 1982].

premotor and prefrontal regions, as well as (4) visual and (5) paravisual areas. Reading aloud activates in addition (6) the rolandic mouth area and (7) the auditory as well as para-auditory areas. The pattern described was similar in both hemispheres [Lassen et al., 1978; Lassen and Larsen, 1980].

In this connection it should be recalled that Roland and Skinhöj [1981] showed that *visual discrimination* of geometrical figures (with verbal reports) activated (1) visual and paravisual areas bilaterally, (2) the two areas 44, (3) parietal areas, as well as (4) a number of prefrontal areas of the upper prefrontal region over the frontal pole to areas 44 and regions anterior to them. The temporal activation in the right hemisphere was more widespread than on the left side.

Reports of memories (performed with closed eyes) gave symmetrical activations of (1) the supplementary motor areas and the prefrontal cortex anterior to it, (2) the mouth areas, possibly including the frontal eye fields, and (3) areas 44, as well as (4) the auditory areas. On the left side there was in addition a more widespread activation of (5) the middle and inferior temporal regions as well as a clear activation of (6) the lower orbitofrontal cortex [Roland et al., 1980].

Humming of a well-known nursery rhyme might be characterized as a nonverbal speech function. In bilateral intravenous rCBF studies, Brådvik et al. [1982] have shown that humming activates both hemispheres rather symmetrically, slightly more on the right than on the left side (Fig. 4). The pattern during humming appears to differ from that of speech in that the lower prefrontal region including Broca's area is not so activated as during speech (Fig. 2).

Resting Consciousness

The findings summarized briefly above might be related to the fact that normally in rCBF studies there is a hyperfrontal distribution of the cerebral blood flow, i.e., in resting conscious subjects the activity (blood flow) is significantly higher in frontal and prefrontal regions than in postcentral parts of the cortex. This resting pattern shows interesting side differences. On the left side, the highest flows are recorded over the lower prefrontal and precentral regions corresponding to Broca's area and the regions anterior to it. The high flows on the right side are more widespread [Ingvar,

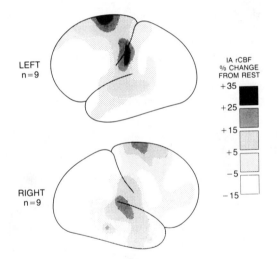

Fig. 2. Automatic speech. Superimposed diagrams of nine right-sided and nine left-sided intra-arterial (IA) rCBF studies in patients without neurological disturbances and with normal speech. The rCBF changes have been calculated in percent relative to the resting state (see Fig. 1). Scale to the right denotes magnitude of flow change. During automatic speech the subjects were asked to count repeatedly from 1 to 20. The subjects had their eyes closed. Note Z-like flow change on the left side with a clear-cut flow peak in the premotor/prefrontal regions, another peak in the mouth/tongue/larynx area, and also an activation of the middle temporal region. On the right side a similar pattern was recorded, but the peaks were not as high and were less well defined, especially in the temporal region. Replotted after color TV display [Larsen et al., 1978, reproduced with permission].

1983] (Fig. 3). This side difference has been confirmed by Hagstadius et al. [1984], and it has also been found in rCMR studies that the metabolism of Broca'a area during resting wakefulness (in silence) is higher on the left side than on the right [Horwitz et al., 1984].

DISCUSSION

Current rCBF and rCMR techniques permit for the first time a quantitative measurement of functional changes in the brain during various types of psychophysiological activation, including those induced by tests of speech functions [Ingvar and Lassen, 1975; Alavi et al., 1982]. This signals a new era in research on speech, since now the hitherto dominating patho-anatomical concepts of localization of speech can be supplemented by actual functional studies in conscious human beings that produce or perceive speech. From the studies related above four main comments can be made.

First, speech performance and speech perception activates the brain in a much more widespread manner than has previously been recognized. Although simple speech tests to not seem to augment the general level of flow (activity) and metabolism of the brain, it has been shown conclusively that speech performance and speech perception activates (redistributes activity to) specific regions in each hemisphere. It should be emphasized that the focal activations are considerable, often with peaks ranging from 20–40% above the resting level.

Second, the speech patterns recorded show important symmetrical features. This appears natural since, for example, the pronunciation of words

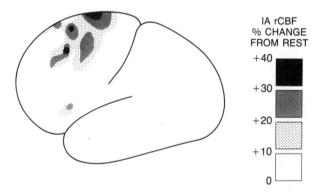

Fig. 3. Silent speech. IA rCBF measurement with a high-resolution instrument with 254 detectors in the left hemisphere in a normal subject. Flow changes displayed in percent related to the resting value for respective region in accordance with the scale to the right. During silent ("inner") speech the subjects were asked to count from 1 to 100 silently. Occasional questions from an observer established how far the subject had come. Note increase of flow in upper prefrontal regions. Replotted from color TV display [Lassen et al., 1978, reproduced with permission].

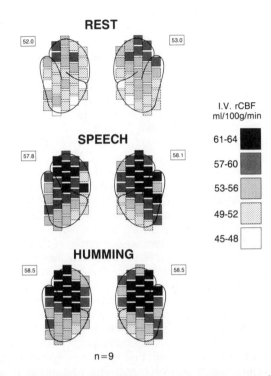

Fig. 4. Speech and humming. IV rCBF measurements in nine male patients who had suffered transient ischemic attacks with minor supratentorial symptoms prior to the flow measurement. At the time of the study all patients showed normal neurological findings, normal speech, and normal prosody. Minor CT abnormalities outside classical speech areas were noted in some of the patients. Some patients also showed slight EEG abnormalities. During *rest* (upper diagram) the noise in the laboratory was kept at a minimum, and the patients were silent, not moving, and had their eyes covered. Note normal mean IV rCBF bilaterally, as well as normal hyperfrontal flow distribution (cf. Fig. 1). During *speech* (middle diagram) the patients were asked to enumerate the weekdays over and over again (automatic speech). In the lower diagram the results are shown during *humming* (without text) a well-known children's song with closed mouth. Note: (1) Normal mean IV rCBF bilaterally at rest with typical hyperfrontal distribution (cf. Fig. 1); (2) an increase of the mean hemisphere flows during both speech and humming of about 10%; (3) great similarity of the speech and humming patterns with marked increase of the prefrontal and lower rolandic flows; (4) increase of rCBF in temporal regions especially on the right side during both speech and humming. This series was used as a reference for IV rCBF studies in patients with right- and left-sided cerebrovascular lesions with aphasia or aprosodia, respectively [Brådvik et al., 1982].

necessitates motor control of mouth, tongue, larynx, etc., from both hemispheres. Also the auditory feedback of spoken words must affect both auditory cortices.

Third, the side differences might be emphasized. Speech perception gave a more widespread temporal activation than on the right side [Nishisawa et al., 1982]. Roland et al. [1981] showed that discrimination of geometrical figures, a sort of "reading," gave a more widespread temporal activation of the right side. Here the side differences in the resting hyperfrontal pattern should also be recalled [Ingvar, 1983] as well as the same asymmetries in the resting pattern seen in rCMR studies [Horwitz et al., 1984].

The classical speech cortices of Broca and Wernicke in the dominant hemisphere do not stand out in the rCBF and rCMR studies made so far in the manner that might have been expected. In the tests used, Broca and Wernicke activations appear limited; i.e., their resting level of activity is often not altered considerably. Further research is necessary to reveal under what circumstances, i.e., during what type of speech tests, these areas become specifically active. The upper speech cortex of Penfield, on the other hand, showed a definite activation in production of speech. Apparently this region plays a role for the temporal organization of spoken words.

Fourth, it should be emphasized that a common denominator of most of the studies related above is the fact that a general activation of prefrontal cortical structures takes place during both speech performance and speech perception. This prefrontal activation, which showed some regional features, supports the idea that the prefrontal cortex is responsible for temporal organization of behavior in general, and insofar as speech is concerned, for the temporal organization of motor patterns pertaining to speech. This conclusion is highly supported by the finding that silent speech, i.e., the inner serial organization of words, selectively activates upper prefrontal cortical regions [Lassen et al., 1978]. The finding of Nishisawa et al. [1982] that speech perception also activates prefrontal fields appears especially relevant. Possibly, the prefrontal cortex plays a much greater role for speech perception than has been known previously. In accordance with the motor theory for speech perception [Liberman et al., 1967] perception of spoken words can only be made in the rapid manner as it takes place by access to motor "templates" for speech, i.e., access to the motor programs for spoken words.

In general the rCBF findings to which the main emphasis has been given above are supported by the few rCMR studies that have been carried out so far [Metter et al., 1982; Phelps et al., 1982]. Thus, there is evidence that rCBF and rCMR studies may in the future reveal a number of unknown features of cortical functions pertaining to speech.

Clinical Comments

rCBF studies in *aphasia* confirm in general classical pathoanatomical findings. Lesions in the Broca area give low flow and metabolism in this region and signs of expressive aphasia. Corresponding findings for the Wernicke region have also been reported, as well as more diffuse rCMR and rCBF abnormalities in patients with global forms of aphasia [Soh et al., 1978]. However, these observations have not been so numerous and detailed. It is, therefore, not possible to give a comprehensive analysis of the complex problems concerning aphasia based upon rCBF and rCMR studies [cf. also Metter et al., 1981].

In chronic *schizophrenia*, a number of speech disturbances have been reported, including a reduction in speech production, a lack of speech fluency as well as peculiar forms of ecolalia, and speech rhythm and abnormal speech melodies, etc. [Chapman, 1979]. In this context it is of interest to recall that in certain types of schizophrenia a low rCBF has been found in prefrontal cortical regions [Ingvar, 1982]. This would in general indicate that the disturbance in the temporal organization of perception and behavior that is so characteristic in the schizophrenic psychosis may also affect speech and that these disturbances are coupled to a dysfunction of prefrontal cortical regions [Ingvar, 1983].

ACKNOWLEDGMENTS

This work was supported by the Swedish Medical Research Council (project no B85-04X-00084-21A) and the Wallenberg Foundation, Stockholm.

REFERENCES

Alavi A, Reivich M, Jones SC, Greenberg JH, Wolf AP (1982): Functional imaging of the brain with positron emission tomography. In Freeman LM, Weissman HS (eds) "Nuclear Medicine Annual." New York: Raven Press, pp 319–372.

Brådvik B, Hedqvist Ch, Ingvar DH, Johnson K, Ryding E (1982): rCBR studies of hemisphere dominance and language functions (Swedish). Swed Assoc Med Sci p 262.

Chapman LJ (1979): Recent advances in the study of schizophrenic cognition. Schizophr Bull 5:568–580.

Greitz T, Ingvar DH, Widén L (eds) (1985): "The Metabolism of the Human Brain Studied with Positron Emission Tomography." New York: Raven Press.

Hagstadius S, Risberg J (1984): Hemispheric asymmetries of rCBF in normal subjects during resting. II Scand Neuropsychol Meeting, Lund, Sweden, August 14–18.

Horwitz B, Duara R, Rapoport SI (1984): Intercorrelations of glucose metabolic rates between brain regions: Application to healthy males in a state of reduced sensory input. J Cereb Blood Flow Metab 4:484–499.

Ingvar DH (1975): Patterns of brain activity revealed by measurements of regional cerebral blood flow. In Ingvar DH, Lassen NA (eds): "Brain Work." Copenhagen: Munksgaard, pp 397–413.

Ingvar DH (1982): Mental illness and regional brain metabolism. TINS 5:199–202.

Ingvar DH (1983): Functional landscapes of the brain pertaining to mentation. Hum Neurobiol 2:1–4.

Ingvar DH, Lassen NA (eds) (1975): "Brain Work." Copenhagen: Munksgaard.

Ingvar DH, Schwartz MS (1974): Blood flow patterns induced in the dominant hemisphere by speech and reading. Brain 97:273–288.

Larsen B, Skinhöj E, Lassen NA (1978): Variation in regional cortical blood flow in the right and left hemispheres during automatic speech. Brain 101:193–209.

Lassen NA, Ingvar DH (1961): The blood flow over the cerebral cortex determined by radioactive Krypton-85. Experientia 17:42–43.

Lassen NA, Ingvar DH (1972): Radioisotopic assessment of regional cerebral blood flow. Progr Nucl Med 1:376–409.

Lassen NA, Hoedt-Rasmussen K, Sörensen SC, Skinhöj E, Cronqvist S, Bodforss B, Ingvar DH (1963): Regional cerebral blood flow in man determined by Krypton-85. Neurology 13:719–727.

Lassen NA, Ingvar DH, Skinhöj E (1978): Brain function and blood flow. Sci Am 239:62–71.

Lassen NA, Larsen B (1980): Cortical activity in the left and right hemispheres during language-related brain functions. Phonetica 37:27–37.

Liberman AM, Cooper FS, Shankweiter DR, Studdert-Kennedy M (1967): Perception of the speech code. Psychol Rev 74:431–461.

Maximilian VA (1982): Cortical blood flow asymmetries during monaural verbal stimulation. Brain Lang 15:1–11.

Mazziotta JC, Phelps ME, Carson RE, Kuhl DE (1982): Tomographic mapping of human cerebral metabolism. Auditory stimulation. Neurology 32:921–937.

Mazziotta JC, Phelps ME, Halgren E (1983): Local cerebral glucose metabolic response to audio-visual stimulation and deprivation: Studies in human subjects with positron CT. Hum Neurobiol 2:1–13.

Metter EJ, Wasterlain CG, Kuhl DE, Hanson WR, Phelps ME (1981): 18-FDG positron emission computed tomography in a study of aphasia. Ann Neurol 10:173–183.

Metter EJ, Riege WH, Hanson WR, Camrus L, Phelps ME, Kuhl DE (1983): Correlations of glucose metabolism and structural damage to language function in aphasia. Am Neurol 10:102.

Nilsson BG, Ryding E, Ingvar DH (1982): Quantitative airway artefact compensation at regional cerebral blood flow measurements with radioactive gasses. J Cereb Blood Flow Metab 2:73–78.

Nishisawa Y, Skyhöj-Olesen T, Larsen B, Lassen NA (1982): Left-right cortical asymmetries of regional cerebral blood flow during listening to words. J Neurophysiol 48:458–466.

Phelps ME, Mazziotta JC, Huang SC (1982): Study of cerebral function with positron computed tomography. J Cereb Blood Flow Metab 2:113–162.

Reivich ME, Kuhl D, Wolf A, Greenberg J, Phelps M, Ido T, Casella V, Fowler J, Hoffman E, Alavia A, Som P, Sokoloff L (1979): The (18F) fluoro-deoxyglucose method for the measurement of local cerebral glucose utilization in man. Circ Res 44:127–137.

Reivich M, Gur R, Alavi A (1983): Positron emission tomographic studies of sensory stimuli, cognitive processes and anxiety. Hum Neurobiol 2:2–9.

Risberg J (1980): Regional cerebral blood flow measurements by 133-Xe inhalation: Methodology and applications in neuropsychology and psychiatry. Brain Lang 9:9–34.

Roland PE, Vaernet K, Lassen NA (1980): Cortical activations in man during verbal report from visual memory. Neurosci Lett 5:478.

Roland PE, Skinhöj E (1981): Extrastriate cortical areas activated during visual discrimination in man. Brain Res 222:166–171.

Roland PE, Skinhöj E, Lassen NA (1981): Focal activations of human cerebral cortex during auditory discrimination. J Neurophysiol 45:1139–1151.

Soh K, Larsen B, Skinhöj E, Lassen NA (1978): Regional cerebral blood flow in aphasia. Arch Neurol 35:625–632.

Stokeley EM, Sveinsdottir E, Lassen NA, Rommer P (1980): A single photodynamic computer-assisted tomograph (DCAT) for imaging brain function in multiple cross-sections. J Comput Assist Tomogr 4:230–240.

Two Hemispheres—One Brain:
Functions of the Corpus Callosum, pages 483–510
© 1986 Alan R. Liss, Inc.

Hemispheric Specialization, Interhemispheric Codes, and Transmission Times: Inferences From Visual Masking Studies in Normal People

MORRIS MOSCOVITCH

Department of Psychology, Erindale College, University of Toronto, Mississauga, Ontario L5L 1C6

The corpus collosum is identified with Roger Sperry as much as the third left frontal convolution is identified with Broca. Indeed, had Sperry lived in the nineteenth century the corpus callosum may have been renamed Sperry's tract in honor of the work he has done to elucidate its function.

Despite a great deal of research that has been conducted on the corpus callosum since Sperry's initial publications with Myers in 1953 [Myers and Sperry, 1953], little is known about the form or code in which information is transmitted across it in normal people. Some researchers have proposed that low-level, but highly local, information is transmitted from which the receiving hemisphere constructs a complete percept [Milner and Lines, 1982]; others have suggested that the information transferred is of a higher order, but still modality specific [Studdert-Kennedy and Schankweiler, 1970; Berlucchi, 1972; Berlin and McNeil, 1976; Moscovitch, 1979] and still others have stated that the information transmitted is more abstract in the sense that it no longer retains even the modality-specific qualities of the original input [Berlucchi et al., 1971, 1977; Milner and Lines, 1982]. Although the evidence from anatomical, electrophysiological, and behavioral lesion studies on the corpus callosum generally favor the latter two alternatives, support for all three of them can be found in the literature [Trevarthen, 1968; Sperry et al., 1969; Gazzaniga, 1970; Pandya et al., 1971; Berlucchi et al., 1979; Berlucchi, 1981; Hamilton, 1982; Lepore and Guillemot, 1982; Van Essen et al., 1982; Seagraves and Rosenquist, 1982a,b]. As yet, however, little has been done to investigate these possibilities systematically. In this paper, I will present some experiments that combine techniques used to study visual perceptual asymmetries with those of visual masking to try to determine the nature of interhemispheric transfer of complex information in normal people.

I wish to emphasize at the outset that this paper is concerned with interhemispheric transfer of information only as it relates to stimulus discrimination, recognition, and identification. The cortical commissures may serve other visual functions as well, such as fusing the visual fields and maintaining perceptual continuity across the midline or aiding in binocular depth perception (see articles in this review). It is possible, and indeed likely, that the type and locus of information transfer will be different for different functions [see Berlucchi et al., 1979]. Therefore, the evidence presented in this paper and the discussions that follow are meant to apply only to those functions associated with the discrimination, recognition, and identification of visual stimuli. Departures from this restricted point of reference will be clearly noted.

Studies of perceptual asymmetry in normal people have been used since the 1950s to investigate the nature of hemispheric specialization. One of the basic assumptions of these studies is that information presented to one sensory field, be it visual, auditory, or somesthetic, is projected initially to the contralateral hemisphere. Differences between sensory fields in the speed or accuracy of information processing arises when one hemisphere is superior to the other in processing that information [Kimura, 1961]. In those cases in which one of the components required to complete a task successfully is *functionally localized* [Moscovitch, 1973,1976,1986] to only one hemisphere, it is assumed that input to the other hemisphere must cross the hemispheric commissures for processing in the superior hemisphere [Kimura, 1967; Moscovitch, 1973; Berlucchi, 1975; Zaidel, 1983]. This makes such tasks ideal for studying the nature of interhemispheric transfer of complex information in normal people. Despite this, few if any investigators have taken advantage of the opportunity. One reason may be that not everyone subscribes to the theory that transfer of information from the inferior to the superior hemisphere underlies the observed perceptual asymmetries. Although alternative accounts of the bases of perceptual asymmetries have been offered, interhemispheric transfer still provides the best explanation for the asymmetries observed in a substantial number of cases [see Moscovitch, 1979, for review].

The more likely reason for the dearth of research on this topic is that laterality studies, contrary to one's expectations, do not lend themselves easily to investigations of the nature of interhemispheric transfer. They are best suited for investigating functional differences between the hemispheres. Although the differences may be due, in part, to interhemispheric transfer of information, it is not immediately apparent how one can determine what sort of information gets transferred. Studdert-Kennedy and Schankweiler [1970], for example, chose to look at error patterns and blends of left and right ear stop consonants in a dichotic listening talk. Their results led them to conclude that phonetic features, rather than some lower-level acoustic information, gets transferred between the hemispheres. Similar conclusions were reached by Berlin and his colleagues using different techniques [reviewed in Berlin and McNeil, 1976]. Comparable studies, however, have not been conducted in the visual domain except on inter-hemispheric transfer of simple, unpatterned stimuli. In a series of experi-ments, Berlucchi and his colleagues [1971,1977] and Milner and Lines [1982] confirmed Poffenberger's [1912] results that the reaction time advan-tage for stimuli in the same visual field as the response hand (uncrossed) over those in the opposite field (crossed) reflect interhemispheric transfer time (but see Guiard [1984] for negative evidence). Moreover, the fact that target eccentricity and energy did not change estimates of interhemispheric transfer led to the conclusion that sensory information was not transferred between the hemispheres. Both Berlucchi et al. [1971,1977] and Milner and Lines [1982] suggested that motor commands were transferred between the hemispheres. It is still possible, however, that the information transferred is visual, but of a sufficiently high order so that it is no longer sensitive to lower-level sensory manipulations such as target energy (see below). In any event, despite using simple stimuli and responses, these studies led to conclusions about interhemispheric transfer that are generally consistent with the more complex dichotic studies—the corpus callosum transfers higher-order information. The generalizability of this conclusion would be reinforced if confirmatory evidence could be obtained with *complex* visual stimuli.

It was partly with this goal in mind that my students and I began a series of making experiments on perceptual asymmetries for words and faces. Visual masking is a form of perceptual interference caused by pre-senting two or more stimuli in close spatial and temporal contiguity. Its appeal to us was that we could use it to interfere selectively with various aspects of target perception at different stages of processing [Turvey, 1973; Michaels and Turvey, 1979; Breitmeyer, 1984]. As such it is a very useful, but little used, technique for investigating the early stages of information processing in tachistoscopic recognition of complex lateralized stimuli [Mi-chaels and Turvey, 1973; Oscar-Berman et al., 1973; McKeever and Suberi, 1974; Cohen, 1976; Ward and Ross, 1977; Polich, 1978; Hellige and Webster, 1979; Marzi et al., 1979; Proudfoot, 1982; Hellige, 1983]. In particular, we used it to try to determine at which stage of processing visual field differ-ences to words and faces emerged in normal people. From this evidence we hoped to infer what type of information gets transferred across the corpus callosum during visual perception and how long it takes for the transfer to occur. The steps involved in making these inferences will become apparent as the studies are described.

WORD IDENTIFICATION

In the first series of experiments we had subjects identify vertically presented three-letter words that appeared in either the right or left visual field. Because most of the words were abstract or grammatical functors, we reasoned that it was very likely that identification of these words was *functionally localized* to the left hemisphere. By functional localization we mean that under normal conditions the individual behaves as if the function is represented exclusively in one hemisphere. We used a backward masking technique to examine visual field differences in word identification. Backward masking is a procedure in which perception of an initial stimulus, the target, is impaired by presenting a second visual stimulus, the mask, after a short temporal interval. As the temporal interval between the target and the mask is increased, the target eventually evades the effects of the mask and is identified correctly. The interval at which target identification exceeds a certain criterion is termed the critical interstimulus interval (ISI). It is assumed that targets presented to the superior hemisphere for that task will be able to evade the mask sooner than those presented to the inferior hemisphere if the mask interferes with target processing at a stage where hemispheric asymmetries occur (see below). Since in this case the targets were words, we expected to find a right visual field (RVF) advantage under the appropriate masking conditions.

We used two types of stimuli to mask the targets—patterned, which consisted of letter fragments, and unpatterned, which consisted of either a bright flash or a display of random dots. Our choice of masks was determined by the repeated observation that under specified conditions masking by pattern and by light operate by different mechanisms at different stages of processing [for reviews, see Kahneman, 1968; Kolers, 1968; Turvey, 1973; Breitmeyer and Ganz, 1976; Breitmeyer, 1984]. Unpatterned stimuli such as bright flashes, or random dot displays, typically mask targets only if they are presented to the same eye as the target. The effectiveness of this type of masking also varies with the total energy of the mask or target. When luminance is kept constant, the total stimulus energy varies as a product of target duration such that a multiplicative function is found when target duration (TD) is plotted against critical ISI: $TD \times critical\ ISI = K$ [Turvey, 1973]. For these and other reasons, unpatterned masks are believed to affect target perception peripherally by interfering with the operation of energy-sensitive analyzers that extract sensory features.

Pattern masks, which have features in common with the target, affect both peripheral and central processes. At the central level, they disrupt the operation of a processor that integrates the output of the peripheral sensory analyzers from each eye into relational or categorical features. Thus, pattern masking can occur even though the mask and target are presented to opposite eyes. Central pattern masking is insensitive to stimulus energy but is proportional, instead, to the total time available for processing the target before the mask arrives. The relationship between target duration and critical ISI for central pattern masking is linear: $TD + critical\ ISI = K$ [Turvey, 1973].

The stages of processing at which the two forms of masking are presumed to operate are illustrated in Figure 1, a simplified version of Turvey's [1973]

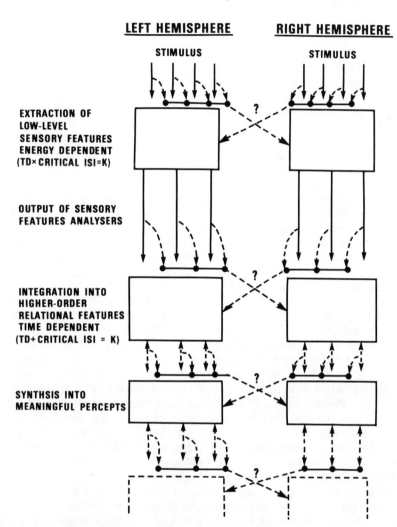

Fig. 1. The stages of processing for stimuli presented initially to the left or right hemisphere. The arrows between the hemisphere represent interhemispheric transfer of information across the commissures. According to Turvey [1973], from whom this model was adopted, each stage does not have to await the end of processing of the previous stage before it receives any information. Instead, it begins processing as soon as *some* information is available from the previous stage. In Turvey's terminology, processing at later stages is concurrent with, yet contingent on, processing at earlier stages (see also McLelland's [1979] cascading processes). The implication for studies of interhemispheric transfer is that estimates of interhemispheric transmission times might vary with the type or amount of information that is required by functionally localized components.

model that has been modified to take lateralized target presentation into account. The temporal interval after target presentation over which a mask is effective is determined by the time it takes for target information to arrive and be processed at the stage at which the mask operates. The critical ISI is a measure of this interval. Visual field differences in critical ISI can occur for one of two reasons. If one hemisphere is simply more efficient than the other at processing information at a particular stage, then the difference in critical ISI will reflect the differences in speed of processing on the two sides. The more interesting case, however, is one in which a particular stage is believed to be functionally localized to one hemisphere. In such a case, stimuli must be transferred via the corpus callosum to that hemisphere for processing. In these instances, the critical ISI will favor stimuli presented initially to the dominant hemisphere by an interval equivalent to the time it takes information to cross the corpus callosum. Under many circumstances visual field differences will be determined by both callosal transfer and hemispheric efficiency. Failure to find differences in critical ISI suggests either that there are no hemispheric differences in processing or that the differences are not detected using critical ISI as a measure [for an extended discussion see Moscovitch, 1986].

By using unpatterned and patterned masks, it is possible to determine at which stage of processing perceptual asymmetries, and by inference hemispheric ones, emerge. If the hemispheres differ in their ability to extract low-level sensory features [Hellige and Webster, 1979; Hellige, 1983], then visual field differences in critical ISI should be found even when an unpatterned mask is used. Moreover, the magnitude of the differences should vary with target duration since that stage of processing is energy dependent. The absence of visual field differences would suggest that both hemispheres are equally efficient at that level of processing. Similarly, hemispheric differences either in integrating the output of sensory analyzers into relational features or in synthesizing those features into meaningful percepts would be reflected in a visual field advantage when a central, pattern mask is used.

In the first experiment, words were presented in either the right or left visual field at exposure durations that ranged from 2–24 msec. Prior to testing, it was determined that identification without a mask was perfect even at the shortest durations. Once testing began, the words were followed immediately by a 50-msec flash or pattern mask. To determine the critical ISI, the interval between target and mask was increased independently for each field by discrete steps after each incorrect response until four consecutive targets were identified correctly [see Moscovitch, 1983, for details]. The trials were blocked by visual field, exposure duration, and mask type.

The results, illustrated in Figure 2, indicate that the critical ISI was significantly shorter by an average of about 4 msec in the pattern mask condition. No perceptual asymmetry was evident in the flash mask condi-

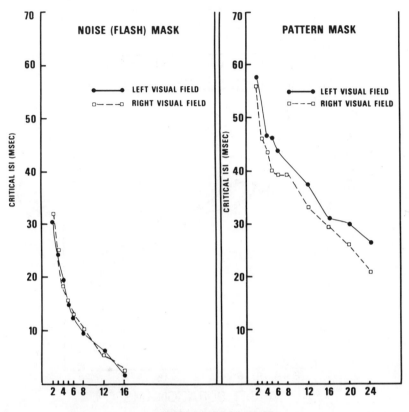

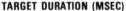

TARGET DURATION (MSEC)

Fig. 2. The critical interstimulus interval (ISI) at which a monocular target word of varying duration in the right (RVF) or left (LVF) visual field escapes a trailing monocular flash or pattern mask.

tion. Because the expected multiplicative relation between the critical ISI and target duration was found in the flash mask condition, the results suggest that hemispheric asymmetries for words are absent at the early, energy-dependent stages of processing. Both hemispheres seem equally efficient at extracting information about sensory features. It is only the later, central stages of processing that are sensitive to pattern masking that hemispheric asymmetries are found (Fig. 2).

This finding was confirmed in later experiments in which target presentation varied randomly between fields (Fig. 3), ruling out the possibility that subjects' expectancies regarding target location led to the asymmetry observed in the initial experiment. In both these studies, but more clearly

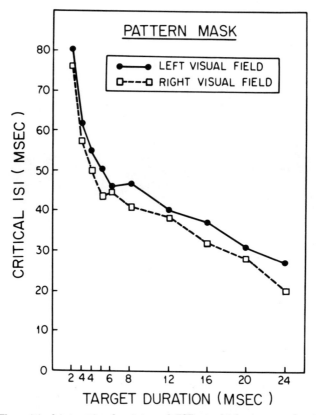

Fig. 3. The critical interstimulus interval (ISI) at which a monocular target word of varying duration in the right (RVF) or left (LVF) visual field escapes a trailing pattern mask. Target location is unpredictable [from Moscovitch, 1983].

in the second, the function relating critical ISI to target duration was additive at the longer durations. This confirmed that the pattern mask acted at a stage of processing where performance was determined by the total time available to the central processor to complete its operation. Whether the hemispheric differences occurred at the stage of processing at which sensory features were integrated into relational units or at later stages in which these units were synthesized into meaningful features cannot be determined by these studies. With the kind of masking procedure we used similar effects are expected regardless of whether the mask interferes with input to the sensory integrator or with readout from it by later stages (see Fig. 1). As we will see later, other, more sensitive masking techniques can distinguish between these possibilities.

In both of the studies that I reported, the criterion that determined the critical ISI was set at a very high level. In effect, the two visual fields were compared at the point at which they first reached asymptotic levels of performance. As a check against the possibility that asymmetries might favor the left visual-right hemisphere at early, sensory stages of processing, as some authors have suggested [Hellige and Webster, 1979; Kimura and Durnford, 1974], a third experiment was conducted in which visual field differences were compared at different levels of accuracy under noise and pattern masking conditions.

To accomplish this, we did not measure critical ISI at a set criterion, but rather monitored accuracy of identification at ISIs ranging from 0 msec, when identification was impossible, to 90 msec, when identification was usually perfect. The results displayed in Figure 4 show clearly that when a pattern mask is used a right visual field/left hemisphere (RVF-LH) advantage emerges as soon as identification accuracy rises above 0. Examination of Figure 4 also shows that when performance is neither on the floor nor approaching ceiling, the ISI at which equivalent levels of performance are reached in the two fields is about 5 msec shorter in the right visual field than in the left, a value that is consistent with that obtained in the previous two experiments. In the noise mask condition, a marginally significant advantage in favor of the left visual field was found that was due almost entirely to performance at target durations of 2 msec. Although this leaves open the possibility that hemispheric differences might occur at peripheral, sensory stages of processing, the three experiments suggest that such asymmetries are weak, fragile, and inconsistent in comparison to those that occur at later, higher-order central stages of processing.

That pattern masking indeed affects central processes that differ between the hemisphere is borne out by other studies that have been conducted. Ron Stringer and I confirmed the observation that in dichoptic studies, where the mask and target are presented to opposite eyes, noise masks are ineffective, whereas pattern masks continue to be potent. Moreover, the critical ISI advantage enjoyed by the RVF when a pattern mask was used was about the same in the dichoptic condition as in the monoptic ones.

In another study, Brenda Linn and I had subjects retain three nonsense syllables while attempting to identify lateralized words in the pattern and noise masking conditions. If pattern masking is a central process, it is likely to demand attentional or cognitive resources. The resources available for target identification under pattern masking conditions should, therefore, be reduced by a concurrent memory task that itself requires similar resources. As a result, the critical ISI for identifying targets should rise in the dual task condition. If the further assumption is made that the left and right hemispheres are partially or fully independent systems, each with its own cognitive resources, then the concurrent memory task, which is distinctly verbal, should deplete primarily left-hemisphere resources. This would be

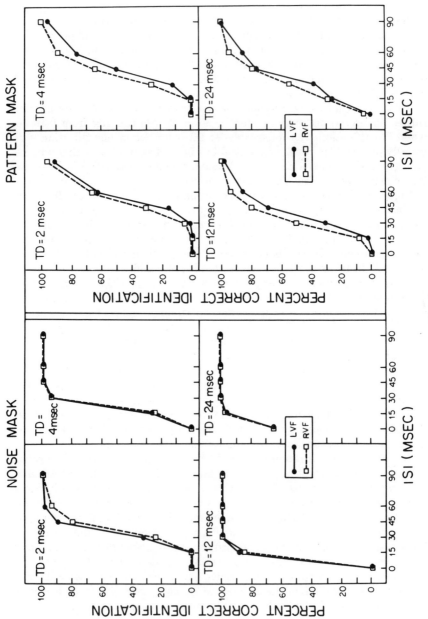

Fig. 4.

reflected in a greater change in critical ISI for identifying right than left field stimuli [Hellige et al., 1979; Moscovitch and Klein, 1980; Friedman and Polson, 1982]. On the other hand, a concurrent memory load is likely to have little effect on performance in the noise mask condition, since that depends on peripheral processes that are relatively automatic. The results generally confirmed our hypotheses (see Fig. 5). The concurrent task had little effect on the noise masking condition when target duration was 2 msec. In the pattern mask condition, however, the concurrent memory load provided an overall increase in critical ISI that was due primarily to a change in RVF performance. These results are consistent with those reported by Hellige et al. [1979], who found similar effects of concurrent memory loads in a lateralized letter-matching task that used response latencies as the dependent measure.

It has been claimed by a number of people that one cause of the cognitive deficits seen in old age is a reduction in attentional capacity or resources necessary for supporting tasks that require some cognitive effort [for review,

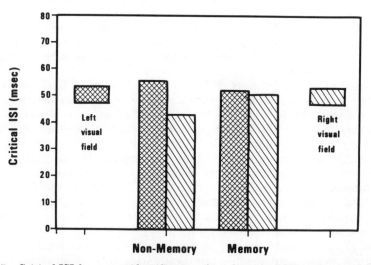

Fig. 5. Critical ISI for correct identification of words in the RVF (right visual field) and LVF (left visual field) under patterned and unpatterned masking conditions with and without a concurrent memory load.

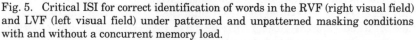

Fig. 4. Percent correct identification of binocular target words of varying durations (TD) in the (RVF) or left (LVF) visual field at different interstimulus intervals (ISI) between the target and a trailing binocular noise or pattern mask [from Moscovitch, 1983].

see Craik, and Byrd, 1982]. It follows from this assumption and the results of our previous study, that old people would be much more vulnerable to masking by pattern than by noise. When visual acuity is equated between young and old people, the predicted pattern of results is seen very clearly [Walsh, 1982; Byrd and Moscovitch, 1984, for review]. Moreover, Mark Byrd and I (see Fig. 6) found that visual field differences in pattern masking are equivalent in young and old people, the only difference being that the elderly require much more time than the young to process the target to the same level.

FACE RECOGNITION

Unlike words, faces are typically recognized better in the LVF [for review, see Moscovitch, 1979; Sergent and Bindra, 1981; Young, 1983], a finding consistent with the observation that deficits in face-recognition are usually associated with right-hemisphere damage, though they may sometimes also accompany left-hemisphere lesions [Benton, 1980; Sergent and Bindra, 1981]. Earlier studies suggested that hemispheric asymmetries for faces, like those for words, emerged at a late stage of processing [Moscovitch et al., 1976; Moscovitch, 1979]. Because face recognition did not seem to be as strongly lateralized as word identification [Moscovitch, 1979; Benton, 1980; Sergent and Bindra, 1981], Myra Radzins and I decided to test the generalizability of the hypothesis that perceptual asymmetries emerge at late stages of processing by applying some of the same masking techniques to faces as to words.

Subjects first studied a set of five male and five female faces until they learned to associate each face with the letter of the alphabet that was assigned to it. This took about 5–10 minutes. The faces were then presented randomly to either the left or right visual field at exposure durations ranging from 2 to 24 msec. Subjects were required to identify the faces by typing the letter associated with them in a computer. In one condition the faces were followed by an array of random dots and in the other by a pattern mask consisting of a collage of cut-up target faces. As in the first word-identification studies, the ISI between mask and target was increased after each incorrect response until a criterion of four consecutive correct answers was reached. This defined the critical ISI.

As Figures 7 and 8 show, the pattern of results was similar to that obtained in the word-identification task except that asymmetries, when they occurred, now favored the left visual field (LVF). As predicted, visual field differences were absent in the noise mask condition but emerged clearly in the pattern mask condition at longer target durations. That the masking function relating target duration to critical ISI was multiplicative when a noise mask was used and additive at longer durations when a pattern mask was used is consistent with the idea that the noise mask acted peripherally and the pattern mask, centrally. The 8-msec advantage in favor

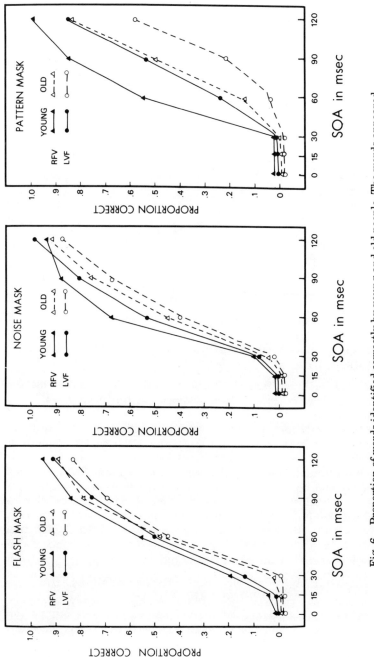

Fig. 6. Proportion of words identified correctly by young and old people. The words appeared in the right (RVF) or left (LVF) visual field and were followed, at various stimulus onset asynchonics (SOA) by either a flash, noise, or pattern mask [from Byrd and Moscovitch, 1984].

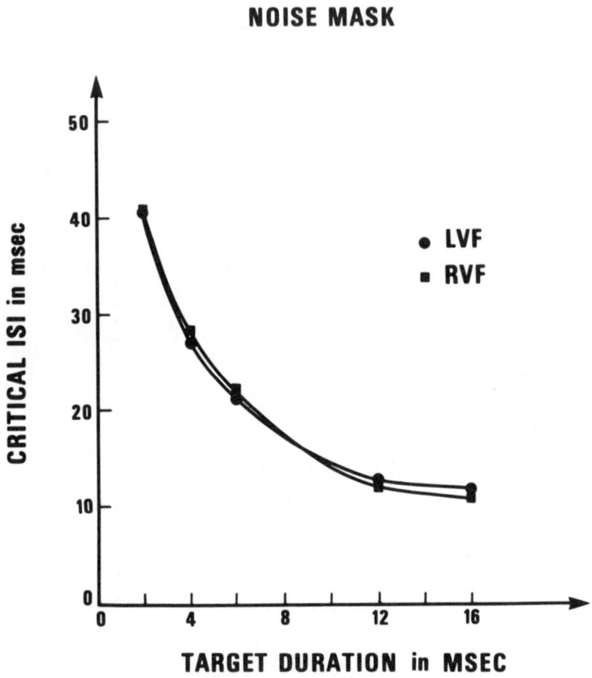

NOISE MASK

Fig. 7. Critical ISI in the left (LVF) and right (RVF) visual field for recognition of faces of various duration (TD) that are followed by a noise mask.

of the LVF-RH in the pattern mask condition, though somewhat high, is still well within the range of values obtained in favor of the RVF-LH in word identification.

Taken together, the experiments on word identification and face recognition support the view that all perceptual asymmetries, and by implication hemispheric ones, emerge at late, higher-order stages of processing. Moreover, the magnitude of perceptual asymmetries remains fairly constant across many conditions, though the direction of such asymmetries may change with stimulus type or processing requirements. In the following sections I will argue, and attempt to demonstrate, that these findings can be used to determine the structural locus at which hemispheric asymmetries emerge, the code in which information is transferred between hemispheres, and the time it takes to transmit this information.

STRUCTURAL LOCUS OF HEMISPHERE ASYMMETRIES IN VISUAL PERCEPTION

The studies reported so far have been concerned with determining only the functional locus at which hemispheric asymmetries emerge. They have

PATTERN MASK

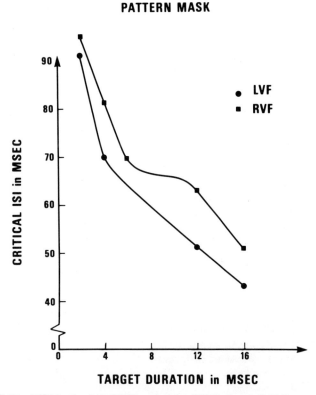

Fig. 8. Critical ISI in the left (LVF) and right (RVF) visual field for recognition of faces of various duration that are followed by a pattern mask.

been consistent in showing that the locus is not at the level of sensory analysis, but beyond it at a central stage of processing that requires attentional resources for its efficient operation. What might be the structural locus at which hemispheric asymmetries emerge? On the basis of the information gathered from our experiments and on neurological evidence that striate cortex lesions have similar effects whether they are on the left or on the right, a reasonable (and safe) guess would be that hemispheric asymmetries emerge anterior to (beyond) the striate cortex. The pattern mask may act at the same level, or alternatively, it may interfere with the target at the striate cortex, but the observable effects may be dependent on the output from that region to later ones.

As an initial test of these predictions, George Schlotterer, Don McLachlan, and I [1984] tested patients in the early or middle stages of Alzheimer's disease. We chose these patients because there was evidence to suggest that the histopathological processes characteristic of the disease initially spared the primary sensory areas of the cortex, which includes the striate [Schenk, 1955; Tomlinson et al., 1968,1970; Crapper, 1976; Benson et al., 1981]. If the striate cortex functions normally in these patients, then they should do well on perceptual tests that are believed to be mediated by it.

We chose first to look at spatial frequency contrast sensitivity. There is evidence that striate neurons in primates are sensitive to black-and-white sinusoidal gratings of different spatial frequencies [DeValois and DeValois, 1980; Lennie, 1980]. Also, damage to striate neurons in humans leads to loss of sensitivity to different spatial frequencies [Bodis-Wollner, 1972, 1977; Regan et al., 1977; Zimmern et al., 1979]. As predicted, on tests of spatial frequency contrast sensitivity, the Alzheimer patients we tested performed no differently from age-matched controls with similar visual acuity (see Fig. 9).

This result encouraged us to test the effects of patterned and unpatterned masks on letter identification in these patients. We were not interested in lateralization of function in these patients, but only in ascertaining whether the neural degeneration associated with the disease makes them much more vulnerable to patterned, than to unpatterned, masks. As Figure 10 shows, Alzheimer patients performed as well as age-matched controls with similar acuity in the flash mask condition but were severely impaired in the pattern mask condition. Having a relatively intact striate cortex seems sufficient to support the extraction of sensory features but not their integration into higher-order units. In a later section, we will review evidence that may help us determine more precisely which areas of the visual cortex mediate the laterality and masking effects we have observed.

INTERHEMISPHERIC TRANSFER TIME

Knowing the stage at which hemispheric asymmetries emerge makes it possible to infer the nature of the callosal code and interhemispheric transfer time from the masking studies. It will be recalled by referring to Figure 1 that such inferences rest on the assumption that one or more components necessary for word identification or face recognition is *functionally localized* to one hemisphere (see pp 6–7). This is a reasonable assumption for word identification, since all but four of the words used in the study were grammatical functors or abstract words, the reading of which is rarely attributable to the right hemisphere [Coltheart, 1980; Marcel and Patterson, 1978; Moscovitch, 1981; Patterson and Besner, 1984; Rabinowicz and Moscovitch, 1985; Young and Ellis, 1985]. To read words presented initially to the right hemisphere, information would have to be transferred via the corpus callosum to the left hemisphere at a stage of processing that precedes the functionally lateralized component [Moscovitch, 1986]. The time it takes to transfer this information will be reflected in an equivalent increase in the

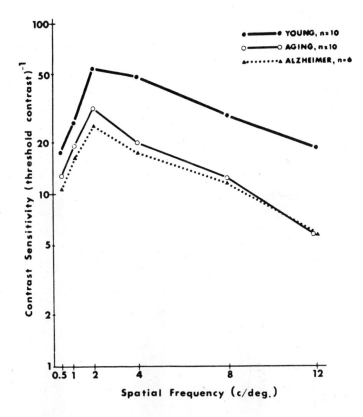

Fig. 9. Spatial frequency contrast sensitivity function for young, aging, and Alzheimer groups [from Schlotterer et al., 1983].

time it takes a LVF target word, as compared to one in the RVF, to escape a mask that interferes with the operation of the functionally lateralized component.

Similar arguments apply for the transfer of information in the opposite direction, from the left to the right hemisphere, in studies of face recognition and other functions that favor the LVF. For simplicity, and because such functions are not always strongly lateralized [Moscovitch, 1979; Moscovitch and Klein, 1980], we will restrict our discussion to word identification. We will assume that a similar pattern of results but with opposite sign will obtain for processes that are functionally localized in the right hemisphere.

As we noted, failure to find visual field differences in the unpatterned mask condition suggests that the extraction of low-level sensory features is

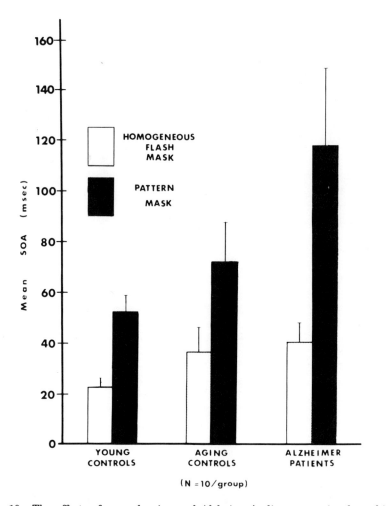

Fig. 10. The effects of normal aging and Alzheimer's disease on visual masking performance. Mean stimulus onset asynchrony in msec when interstimulus interval is zero is compared for young, aging, and Alzheimer groups for homogeneous and pattern masking conditions. The error bars represent standard deviations [Schlotterer et al., 1983].

neither functionally localized nor even lateralized with any consistency to one hemisphere under the conditions tested. This makes it unlikely that relatively raw sensory data, which is the input to that stage of processing, is transferred across the interhemispheric commissures for use in stimulus identification and recognition (see Fig. 1). Sensory feature analysis of the stimulus seems to be computed prior to transfer across the corpus callosum.

When the target is a word and a pattern mask is used, however, a consistent RVF advantage in critical ISI is obtained. The magnitude of the RVF advantage is on the order of 3–5 msec and varies little with predictability of stimulus location, with level of performance, or with masking procedure (monoptic vs. dichoptic). This high degree of consistency lends added support to the assumption that the differences between visual fields in critical ISI reflect the time it takes to transfer information across the interhemispheric commissures from the inferior hemisphere to the functionally localized component(s) in the superior hemisphere. Differences in critical ISI, therefore, provide a measure of interhemispheric transfer time that is well within the range of times predicted by neuroanatomical data, measured by electrophysiological techniques, and inferred from behavioral studies of simple reaction time to unpatterned stimuli [Poffenberger, 1912; Jeeves, 1969; Berlucchi et al., 1971, 1977; Bashore, 1981; Milner and Lines, 1982]. Our studies also replicate and extend Turvey's [1973] findings and support his view that the pattern mask interferes with that central stage of processing at which sensory features are integrated into higher-order units. As we noted earlier, we cannot determine from our studies whether functional localization applies to this stage or to a later stage whose function is to read out information and synthesize it into meaningful percepts or store them in memory. By the first alternative, a RVF advantage is found because the need for interhemispheric transfer of LVF information delays its integration into relational features, whereas by the second alternative, transfer delays the readout of information that is based on these features or is synthesized from them. Examination of Figure 1 suggests that if the first alternative is correct, the corpus callosum transmits information about sensory features, whereas if the second alternative is correct, it transfers higher-order information.

The results of a study by Michaels and Turvey [1979] favor the second alternative. On the basis of a series of clever and elegant masking experiments, they proposed that it was possible to distinguish three types of processes or stages involved in central masking. The first stage involves integration of sensory features into relational units. In the second stage, these units are synthesized into a short-lived visual or iconic representation, and in the third stage, information is read out from this iconic representation into a memory store in which items are represented in terms of higher-order categorical, but presumably still visual, features [see also DiLollo and Moscovitch, 1983].

Figure 11 indicates how the operations of these three stages of processing influence performance of target identification at different temporal asyn-

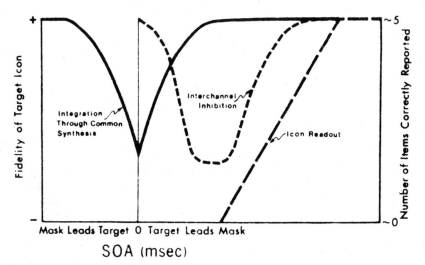

Fig. 11. A three-process model of central, cortical pattern masking, showing hypothetical target fidelity (left ordinate) and number of items correctly reported or readout from icon (right ordinate) as a function of mask SOA. Target pattern fidelity is affected by central integration through common synthesis of target and mask elements at the level of iconic representation, or by prior interchannel inhibition at the level at which sensory features are integrated into higher-order units. Lastly, identification accuracy is affected by the rate at which information is read out from the icon and encoded in terms of relational or categorical features that lead to a meaningful percept [from Michaels and Turvey, 1979].

chronies between the onset of the target and the pattern mask (SOAs) in central masking. If hemispheric asymmetries first emerge during the readout phase, then visual field differences in word identification should only be found at long SOAs, which is when the readout phase operates. As Figure 12 shows, visual field differences were absent at short SOAs only to emerge at longer SOAs. The statistical significance of this finding was marginal, so that the conclusions drawn from this study must be tentative. Nonetheless, they suggest, in line with previous studies [Moscovitch et al., 1976; Marzi et al., 1979; DiLollo, 1981] that the representation of precategorical iconic information is usually characterized by perceptual and hemispheric symmetry, whereas the encoding of iconic information into a more permanent, categorical representation requires the specialized functions of each hemisphere and leads to consistent perceptual asymmetries in target identification and recognition. The possibility exists that slight, but noticeable, hemispheric asymmetries might be found in the integration of sensory features into relational units that are then fed into the icon. Experiments in our laboratory are now under way to answer this question.

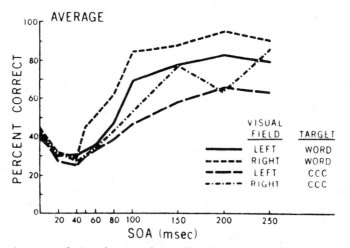

Fig. 12. Average relations between letter identifiability and SOA for three-letter words and consonant trigrams under conditions of dichoptic masking with the target presented to either the left or right visual field [from Michaels and Turvey, 1979].

With Figure 1 in mind, we can now review our argument and summarize our conclusions. Assuming that functional localization holds for the word-identification task, then if hemispheric asymmetries emerge at the stage at which sensory features are integrated, it is information about these features that is transmitted across the cortical commissures. On the other hand, if asymmetries first occur when precategorical iconic information is encoded into meaningful percepts, then what is transmitted is information about relational, but precategorical, features. As we noted earlier, it is too soon to know which of these alternatives is correct. It is possible that both types of higher-order information are transmitted. What has been ruled out by our experiments is that raw sensory information is either not transferred by the interhemispheric commissures or is not functionally useful in target iden-tification.

The nature of the information transferred between the hemispheres as inferred from masking studies is in partial agreement with inferences based on comparing crossed and uncrossed simple reaction times to homogeneous visual stimuli. Like us, Berlucchi et al. [1971, 1977] and Milner and Lines [1982] found that variables that affect stimulus quality or energy, such as retinal eccentricity and stimulus luminance, did not alter the magnitude of the latency difference between crossed and uncrossed pathways. The reader will recall, however, that unlike us, they interpreted the absence of sensory effects on interhemispheric transmission time to mean that a nonvisual code, such as a motor command, is used to transfer information between the two hemispheres. An alternative interpretation consistent with our masking experiments, however, is that the useful signal that is transmitted interhemispherically is still visual but of such a high order that it is usually immune to low-level sensory manipulations.

THE STRUCTURAL LOCUS OF INTERHEMISPHERIC TRANSFER

Where along the extensive network of visual commissural connections from prestriate to posterior temporal cortex does this transfer occur? Some clues can be obtained by comparing the characteristics of backward pattern masking with the neurophysiological properties of cortical neurons. For backward pattern masking to be effective, the target and mask must be in close spatial proximity or, in the case of dichoptic masking, must at least appear to be in close proximity after binocular fusion [Kahneman, 1968; Turvey, 1973; Breitmeyer and Gazz, 1976; Schlotterer et al., 1983]. Although the mask competes with the target for the resources of a central processor, that processor has a narrow field of operation. A separation of as little as one degree between the target and mask, when target presentations are foveal, eliminates the effectiveness of the mask completely [Schlotterer et al., 1983; Breitmeyer, 1984]. This suggests that the neurons that supposedly integrate sensory features into coherent patterns have relatively small receptive fields. Neurons in the extrastriate cortex have these narrow receptive field properties [Berlucchi, 1981], whereas neurons in the inferotemporal cortex do not, since their receptive fields often cover several degrees and extend across the visual midline [Gross et al., 1972; Rocha-Miranda et al., 1975]. The best guess, then, would be that visual information about complex graphemic material is transferred across the corpus callosum at the level of the extrastriate cortex.

It must be emphasized that this conjecture rests on the assumption that hemispheric asymmetries first occur at the stage of sensory-feature integration. As I stated earlier, it is entirely possible, and even likely, that it is only when these features are synthesized into meaningful percepts that hemispheric differences in processing emerge. If that is the case, information necessary for target identification is probably transmitted across the callosum from structures beyond the extrastriate cortex. A third possibility is that interhemispheric transfer of relevant information occurs at many places along the network of cortical commissures from extrastriate to the posterior temporal lobes. Although it is not possible now to decide conclusively among these alternatives, I hope the discussion has indicated how, given a few simplifying assumptions, masking techniques can be used to elucidate both the functional and structural properties of the cerebral hemispheres and its commissures.

As a final example of the use to which masking can be put, I wish to consider a recent suggestion that the hemispheres are sensitive to different spatial frequencies [Broadbent and Broadbent, 1976; Martin, 1979; Sergent, 1982]. The left hemisphere is considered to be more efficient at processing the output of high spatial frequency analyses, whereas the right is specialized in processing low spatial frequency output. Couched in these terms, the locus at which these hemispheric differences would be detected is at the stage at which sensory features, such as spatial frequency, are integrated into the higher-order relational units [see also Michaels and Turvey, 1979]. Accordingly, since masking is spatial frequency specific [Legge, 1978], masking a target with high spatial frequencies should allow low spatial frequency information to escape and bias target identification in favor of the right hemisphere. Similarly, the left hemisphere would be favored if low spatial frequency masks were used. Moreover, since neural transmission is slower for high than for low spatial frequencies [Breitmeyer, 1975; Breitmeyer and Ganz, 1976], estimates of interhemispheric transmission times should vary with the type of spatial frequency information that is being transferred.

Myra Radzins and I are currently examining the effects of spatial-frequency masking on identification of faces to the right and left hemisphere. Preliminary evidence argues against the spatial frequency hypothesis in that we found no relation between mask frequency and visual field differences. If the results hold up it would further support the suggestion that hemispheric asymmetries emerge beyond the stage of sensory integration and that identification of complex stimuli requires commissural transmission of posticonic relational information rather than sensory features. Neurophysiological data regarding the spatial-frequency sensitivity of visual callosal neurons involved in pattern recognition would be helpful here. According to our findings, these neurons should show reduced sensitivity to spatial frequency in comparison to neurons earlier in the system.

SUMMARY AND CONCLUSIONS

The experiments reported in this paper used masking techniques to interfere with different stages of processing in the identification and recognition of lateralized words and faces. The results suggested that hemispheric asymmetries of processing first appear beyond the stage of extraction of stimulus features, either at the point at which these features are integrated into relational units or at which higher-order information is encoded from a visual icon that is represented in terms of the relational features. It was also suggested that differences in critical ISI between visual fields provides an estimate of interhemispheric transmission time of complex information that is in the range of 3–9 msec. On the basis of these results, it was inferred that the cortical commissures transmit visual information regarding either sensory features or higher-order relational or categorical features involved in forming meaningful percepts. The structural locus at which hemispheric asymmetries first occur could not be determined precisely with a high degree of confidence. Although the locus might exist at a number of areas from the extrastriate to posterior temporal cortex, it was suggested that the most likely regions was closer to the posterior temporal lobes than to earlier visual processing areas.

The paper deliberately refrained from considering the nature of inter-hemispheric transmission both of lower-level information, such as might be involved in depth perception, and of higher-level information, such as might occur when images or propositions are brought to mind. With respect to the latter examples, there is little evidence of how much of this information, or what aspect of it is transmitted interhemispherically, or even that the cortical commissures are necessary for this type of transfer to occur. Recent work from Gazzaniga and Zaidel's laboratories [Gazzaniga and LeDoux, 1978; Gazzaniga, 1983; Sidtis and Gazzaniga, 1983; Zaidel, 1983; Farah, 1984; Farah et al., 1985] makes for very tantalizing reading and holds out the hope that we can begin to answer new and more difficult questions even as we work to solve older and seemingly simpler probems.

REFERENCES

Bashore TR (1981): Vocal and manual reaction time estimates of interhemispheric transmission time. Psychol Bull 89:352–368.

Benson DF, Cummings JL, Kuhl DE (1981): Dementia: cortical-subcortical. Paper presented at the 33rd Annual Meeting of the Academy of Neurology. Toronto, Canada. Neurology 31:101 (Abstract).

Benton AL (1980): The neuropsychology of facial recognition. Am Psychol 35:176–186.

Berlin CI, McNeil MR (1976): Dichotic listening. In Lass NJ (ed.): "Contemporary Issues in Experimental Phonetics." New York: Academic Press.

Berlucchi G (1972): Anatomical and physiological aspects of visual functions of the corpus collosum. Brain Res 37:371–392.

Berlucchi G (1975): Some features of interhemispheric communication of visual information in brain damaged cats and normal humans. In Michel F, Scott B (eds): "Les Syndromes des Disconnexion Calleuse Chez l'Homme." Lyon: Colloque International de Lyon.

Berlucchi G (1981): Recent advances in the analysis of the neural substrates of interhemispheric communication. In Pomepeiano O, Marsan AC (eds): "Brain Mechanisms and Perceptual Awareness." New York: Raven Press, pp 133–152.

Berlucchi G, Crea F, DiStefano M, Tassinari G (1977): Influence of spatial stimulus-response compatibility on reaction time of ipsilateral and contralateral hand to lateralized light stimulus. J Exp Psychol [Hum Percept] 3:506–517.

Berlucchi G, Hero W, Hyman R, Rizzolatti G, Umilta C (1971): Simple reaction times of ipsilateral and contralateral hand to lateralized visual stimuli. Brain 94:419–430.

Berlucchi G, Sprague JM, Antonini A, Simoni A (1979): Learning and interhemipheric transfer of visual pattern discriminations in split chiasm cats. Exp Brain Res 34:551–574.

Bodis-Wollner I (1972): Visual acuity and contrast sensitivity in patients with cerebral lesions. Science 178:769–771.

Bodis-Wollner I (1977): Recovery from cerebral blindness: evoked potentials and psychophysical measurements. Electroencephelography and Clinical Neurophysiology 42:179–184.

Breitmeyer BG (1975): Simple reaction time as a measure of the temporal response properties of transient and sustained cells. Vision Res. 15:1411–1412.

Breitmeyer BG (1984): "Visual Masking: An Integrative Approach." New York: Oxford University Press.

Breitmeyer BG, Ganz L (1976): Implications of sustained and transient channels for theories of visual pattern masking, saccadic suppression, and information processing. Psychol Rev 83:1–36.

Broadbent DE, Broadbent MHP (1976): General shape and local detail in word perception. In Dornic S (ed): "Attention and Performance VI." Hillsdale, NJ: Erlbaum.

Byrd M, Moscovitch M (1984): Lateralization of peripherally and centrally masked words in young an elderly people. J Geront 39:699–703.

Cohen G (1976): Components of the laterality effet in letter recognition: Asymmetries in iconic storage. Q J Exp Psychol 28:105–114.

Coltheart M (1980): Deep dyslexia: A right hemisphere hypothesis. In Coltheart M, Patterson K, Marshall JC (eds): "Deep Dyslexia." London: Routledge and Kagen Paul, pp 326–380.

Craik FIM, Byrd M (1982): Aging and cognitive deficits: The role of attentional resources. In Craik FIM, Trehub S (eds.): "Aging and Cognitive Processes." New York: Plenum Press.

Crapper DR (1976): Functional consequences of neurofibrillary degeneration. In Terry RD, Gershon S (eds.): "Neurobiology of Aging." New York: Raven Press.

DeValois RL, DeValois KK (1980): Spatial vision. Annu Rev Psychol 31:309–341.

DiLollo V (1981): Hemispheric symmetry in visible persistence. Percept Psychophys 29:21–25.

DiLollo V, Moscovitch M (1983): Perceptual interference between spatially separate sequential displays. Can J Psychol 37:414–428.

Farah MJ (1984): The neurological basis of mental imagery: A componential analysis. Cognition 18:245–272.

Farah MJ, Gazzaniga MS, Holtzman JD, Kosslyn SM (1985): A left hemisphere basis for visual imagery. Neuropsychologia 23:115–118.

Friedman A, Polson MC (1982): The hemispheres as independent resource systems: Limited-capacity processing and cerebral specialization. J Exp Psychol [Hum Percept] 8:146–157.

Gazzaniga MS (1970): "The Bisected Brain." New York: Appleton-Century-Crofts.

Gazzaniga MS (1983): Right hemisphere language following brain bisection: A 20-year perspective. Am Psychol 38:525–537.

Gazzaniga MS, LeDoux JE (1978): "The Integrated Mind." New York: Plenum Press.

Gross CG, Rocha-Miranda CE, Bender DB (1972): Visual properties of neurons in inferotemporal cortex of the macaque. J Neurophysiol 35:96–111.

Guiard Y (1984): Spatial compatibility effects in the writing page: A comparison of left-handed inverters and noninverters. Acta Psychol 57:17–28.

Hamilton CR (1982): Mechanisms of interocular equivalence. In Ingle D, Goodale M, Mansfield R (eds): "Advances in the Analysis of Visual Behavior." Cambridge: MIT Press, pp 693–717.

Hellige JB (1983): Feature similarity and laterality effects in visual masking. Neuropsychologia 21:633–639.

Hellige JB, Cox PJ, Litvac L (1979): Information processing in the cerebral hemispheres: Selective hemispheric activation and capacity limitations. J Exp Psychol: Gen 108:251–279.

Hellige JG, Webster R (1979): Right hemisphere superiority for initial stages of letter processing. Neuropsychologia 17:653–660.

Jeeves MA (1969): A comparison of interhemispheric transmission times in acollosals and normals. Psychonom Sci 16:245–246.

Kahneman D (1968): Method, findings, and theory in studies of visual masking. Psychol Bull 70:404–426.

Kimura D (1961): Cerebral dominance and the perception of verbal stimuli. Can J Psychol 23:445–458.

Kimura D (1967): Functional asymmetry of the brain in dichotic listening. Cortex 3:163–178.

Kimura D, Durnford M (1974): Normal studies on the function of the right hemisphere in vision. In Dimond SJ, Beaumont JG (eds): "Hemispheric Function in the Human Brain." London: Elek Scientific Books.

Kolers PA (1968): Some psychological aspects of pattern recognition. In Kolers PA, Eden M (eds): "Recognizing Patterns." Boston: MIT Press.

Legge GE (1978): Sustained and transient mechanisms in human vision: Temporal and spatial properties. Vision Res 18:69–81.

Lennie P (1980): Parallel visual pathways: A review. Vision Res 20:561–594.

Lepore F, Guillemot JP (1982): Visual receptive field properties of cells innervated through the corpus callosum. Exp Brain Res 46:413–424.

Marcel T, Patterson K (1978): Word recognition and production: Reciprocity in clinical and normal studies. In Requim J (ed): "Attention and Performance VII." Hillsdale, NJ: Erlbaum, pp 209–226.

Martin M (1979): Hemispheric specialization for local and global processing. Neuropsychologia 17:33–40.

Marzi CA, Di Stefano M, Tassinari G, Crea F (1979): Iconic storage in the two hemispheres. J Exp Psychol: Hum Perc Perf 5:31–41.

McKeever WF, Suberi M (1974): Parallel but temporally displaced visual half field metacontrast function. Q J Exp Psychol 26:258–265.

Michaels CF, Turvey MT (1973): Hemiretinae and nonmonotoic masking functions with overlapping stimuli. Bull Psychonom Soc 2:163–164.

Michaels CF, Turvey MT (1979): Central sources of visual masking: Indexing structures supporting seeing at a single, brief glance. Psychol Res 41:1–61.

Milner AD, Lines C (1982): Interhemispheric pathways in simple reaction time to lateralized light flash. Neuropsychologia 20:171–179.

Moscovitch M (1973): Language and the cerebral: Reaction-time studies and their implication for models of cerebral dominance. In Pliner P, Alloway TA, Krames L (eds): "Communication and Affect: Language and Thought." New York: Academic Press, pp 89–126.

Moscovitch M (1976): On the representation of language in the right hemisphere of right-handed people. Brain Lang 3:47–71.

Moscovitch M (1979): Information processing and the cerebral hemispheres. In Gazzaniga MS (ed): "Handbook of Behavioral Neurobiology: Neuropsychology," Vol 2. New York: Plenum Press, pp. 379–446.

Moscovitch M (1981): Right-hemisphere language. Topics Lang Dis 1:41–61.

Moscovitch M (1983): Laterality and visual masking: Interhemispheric communication and the locus of perceptual asymmetries for words. Can J Psychol 37:85–106.

Moscovitch M (1986): Afferent and efferent models of visual perceptual asymmetry: Theoretical and empirical implications. Neuropsychologia. Volume 24.

Moscovitch M, Klein D (1980): Material-specific perceptual interference for visual words and faces: Implications for models of capacity limitations, attention, and laterality. J Exp Psychol [Hum Percept] 6:590–504.

Moscovitch M, Scullion D, Christie D (1976): Early vs late stages of processing and their relation to functional hemispheric asymmetries in face recognition. J Exp Psychol [Hum Percept] 2:401–416.

Myers RE, Sperry RW (1953): Interocular transfer of a visual form discrimination habit in cats after section of the optic chiasm and corpus callosum. Anat Rec 175:351–352.

Oscar-Berman M, Goodglass H, Cherlow (1973): Perceptual laterality and iconic recognition of visual materials by Korsakoff patients and normal adults. J Comp Physiol Psychol 82:216–231.

Pandya DN, Karol EA, Heilbronn D (1971): The topographical distribution of inter-hemispherical projections in the corpus callosum of the rhesus monkey. Brain Res 32:31–43.

Patterson K, Besner D (1984): Is the right hemisphere literate? Cognitive Neuropsychol 1:315–341.

Poffenburger AT (1912): Reaction time to retinal stimulation with special reference to the time lost in conduction through nerve centres. Arch Psychol 13:1–73.

Polich JM (1978): Hemispheric differences in stimulus identification. Percep Psychophys 24:49–57.

Proudfoot RE (1982): Hemispheric asymmetry for face recognition: Some effects of visual masking, hemiretinal stimulation and learning task. Neuropsychologia 20:129–144.

Rabinowicz B, Moscovitch M (1983): Right hemisphere literacy: A critique of some recent approaches. Cognitive Neuropsychol 1:343–350.

Regan D, Silver R, Murray TJ (1977): Visual acuity and contrast sensitivity in multiple sclerosis: hidden visual loss: an auxiliary diagnostic test. Brain 100:563–579.

Rocha-Miranda CE, Bender DB, Gross CG, Mishkin M (1975): Visual activation of neurons in inferotemporal cortex depends on striate cortex and forebrain commissures. J Neurophysiol 38:475–491.

Schenk WVD (1955): Syndrome d'Alzheimer: etude anatamoclinique de 35 cas. Folia Psychiat Neurol Neurochir 58:422–437.

Schlotterer B, Moscovitch M, Crapper-McLachlan D (1984): Visual processing deficits as assessed by spatial frequency contrast sensitivity and backward masking in normal aging and Alzheimer disease. Brain 107:309–325.

Seagraves MA, Rosenquist AC (1982a): The distributions of cells of origin of callosal connections of retinotopically defined areas in cat cortex. J Neurosci 2:1074–1089.

Seagraves MA, Rosenquist AC (1982b): The afferent and efferent callosal connections of retinotopically defined areas in cat cortex. J Neurosci 2:1090–1107.

Sergent J (1982): Theoretical and methodological consequences of variations in exposure duration in visual laterality studies. Percept Psychophys 31:451–461.

Sergent J, Bindra D (1981): Differential hemispheric processing of faces: Methodological considerations and reinterpretation. Psychol Bull 89:541–554.

Sidtis JJ, Gazzaniga MS (1983): Competence versus performance after callosal section: Looks can be deceiving. In Hellige JB (ed): "Cerebral Hemisphere Asymmetry: Method, Theory, and Application." New York: Praeger.

Sperry RW, Gazzaniga MS, Bogen JE (1969): Interhemispheric relationships: The neocortical commissures syndromes of hemispheric disconnection. In Vinken PJ, Bruyn GW (eds): "Handbook of Clinical Neurology." Amsterdam: North Holland Publishing Co., Vol 4, 1969, pp 273–290.

Studdert-Kennedy M, Schankweiler D (1970): Hemispheric specialization for speech perception. J Acoust Soc Am 48:579–594.

Tomlinson BE, Blessed GL, Roth M (1968): Observations on the brains of nondemented old people. J Neurol Sciences 7:331–356.

Tomlinson BE, Blessed GL, Roth M (1970): Observations on the brains of demented old people. J Neurol Sciences 11:205–242.

Trevarthen CB (1968): Two mechanisms of vision in primates. Psychol Forsch 31:299–337.

Turvey MT (1973): On peripheral and central processes in vision: Inferences from an information-processing analysis of masking with patterned stimuli. Psychol Rev 80:1–52.

Van Essen DC, Newsome WT, Bixby JL (1982) The pattern of interhemispheric connections and its relationship to extrastriate visual areas in the Macaque monkey. J Neurosci 2:265–283.

Walsh DA (1982): The development of visual information processes in adulthood and old age. In Craik FIM, Trehub S (eds.): "Aging and Cognitive Processes." New York: Plenum Press.

Ward TB, Ross LE (1977) Laterality differences and practice effects under central backward masking conditions. Memory Cognition 5:221–226.

Young AW (1983): "Functions of the Right Cerebral Hemisphere." New York: Academic Press.

Young AW, Ellis AW (1985): Different methods of lexical access for words presented in the left and right visual hemifields. Brain Lang 24:326–358.

Zaidel E (1983): Disconnection syndrome as a model for laterality effects in the normal brain. In Hellige JB (ed): "Cerebral Hemisphere Asymmetry." New York: Praeger.

Zimmern RL, Campbell FW, Wilkinson IMS (1979): Subtle disturbances of vision after optic neuritis elicited by studying contrast sensitivity. J Neurol Neurosurg Psychiat 42:407–412.

Two Hemispheres—One Brain:
Functions of the Corpus Callosum, pages 511–521
© 1986 Alan R. Liss, Inc.

Two Hemispheres Are Better Than One: Manual Regulation in Some Left-Handers

JERRE LEVY

Department of Behavioral Sciences, University of Chicago, Chicago, Illinois 60637

In December 1969, during my doctoral dissertation defense, the question of brain organization in left-handers was under discussion. I described the evidence from the neurological literature that indicated a great heterogeneity in cerebral asymmetry patterns among sinistrals. A majority appeared to have a left-hemisphere specialization for language; in others, the predominant language processes seemed to be right-hemisphere specialized, and in one or both groups, some fraction had at least a partial bilateral representation of linguistic functions. At this point, Roger Sperry interrupted and asked, "How do left-handers with verbal processes in the left hemisphere regulate writing with the left hand?"

Although in retrospect the question is obvious, it was one that had never occurred to me, and one that I had not seen discussed in the literature. It was typical of Sperry to ask simple, but central, questions that others had failed to consider. After some period of silence, I gave the only answers possible, namely, that this regulation either was mediated via transcallosal pathways or via the uncrossed motor tracts. "But which?" asked Sperry, "and why would such abnormal regulatory systems be used?" I was then unable to offer even the most speculative answers, but now, some 15 years later, strong clues are beginning to emerge.

THE HANDWRITING-POSTURE DIMENSION

Although people vary considerably in many aspects of handwriting posture, the vast majority of right-handers position the hand below the line of writing and orient the pen so that its tip points toward the top of the page. Indeed, in a survey of some 2,000 people, Tapley and Bryden [1983] found that over 99% had the typical noninverted posture (RN individuals), whereas less than 1% of right-handers positioned the hand above the line of writing, with the tip of the pen pointing toward the bottom of the page in the inverted posture (RI individuals).

Among left-handers, in contrast, the inverted handwriting posture is extremely common, and more frequent in male than in female sinistrals.

Table 1 displays data from four studies of North American adult left-handers whose handwriting postures were evaluated by the experimenter with respect to hand and pen position relative to the line of writing and edges of the sheet. The distributions do not differ significantly between studies [see Levy, 1984], and 77.8% of male left-handers and 48.1% of female left-handers employ the inverted posture (LI individuals). Only a minority of male sinistrals and about half of female sinistrals use the standard noninverted posture (LN individuals) that is characteristic of right-handers.

A common assumption had been that inversion of the handwriting posture was specific to left-handers and was an adaptation to the necessity to write from left to right with the left hand. Until Levy [1974] described an RI individual, there was no reason to doubt this explanation of the peculiar handwriting posture seen in so many left-handers. The peripheral explanation of inversion in left-handers, however, cannot explain its occurrence in right-handers, and the question arose as to whether handwriting posture might reflect aspects of central brain organization [Levy, 1974].

HANDWRITING POSTURE AND BRAIN ORGANIZATION

Levy and Reid [1976, 1978] pointed out that motor programs for the control of writing would vary depending on the relation of the hand and pen to the line of writing, and it seemed possible that if unusual regulatory routes for manual control were necessitated in those left-handers in whom programs for writing were specialized to the ipsilateral left hemisphere, this would be correlated with unusual hand postures during writing. They found that on a verbal tachistoscopic task, LI and RN people had a right-visual-field/left-hemisphere (RVF/LH) advantage, whereas LN people had a left-visual-field/right-hemisphere (LVF/RH) advantage. Smith and Mosco-

TABLE 1. Distributions of Handwriting Posture Among North American Adult Left-Handers, Assessed by the Experimenter for Hand Position Relative to the Line of Writing and Pen Orientation Relative to the Edges of the Sheet

	Male		Female	
Investigator	% LI[1]	Total number	% LI	Total number
Herron et al., 1979	87.5	24	54.6	22
Levy et al., 1983	75.5	49	52.2	46
McKeever, 1979	78.9	38	44.4	45
McKeever and VanDeventer, 1980	70.8	24	43.9	41
Total	77.8	135	48.1	154

[1]LI = left-handers with the inverted handwriting posture in which the hand is above the line of writing and the tip of the pen points toward the bottom of the page.

vitch [1979] confirmed these relations on a similar verbal tachistoscopic task but found no relation between handwriting posture in left-handers and ear asymmetries on a verbal dichotic-listening test. They proposed that handwriting posture in left-handers was related to the lateralization of visuo-verbal processes, but not to the lateralization of audioverbal processes.

Herron et al. [1979] reached the same conclusion based on electroen-cephalographic (EEG) asymmetries of RN, LN, and LI subjects as they performed cognitive tasks. The RN and LI subjects manifested the same asymmetries, which were opposite to those of LN subjects, for activity recorded from occipital leads, but there was no effect of hand posture on asymmetries recorded from central or parietal leads. The evident lack of relation between the lateralization of visuoverbal versus audioverbal pro-cesses in left-handers is consistent with observations of Gloning et al. [1969]. They found that speech and speech comprehension were usually lateralized to the same hemisphere in their non-right-handed neurological patients, and similarly, that reading and writing were also usually specialized to the same hemisphere. However, the lateralization of speech and speech compre-hension, on the one hand, was unpredictive of the lateralization of reading and writing, on the other [see Levy, 1982].

A number of studies have verified the lack of any relation between handwriting posture in left-handers and ear asymmetries on verbal dichotic-listening tasks [see reviews of Weber and Bradshaw, 1981; Levy, 1982]; and recently, Ajersch and Milner [1983] have shown that handwriting posture in left-handers is unrelated to the lateralization of speech. When differences in hemispheric asymmetry between LI and LN people have been found, they are confined to processes in the visual or visuomotor domains [see Levy, 1982].

In any case, the available evidence suggests that certain aspects of visuoverbal processes are left-hemisphere specialized in LI people and right-hemisphere specialized in LN people. If so, the LI population would repre-sent that subgroup of left-handers in whom the neural programs for the control of writing are ipsilateral to the writing hand. The question is whether manual regulation is achieved via transcallosal pathways or di-rectly via uncrossed motor tracts. A second question is why such people did not develop as right-handers, with direct control over the right hand by the normal crossed motor tracts.

REACTION TIME AND MANUAL REGULATION

These issues can be addressed by examining manual reaction times (RTs) to lateralized sensory signals on either the simple or go/no-go RT paradigm. As Poffenberger [1912] originally showed, and as has been verified and clarified by others [Anzola et al., 1977; Berlucchi et al., 1977], conduction time through neural centers can be detected from RT responses. If a later-alized sensory signal is presented, responses by the hand homolateral to the signal are faster by a few milliseconds than are responses by the hand heterolateral to the signal. In the first case, the same hemisphere that receives the signal controls the motor response, but in the second case, one hemisphere receives the signal, but the opposite hemisphere controls the response, necessitating a relay of information across the corpus callosum. That it is anatomical-pathway factors that generate the homolateral hand-signal advantage in speed of response is shown by the fact that the advantage favoring homolateral hand-signal combinations still appears even when the right hand responds to a button located on the left or the left hand responds to a button located on the right [Anzola et al., 1977; Berlucchi, et al., 1977]. The absence of spatial-compatibility effects is specific for the simple and go/no-go RT paradigms; on the two-choice discriminative RT paradigm, it is the compatibility of signal and response-button locations that determines speed of response, not anatomical pathways [Anzola et al., 1977].

Based on the foregoing relations, Smith and Moscovitch [1979] used the go/no-go paradigm to investigate RTs of RN, LN, and LI subjects to lateralized visual signals. They reasoned that if LI people actually rely on the uncrossed motor pathways for manual regulation, they should display a heterolateral hand-signal advantage, instead of the normal homolateral hand-signal advantage. Indeed, just such a heterolateral advantage appeared in LI subjects, contrasting with RN and LN subjects, who displayed the expected homolateral advantage. However, Moscovitch and Smith [1979] examined a new sample of subjects for go/no-go RT responses to lateralized auditory, tactile, and visual signals, and although they confirmed the anomalous heterolateral advantage in LI subjects for responses to visual signals, the LI subjects had a normal homolateral advantage for audiomotor and tactomotor responses. These latter observations ruled out the possibility that LI people have any general reliance on uncrossed motor pathways, and Moscovitch and Smith [1979] proposed that left-handers with the inverted handwriting posture suffer from some type of disorder in visuomotor integration. There was, of course, the possibility that LI people rely on the uncrossed motor pathways specifically and only in response to visual signals, but this was disconfirmed in three separate studies that used a simple RT paradigm.

McKeever and Hoff [1979] compared LN and LI subjects on a simple RT paradigm for manual responses to lateralized visual signals. The LN subjects had the expected homolateral advantage, but the LI subjects, instead of displaying a heterolateral advantage, simply showed equal response speeds for homolateral and heterolateral hand-signal combinations and differed significantly from LN subjects. Thus, the LI subjects were anomalous in failing to manifest a homolateral advantage, but the absence of a heterolateral advantage is inconsistent with a reliance on uncrossed motor pathways for visuomotor reactions. With a slightly different simple RT paradigm, McKeever and Hoff [1983] replicated their earlier results, and using still a third variation on the simple RT paradigm, Levy and Wagner [1984] confirmed the results of McKeever and Hoff [1979, 1983]. In all three simple RT studies [McKeever and Hoff, 1979, 1983; Levy and Wagner, 1984] LI subjects failed to display the homolateral hand-signal advantage in response to visual signals that was present in other subjects, and were equal in speed of responses for homolateral and heterolateral hand-signal combinations. Briefly, in five separate studies, all using RT paradigms known to be sensitive to anatomical-pathway factors, LI subjects manifested anomalous visuomotor RT patterns in their failure to demonstrate a homolateral hand-signal advantage (see Table 2), but they were also anomalous in showing a dissociation between response patterns for the go/no-go versus the simple RT paradigm. Further, Levy and Wagner [1984] showed that on their simple RT task, auditory and tactile signals elicited a general homolateral advantage that was unaffected by handedness or handwriting posture, confirming the results that Moscovitch and Smith [1979] found on their go/no-go tasks.

Both McKeever and Hoff [1983] and Levy and Wagner [1984] concurred with Moscovitch and Smith [1979] that LI individuals suffer from a disorder of visuomotor integration. But what is the nature of this disorder? How does it generate the response patterns that LI subjects display? How can it account for the heterolateral advantage of LI subjects on the go/no-go paradigm, but not on the simple RT paradigm?

TABLE 2. A Summary of Data From Five Studies on Speed of Manual Reaction Times (RTs) to Lateralized Visual Signals in Which Handwriting Posture in Left-Handers Was an Independent Variable and a Go/No-Go or Simple RT Paradigm Was Used

	Homolateral advantage in msec (frequency of Ss with homolateral advantage)		
	RN subjects	LN subjects	LI subjects
Go/no-go paradigm			
A[1]	33.0 (13/15)*	6.0 (11/15)*	−18.0 (1/15)*
B	9.3 (10/12)*	10.6 (9/12)*	−8.7 (3/12)*
Simple RT paradigm			
C	—	2.6 (10/12)*	−0.5 (8/15)
D	2.5 (?/12)*	4.2 (9/12)*	0.6 (9/18)
E	2.0 (22/32)*	2.3 (26/32)*	−0.8 (11/32)

[1]Only right-hand responses were used in this study. An asterisk indicates that the homolateral or heterolateral advantage was statistically significant. A = Smith and Moscovitch, 1979; B = Moscovitch and Smith, 1979; C = McKeever and Hoff, 1979; D = McKeever and Hoff, 1983; E = Levy and Wagner, 1984.

THE VISUOMOTOR INTEGRATIVE DISORDER OF LI PEOPLE
The Proposed Model

Figure 1 shows a schematic of possible neural systems for visuomotor integration needed for manual regulation. A functional distinction is made between visuomotor integrative pathways that are used for contralateral hand regulation versus those that are used for ipsilateral hand regulation via a transfer of information across the corpus callosum. The fact that right-handers can write with the left hand without simultaneous synkinetic movement of the right hand means that visuographic programs of the left hemisphere can be callosally relayed to the right hemisphere for left-hand control without activating the contralateral hand. Similarly, of course, when right-handers write with the right hand, they do not show synkinetic left-hand movement. It must be concluded, therefore, that left-hemisphere programs for writing become functionally separated at some point for either direct contralateral hand regulation or for transfer across the callosum for indirect ipsilateral hand regulation, and this is shown in the figure.

Levy and Wagner [1984] suggest that within-hemisphere visuomotor integration for contralateral hand regulation, specifically, is disordered in LI people, but that within-hemisphere visuomotor integration of programs to be relayed across the corpus callosum for ipsilateral hand regulation is normal. This contrasts with the idea that LI people suffer from a completely general within-hemisphere visuomotor integrative pathology [McKeever and Hoff, 1983] for manual regulation, and the more specific model is necessary in order to account for the observed findings.

Why? Milner and Lines [1982] demonstrated that manual RTs for heterolateral hand-signal combinations do not involve a callosal transfer of visual information, but rather a callosal transfer of motoric information. This means that even with heterolateral hand-signal combinations, there must be a within-hemisphere visuomotor integration prior to callosal information transfer. Were there some completely general within-hemisphere visuomotor integrative disorder in LI people, this would slow responses equally for homolateral and heterolateral hand-signal conditions, and a homolateral hand-signal advantage would still emerge.

If it is postulated that in LI people, visual and not motoric information is callosally transferred for heterolateral hand-signal conditions, a within-hemisphere visuomotor integration would still be required prior to response, but based on callosally received visual information for heterolateral conditions as contrasted with directly received visual information for homolateral conditions. In both cases, within-hemisphere visuomotor integration would be required, and any disorder of the integrative system in general would affect homolateral and heterolateral responses equally. Again, a homolateral advantage would be present in LI people. It is possible that there could be a disorder in LI people for integrating directly received visual information with a motor response, but no disorder for integrating callosally re-

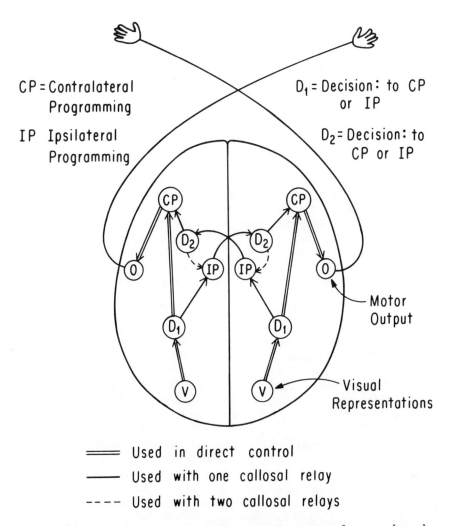

CP = Contralateral Programming

IP Ipsilateral Programming

D_1 = Decision: to CP or IP

D_2 = Decision: to CP or IP

Motor Output

Visual Representations

═══ Used in direct control

——— Used with one callosal relay

– – – – Used with two callosal relays

Fig. 1. Schematic of proposed visuomotor integrative systems for manual regulation. In left-handers with the inverted handwriting posture (LI individuals), it is hypothesized that the system D_1 to CP is disordered, but not the system D_1 to IP. Contralateral visuomotor regulation of the hand proceeds by the within-hemisphere pathways V to D_1 to CP to O and then down the crossed motor pathway to the hand. Ipsilateral visuomotor regulation of the hand proceeds by the within-hemisphere pathways from V to D_1 to IP, across the corpus callosum to D_2 of the opposite hemisphere, to CP, then O, of that hemisphere, and then down the crossed motor pathway to the hand. The dashed line from D_2 to IP is included as a possible regulatory route involving two callosal relays.

ceived visual information with a motor response, but such a model has little to motivate it. It is at variance with data of Milner and Lines [1982], and additionally, when complex tasks such as writing are considered, it is difficult to see how a callosal transfer of purely visual representations would be adequate to regulate precision movements of the hand by a hemisphere that is not specialized for such regulation.

Levy and Wagner [1984] therefore believe that the most reasonable hypothesis is that LI individuals have a specific within-hemisphere disorder of visuomotor integration for direct regulation of the contralateral hand, and normal visuomotor integrative functions for programs to be callosally relayed for ipsilateral hand regulation. Consequently, there is a relative slowing of RTs in LI subjects for homolateral conditions, which require reliance on the disordered system (unless two callosal relays are used), as compared to RTs for heterolateral conditions, where the abnormal integrative system is bypassed. But other than the evidence that motivated its formulation, what predictions follow from the idea that LI people have a disorder of within-hemisphere visuomotor integration, and how would such an integrative deficit account for the heterolateral advantage of LI subjects on the go/no-go paradigm and its absence on the simple RT paradigm?

The Integrative Deficit: A Test

The go/no-go RT paradigm is more complex than the simple RT paradigm and places a greater burden on integrative systems. This is indicated not only by the fact that RTs are longer on the go/no-go task (an average of 270 msec for visual responses in Moscovitch and Smith [1979]) than on the simple RT task (an average of 214 msec for visual responses in Levy and Wagner [1984]), but also by the fact that there is a monotonic increase in the magnitude (negative) of the correlation between RT and IQ as the number of decision processes in the RT tasks increases, up to about 4 bits [Jensen, 1982]. If LI people suffer from an integrative disruption, the effects of this would be expected to be magnified for an RT parameter that has greater sensitivity to integrative function as compared to one with lesser sensitivity. Thus, for the go/no-go task, the disordered system, used for homolateral conditions, may be less efficient than the indirect, but normal, transcallosal system, used for heterolateral conditions, generating a heterolateral advantage. On the simple RT task, the disordered and direct system may be able to achieve the same level of efficiency as the indirect transcallosal system, which is normal, resulting in equality of response speeds for homolateral and heterolateral hand-signal combinations.

If so, this predicts that any RT parameter with sufficient sensitivity to integrative function and that is also sensitive to callosal-relay effects should yield a heterolateral advantage in LI subjects for visuomotor reactions. Although speed of response on the simple RT task is uncorrelated with IQ in normal populations, trial-to-trial consistency of response on the same task, as measured by the intraindividual standard deviation (ISD), is correlated (negatively). Levy and Wagner [1984] therefore not only examined speed of reactions, but also consistency of reactions. In RN and LN people, the integrative load is higher for transcallosal (heterolateral) responses than for direct (homolateral) responses, so that consistency should be better for the latter than the former. If LI people have an integrative disorder for direct (homolateral) responses, the reverse should be true for them, and consistency should be superior for heterolateral conditions.

Precisely these results were found. The RN and LN subjects had a homolateral advantage in the ISD, of the same magnitude as their homolateral advantage for speed. In contrast, LI people had a heterolateral advantage in the ISD that was significantly larger than their nonsignificant heterolateral advantage for speed of responses to visual signals. This heterolateral advantage of the LI subjects was highly significant, since it appeared in 27 of the 32 subjects. Both speed on the go/no-go task and consistency of response on the simple RT task are sensitive to integrative function, and both yield a clear heterolateral hand-signal advantage in LI subjects for responses to visual signals. Speed of responses on the simple RT task is insensitive to integrative function, and three separate studies show that LI subjects respond equally fast for homolateral and heterolateral hand-signal combinations.

COMPLEX MANUAL REGULATION IN LI PEOPLE

It is now possible to offer Sperry at least tentative answers to his questions. Only under the artificial conditions of the RT task are people compelled to use a direct-control system (when homolateral conditions occur). Under normal circumstances, visuomotor regulation of a hand can bypass a direct-control route in favor of a transcallosal route, and one must assume that this is what occurs when right-handers write with the left hand. If, as the RT studies suggest, transcallosal regulation is more efficient in LI people than direct regulation when the integrative demand exceeds even a minimum level, it would be reasonable to suppose that visuomotor manual regulation in LI people normally is mediated via a transcallosal pathway. They develop as left-handers because a transcallosal regulation from the left hemisphere to the left hand permits superior manual control on complex tasks as compared to direct regulation of the right hand. For the LI individual, two hemispheres are better than one in guiding manual control in accordance with visual representations, and because human beings are adaptive and plastic, the child suffering from a visuomotor integrative disorder for direct regulation of the contralateral hand bypasses this disordered system in favor of a more indirect, yet more efficient, control route.

Although the ideas offered still remain speculative and require much more research to determine their validity, they appear to be correct for at least one LI individual in the world. Gur et al [1982] described an LI callosotomy patient in whom all language functions were specialized to the left hemisphere. Following callosotomy, he became completely agraphic with the left hand, and in the several years since surgery, had been unable to regain left-hand writing . He has, however, now learned to use the right hand for writing, showing that the direct control system had always been available for use, but had been bypassed, presurgically, in favor of transcallosal regulation of the left hand. The use of the transcallosal pathway prior to callosotomy would be difficult to explain unless it were more efficient than the direct-control system that this patient is compelled to use postsurgically.

CONCLUSIONS

I apologize to Sperry for waiting 15 years before offering possible answers to his questions, but until he asked them, the issues had never been given serious consideration. No doubt, Sperry will now ask me, But what is the precise neurological pathology of visuomotor integration? How did it develop? What is its cause? And why, in any case, should a transcallosal regulation of writing produce inversion of the hand posture? I am as unable to answer these new questions now as I was when confronted with the older ones many years ago, and must simply hope that Sperry will be as generous with his patience in the future as he has been in the past.

ACKNOWLEDGMENTS

The support of the Public Health Service (DHEW RO1 HD 13010) and of the Spencer Foundation is gratefully acknowledged. Appreciation is expressed to volunteers in the experiments, who gave their informed, signed consent.

REFERENCES

Ajersch MK, Milner B (1983): Handwriting posture as related to cerebral lateralization, sex, and writing hand. Hum Neurobiol 2:143–145.
Anzola GP, Bertoloni G, Buchtel HA, Rizzolatti G (1977): Spatial compatibility and anatomical factors in simple and choice reaction time. Neuropsychologia 15:295–302.
Berlucchi G, Crea F, Di Stefano M, Tassinari G (1977): Influence of spatial stimulus-response compatibility on reaction time of ipsilateral and contralateral hand to lateralized light stimuli. J Exp Psychol [Hum Percept] 3:505–517.
Gloning I, Gloning K, Haub G, Quatember R (1969): Comparison of verbal behavior in right-handed and non-right-handed patients with anatomically verified lesion of one hemisphere. Cortex 5:43–52.
Gur RE, Sussman NM, O'Connor M, Vey MM, Gur RC (1982): The effects of corpus callosotomy on writing in a left-hander with left hemisphere language. Neurology 12:A–188.
Herron J, Galin D, Johnstone J, Ornstein RE (1979): Cerebral specialization, writing posture, and motor control of writing in left-handers. Science 205:1285–1289.

Jensen A (1982): Reaction time and psychometric g. In Eysenck HJ (ed): "A Model for Intelligence." New York: Springer, pp 93–132.

Levy J (1974): Psychobiological implication of bilateral asymmetry. In Dimond SJ, Beaumont JG (eds): "Hemisphere Function in the Human Brain." New York: John Wiley & Sons, pp 121–183.

Levy J (1982): Handwriting posture and cerebral organization: How are they related? Psychol Bull 91:589–608.

Levy J (1984): A review, analysis, and some new data on hand-posture distributions in left-handers. Brain Cognition 3:105–127.

Levy J, Heller W, Banich M, Burton L (1983): Asymmetry of perception in free viewing of chimeric faces. Brain Cognition 2:404–419.

Levy J, Reid M (1976): Variations in writing posture and cerebral organization. Science 194:337–339.

Levy J, Reid M (1978): Variations in cerebral organization as a function of handedness, hand posture in writing, and sex. J Exp Psychol: [Gen] 107:119–144.

Levy J, Wagner N (1984): Handwriting posture, visuomotor integration, and lateralized reaction-time parameters. Hum Neurobiol 3:157–161.

McKeever WF (1979): Handwriting posture in left-handers: Sex, familial sinistrality and language laterality correlates. Neuropsychologia 5:429–44.

McKeever WF, Hoff AL (1979): Evidence of a possible isolation of left hemisphere visual and motor areas in sinstrals employing an inverted handwriting posture. Neuropsychologia 17:445–454.

McKeever WF, Hoff AL (1983): Further evidence of the absence of measurable interhemispheric transfer time in left-handers who employ an inverted handwriting posture. Bull Psychonom Soc 21:255–258.

McKeever WF, VanDeventer AD (1980): Inverted handwriting position, language laterality, and the Levy-Nagylaki genetic model of handedness and cerebral organization. Neuropsychologia 18:99–102.

Milner AD, Lines CR (1982): Interhemispheric pathways in the simple reaction time to lateralized light flash. Neuropsychologia 20:171–179.

Moscovitch M, Smith LC (1979): Differences in neural organization between individuals with inverted and non-inverted hand posture during writing. Science 205:710–713.

Poffenberger AT (1912): Reaction time to retinal stimulation with special reference to the time lost in conduction through nervous centers. Arch Psychol 23:1–73.

Smith LC, Moscovitch M (1979): Writing posture, hemispheric control of movement and cerebral dominance in individuals with inverted and noninverted hand postures during writing. Neuropsychologia 17:637–644.

Tapley SM, Bryden MP (1983): Handwriting position and hemispheric asymmetry in right-handers. Neuropsychologia 21:129–138.

Weber AM, Bradshaw JL (1981): Levy and Reid's neurological model in relation to writing hand/posture: An evaluation. Psychol Bull 90:74–88.

Two Hemispheres—One Brain:
Functions of the Corpus Callosum, pages 523–540
© 1986 Alan R. Liss, Inc.

The Role of Cortico-Cortical Connections

KARL H. PRIBRAM

Departments of Psychology and Psychiatry and Behavioral Sciences, Stanford University, Palo Alto, California 94305

THE PROBLEM

At the end of a conference such as this, in which the flow of data was almost inundating, it would be foolish to try to "summarize" the reports. What I wish to do instead is to address a problem central to all of the reports: How do the cerebral commissures in particular, and cortico-cortical connections in general, function? In order to discuss this problem I will focus on two presentations: briefly on that of Maryse Lassonde, and at greater length, the one by Mortimer Mishkin.

First, a few words about Lassonde's beautiful presentation, which made a most convincing case for the proposition that the corpus callosum functions as an excitatory and not as an inhibitory pathway. This proposition received ample support from several of the other presentations given over the following days. However, I wish to point out that excitation may well function to produce inhibition, as shown by Lassonde's own data, which constituted her doctoral thesis [1977]. She performed an experiment in which she investigated the effects of electrical stimulation of the basal ganglia and cerebral cortex on the organization of receptive fields of single neurons in the primary visual cortex. She found, among other results, that contralateral cortical stimulation, irrespective of location (frontal or posterior), decreased the size of the receptive field. No direct test was made as to whether the effect of stimulation was mediated by the corpus callosum. Nonetheless, there was no callosal excitation evident as an end result in these experiments.

I mention this because I believe that statements regarding the inhibitory or excitatory functions of the commissures and cortico-cortical connections in general need to be qualified. There may be in fact an overall inhibitory or excitatory effect of commissural or other cortico-cortical activity. Often, however, as in the Lassonde physiological experiments, excitation leads to inhibition at the microneurological (receptive field, dendritic) level as an end result. The effects on behavior and on perception of such changes would not appear simply as inhibition or excitation, but as changes in *patterns* of processing. It is the organization of these processing patterns that I next want to discuss.

DISCONNECTION SYNDROMES IN MONKEYS

Within the framework of this conference, the theme of my presentation may seem misplaced: I will focus on some intrahemispheric connections as well as on the interhemispheric. In part, this is because my expertise lies in the distinctions in functions between the frontal and posterior cortex, and the relationship between the frontal cortex and the limbic forebrain. At the same time, I am no stranger to studies using callosotomy to solve specific problems—although my name has not appeared on these studies, since they were performed primarily by graduate and postdoctoral students in the laboratory. Some have not been published. The first of the experiments was reported by Ettlinger [1959b]. Mishkin and I helped design the experiment and carried out the surgery. It is this line of research that Mishkin has pursued in the work reported here.

Another use made in the laboratory of the "split-brain" preparation has been to ascertain whether the effects of amygdalectomy are more related to the processing of sensory input or to a defective response mechanism [Minturn, 1952; Barrett, 1969]. The results were in accord with the theme of this conference: When using the amygdalectomized hemisphere, the monkeys failed to utilize information gained by using the other, normal hemisphere, but were able to learn visual discriminations normally. Thus the effect of amygdalectomy (e.g., taming, oral behavior) was inferred to influence a *pre*decisional or relatively independent (parallel) stage of visual processing. This result, as will become evident below, runs counter to Mishkin's proposal for the serial operation of a striate → prestriate → temporal cortex → amygdala circuit.

In still another set of experiments with callosectomized monkeys [Reitz-Blehert, 1968] additional difficult-to-explain findings resulted that make worthwhile a reevaluation of the entire program of experiments so ably performed and described here and elsewhere by Mishkin. So please bear with me while I delve into the problems raised by disconnection syndromes, those produced by severing intrahemispheric cortico-cortical tracts as well as interhemispheric commissures.

ALTERNATIVE MODELS OF HIERARCHICAL PROCESSING SYSTEMS

Mishkin has presented a carefully documented brain model of visual processing, pointing out not only the evidence in support of his model but also points where the model runs into some difficulty. I now want to make a case for an alternative that had its inception one evening more than 30 years ago when Mishkin, Lashley and I were discussing how the sensory mode specificity of the inferotemporal (and in fact much of the posterior intrinsic "association") cortex of monkeys comes about. We had discovered these sensory mode-specific functions some years earlier [Blum et al., 1950; Pribram and Bagshaw, 1953; Mishkin and Pribram, 1954; Pribram, 1954, 1958a,b; Pribram and Barry, 1956; Dewson et al., 1969] and Evarts [1952] had made extensive removals of the prestriate cortex with no lasting effect on visual discrimination learning and performance, such as that which follows resections of the inferotemporal cortex. There is no known direct input to the inferotemporal cortex from the primary visual cortex or from the lateral geniculate nucleus of the thalamus, so how does the inferotemporal cortex receive the visual information necessary to allow the monkey to make visual discriminations when the indirect paths through the prestriate cortex have been removed?

I suggested that perhaps visual input was not the critical factor in visual discrimination learning and performance; that instead, it was the output from the inferotemporal cortex to the visual system that is critical. Neither Lashley nor Mishkin thought much of the suggestion, dismissing the issue as being the result of incomplete removal of prestriate tissue. Thus the model that Mishkin presented here is a result of many years of effort to trace visual input to the inferotemporal cortex. Meanwhile, I pursued the possibility that the visual specificity of the inferotemporal cortex could be due to its output rather than to its input characteristics.

Some Evidence

First I had to establish the fact that more complete resections of the prestriate cortex would still leave the monkeys able to perform the visual discrimination tasks. Several experiments accomplished this [Pribram et al., 1969; Ungerleider et al., 1977; Cardu et al., in preparation]. All of these monkeys were able to perform visual discriminations, most without deficit despite deep cuts into the optic radiations that course just below the prestriate cortex, cuts that resulted in considerable degeneration of the lateral geniculate nucleus with resulting scotomata and often long periods of postoperative blindness. The important consideration has been to delay postoperative testing until the effects of geniculostriate damage has been overcome. Sometimes this takes as long as 6 months, during which the monkeys are trained to respond to peanuts suspended by a thread and dangled within the remaining functional visual field. If this is done, performance on formal tests has shown surprisingly little if any effect of the lesion (except as noted below, in size constancy).

There was still the possibility of an indirect visual input from the lateral geniculate nucleus to the pulvinar and then to the inferotemporal cortex. This possibility was ruled out by Mishkin [1973], who made large pulvinar lesions in some 27 monkeys and found no effect on visual discrimination behavior. (More recently Lindsley [1984] has found such effects but only when the cues are presented tachistoscopically.) Charles Gross [1973] pointed out that the possibility still remained that either the direct cortical or the indirect thalamic route could function in the absence of the other. This last alternative was also ruled out in a study in which both extensive prestriate and pulvinar lesions were made without impairing visual discrimination performance [Ungerleider et al., 1977].

Next, the possibility that there were in fact corticofugal pathways from the inferotemporal cortex to the visual system had to be explored. Tracts ending in the lateral geniculate nucleus would have solved our problem, but silver stains failed to show any input from the inferotemporal cortex to thalamus except to the pulvinar, from which the corticopetal fibers to the inferotemporal cortex arise. Instead, the deeper layers of the superior colliculus and the pretectal region turned out to be the prime corticofugal targets [Whitlock and Nauta, 1956].

More surprising was a heavy projection from the inferotemporal cortex to the putamen, which was demonstrated both by anatomical and electrophysiological techniques [Reitz and Pribram, 1969; Pribram, unpublished]. How these connections influence the visual system remains to be determined, but I have some preliminary evidence that the pathway—putamen to globus pallidus to reticular nucleus to the thalamus—might be critical. What is known is that cross-hatching of the inferotemporal cortex results in no deficit in visual discrimination learning or performance, while undercutting this cortex or making lesions in the neighborhood of the tail of the caudate nucleus and putamen do [Pribram et al., 1966; Buerger et al., 1974].

A Cortico-Subcortical Hierarchy

Despite these differences, there are many similarities between the models that Mishkin and I have developed. In an invited address at the Eastern Psychological Association Meetings in 1954, I pointed out that the sensorimotor systems must be hierarchically organized in the sense that resections of each succeeding processing stage leave more and more of the sensory-guided behavior intact. This was not a novel idea. Henry Head and Carl von Monikov, among others, had made the point previously, and Alexander Romanovitch Luria has emphasized it more recently. In my own writing, the idea was central in "The Intrinsic Systems of the Forebrain," my contribution to the *Handbook of Physiology* [1960].

This contribution also made the point about which Mishkin and I are at odds. The subtitle to that chapter was "An Alternative to the Transcortical Reflex," but unfortunately the editors decided to delete it, perhaps for the same reason that Lashley and Mishkin felt uncomfortable with the proposal. Let me therefore once again describe the data that make me challenge the transcortical model, with which, by the way, I would also feel most comfortable were there not so much evidence against it.

The hierarchical model is based on the fact that excision of the eyes leaves the organism totally blind, while after resections of the primary visual cortex there remains considerable residual vision [see Weiskrantz and Cowey, 1970; Weiskrantz et al. 1974]. And as has been pointed out, resection of the prestriate cortex leaves the monkey still more intact. However, this does not mean that no visual deficit occurs: size constancy is impaired; the monkeys respond to retinal image size, ignoring the cues that ordinarily relate size to distance [Ungerleider et al., 1977].

Inferotemporal resections also leave the organism with considerable visual skills. As Mishkin pointed out, the relation of the visual system to space is carried out cortically in proximity to the somatosensory systems in the parietal lobe [Pribram and Barry, 1956; Wegener, 1968; Wilson, 1975; Mountcastle et al., 1975]. Only visual form (and color) discrimination is impaired after bilateral resection of the inferior portion of the temporal lobe [Blum et al., 1950; Chow, 1951; Mishkin and Pribram, 1954]. This deficit is proportional to the difficulty of the task: easy discriminations such as color and three-dimensional objects are discriminated, albeit always with some deficit in the number of learning or retention trials when compared with control performance.

In natural settings the discrimination deficit is hard to observe. Monkeys with inferotemporal lesions will track moving objects such as gnats and appear to respond normally to food, their conspecifics, and to foreign intrusions [Reynolds and Pribram, unpublished observations]. Even in the laboratory, when choice is not involved, the monkeys can track changes in luminance [Ettlinger, 1959a].

Sensory-Mode-Specific Regions Within the Posterior Cortical Convexity

The deficit in visually guided behavior following resections of the inferotemporal cortex becomes manifest whenever choices among stimuli that have a consistent reinforcement history are required. This deficit is restricted to the visual modality; resections of other portions of the parietotemporal-preoccipital convexity impair somatosensory, gustatory, and auditory discriminations [Blum et al., 1950; Bagshaw and Pribram, 1953; Pribram and Bagshaw, 1953; Pribram and Barry, 1956; Dewson et al., 1969]. Within the visual mode, the deficit depends on a variety of factors. Some are sensory, e.g., size or luminance [Mishkin and Hall, 1955]. Other factors are situational, however, and have little to do with visual sensory input per se. As an example, a monkey can show excellent discrimination between an ashtray and a tobacco tin when these are presented simultaneously. When, however, the same cues are presented successively and it has to make differential responses in the absence of the second cue, it fails miserably. The monkey shows that it is able to tell the difference between the two cues (in the simultaneous situation) but that it is unable to apply this ability to the somewhat harder successive task [Pribram and Mishkin, 1955].

The Non-Sensory Aspect of Modal Specificity

The finding that the visual impairment following inferotemporal resections is not always related to visual sensory factors, per se, alerts us to the possibility that the essence of the deficit may lie elsewhere than in visual input. On the other hand, the fact that visual generalization gradients are flattened [Butter et al., 1965], that the monkeys with such lesions process fewer features of the cues to be discriminated [Butter, 1968], or fewer of the cues of a set that needs to be discriminated [Pribram, 1960], indicates that whatever the impairment might be it impinges critically on the visual process.

Mishkin has handled this dilemma by subdividing the inferotemporal cortex into posterior and anterior parts, and has shown that the more posterior resections result in sensory-perceptual difficulties, while anterior lesions interfere with the memory-based performance aspects of these tasks [Iwai and Mishkin, 1968, 1969]. Furthermore, he has made a good case that the anterior lesions produce their effects because the pathways to such limbic structures as the amygdala and hippocampus are destroyed [Mishkin, 1982]. This recourse to hierarchy flows naturally from the earlier, less-refined conceptualizations.

The Limbic Connection: Some Problems

Though attractive and perhaps partially correct, Mishkin's formulation runs into severe difficulties. If, indeed, visual learning and performance are dependent on amygdala and hippocampal function, then resections of the medial temporal region (i.e., of the amygdala and hippocampus) should result in deficits when such tasks are given. This is not the case. Mishkin and I showed, in our early work together, that visual discrimination performance remains intact after such resections and that original learning of a visual discrimination is only slightly affected [Mishkin and Pribram, 1954; Pribram and Mishkin, unpublished results]. More recently, Mishkin has shown that a deficit in recognition tasks can be produced by medial temporal resections [Mishkin, 1982]. But these tasks employ trial-unique stimuli, which change them into one-trial learning tasks, more akin to delayed alternation and delayed response than to the discrimination tasks affected by inferotemporal lesions [Jacobsen and Nissen, 1937; Nissen, 1951]. And one-trial learning tasks are well known to be affected by medial temporal and other frontolimbic lesions [Pribram et al., 1952; Mishkin and Pribram, 1954; Pribram et al., 1962].

A word about such one-trial recognition tasks. They are highly sensitive to distractors, especially spatial distractors and to those which produce retroactive and proactive interference. Malmo [1942], Pribram [1961], Douglas and Pribram [1969], Grueninger and Pribram [1969], and Anderson et al. [1976] have presented a considerable body of evidence to this point. While resections of various frontolimbic formations make monkeys more sensitive to such changing cue presentations, performance after inferotemporal lesions is actually enhanced by changing presentations [Brody et al., 1977].

These facts do not detract from the importance of the finding that medial temporal lobe resections interfere with the performance of recognition tasks presented in this fashion [Gaffan, 1974; Mishkin, 1982]. The results of such experiments on monkeys have gone a considerable way to relating the work with nonhuman primates to that on humans with such lesions in whom Milner [1958] has described a particular memory deficit restricted to recall of events which have occurred since surgery, but which does not involve immediate short-term memory. However, once again I would emphasize the fact that short-term memory is intact in these patients until distraction intervenes, at which point interference disrupts the coding necessary to proper retrieval [Weiskrantz and Warrington, 1975]. Susceptibility to interference rather than recognition, per se, characterizes the medial temporal lobe deficit, since events that occurred preoperatively are readily recognized, and furthermore, perceptual and motor skills are readily mastered postoperatively. Thus, if one applies a behavioral, instrumental indicator, task recognition remains intact.

The Basal Ganglia

Mishkin [Mishkin et al., 1984; Mishkin and Petri, 1984] in two recent reviews handles the sparing of visual discrimination performance following medial temporal resection by a proposal that there are at least two different processes leading to retention in memory. As is pointed out in the reviews, similar proposals have also been made by Hirsh [1969], Gaffan [1974], Kinsbourne and Wood [1975], Huppert and Piercy [1976], O'Keefe and Nadel [1978], Cutting [1978], Olton et al. [1979], Wickelgren [1979], Cohen and Squire [1980], Cormier [1981], Stern [1981], Hirst [1982], Warrington and Weiskrantz [1982], and Graf et al. [1982].

Further, Mishkin suggests that the incentive form of retention necessary to trial-unique learning is mediated limbically, while choices among stimuli with consistent reinforcement histories depend on the integrity of the basal ganglia. These proposals are consistent with those that I and my laboratory colleagues, including Mishkin, have put forward over the past 30 years [Pribram, 1954, 1958a; Kimble and Pribram, 1963; Douglas and Pribram, 1966; Douglas, 1966; Hirsh, 1969; Kimble, 1969; Pribram, 1969; Pribram, 1977; Pribram, 1984]. For instance, evidence for the idea that the limbic formations are involved in learning based on incentive is presented in Douglas and Pribram [1966] (though the term "impellence" rather than "incentive" was used). As noted by Mishkin, he adopted Hirsh's nomenclature, which he developed in his Stanford doctoral thesis. In a paper entitled "The Amnestic Syndromes," the distinction between two types by retention was made by Pribram in a contribution to a volume by Talland and Waugh

[1969]. The importance of the basal ganglia to the functions of inferotem-poral cortex was delineated in an address entitled "New Dimensions in the Function of the Basal Ganglia" [Pribram, 1977]. The difficulty with Mish-kin's otherwise superbly illuminating formulation comes when the trial-unique type of process is identified with "recognition." In neurology and ordinary discourse, the term "recognition" is used to denote what in psy-chology is called "identification." In psychology, the term "recognition" is used to denote what in ordinary discourse and neurology is called "familiar-ity." Furthermore, for me, the distinction made by Tulving [e.g., Tulving and Donaldson, 1972] of episodic vs. semantic processing, or that of Olton [e.g., Olton et al., 1979], which teases apart the processes of working from reference memory, are more cogent. [But this is a matter of terminology, not of substance. These findings and their immediate interpretation seems securely established.]

A CORTICO-SUBCORTICAL, SENSORIMOTOR RECIPROCITY MODEL

The outlines of an alternative to the transcortical model are as follows: image processing and the perception of objects are sharply distinguished, and these in turn are differentiated from categorizing. Image, object, and category stand in hierarchical relationship to one another. The hierarchy is characterized by a progressive loss of detail in the patterns being processed. Thus, the model is, in a nontrivial sense, the reverse of the "initial sketch pad" theory proposed by David Marr [1982] and his MIT colleagues, [Marr et al., 1978]. However, the model is consonant with the psychophysical observations of S.S. Stevens [1951] and the neurophysiological proposals made by Horace Barlow [1961].

Image processing is a function of the primary retinogeniculostriate sys-tem. By contrast, object perception depends on interactions between the geniculostriate system and a set of visual motor mechanisms located in the prestriate-superior collicular connectivity. Categorizing is a function of op-erations of an inferotemporal-pretectal system, as it influences geniculostri-ate and/or prestriate-collicular activity. In this model, therefore, the operations that lead to both object perception and categorizing are prepro-cessing the input so that image, object, and category are simultaneously perceived.

The mechanisms of retinal, geniculostriate, and prestriate processing have been detailed in three other manuscripts by Pribram and Carlton [Carlton, 1985; Pribram and Carlton, 1985a,b]. Essentially, the first of these papers presents evidence for the formation of a retinal space-time image by the pupil-lens system, which performs a Fourier transform on the distrib-uted incident spectrum of electromagnetic energy. The second paper ad-dresses the functional microstructure of the striate cortex. While the gross overall organization of receptive fields reflects the topology of the space-time image of the retina, the output of each single neuron responds to the

Gabor transform of its receptive field. The Gabor transform is a Fourier transform that is essentially limited by a Gaussian envelope. Thus the distributed pattern which, were it produced by a Fourier transform, would reach infinity, becomes restricted to the boundaries of the dendritic receptive field of the neuron, most likely by way of lateral inhibition. Distributed processing has the advantage that correlations are readily achieved.

Correlations become the critical operation to achieve object constancy. These correlations are formed when eye movements scan an object to establish a center of symmetry from which the Fourier descriptors (the outlines) of the object can be computed. Input from the striate to the prestriate cortex becomes segregated to some extent according to features (e.g., color, shape) and figure-ground relations are enhanced by the stopped (hypercomplex) and opponens (and double opponens) nature of the receptive fields, which reflects an increase in the amount of lateral inhibition. Feature segregation aids in establishing centers of symmetry, which serve as foci for the eye movement patterns, which are organized by the pathways from the prestriate cortex to the superior colliculus. The correlations that are computed on the basis of the scan of the object then form a local context that is imposed on the striate cortex, and therefore on image processing, by collicular-striate connections.

The Inferotemporal System

According to this model, the functions of the inferotemporal system are another step in abstraction that segregates portions of the image from one another. However, the rules of operation of segregation are different from those that function in object perception. Categories are established on the basis of generalization gradients that differentiate among inputs. Butter et al. [1965] have shown that generalization gradients are dramatically flattened after bilateral resections of the inferotemporal cortex, and Martha Wilson [1975] has presented evidence that such resections interfere with categorizing. She proposes that the impairment is due to an interference with the formation of separate adaptation levels to each of the features or objects to be segregated. Roger Shepard (personal communication) is developing a multidimensional scaling approach that takes into account both adaptation level and generalization. Shepard distinguishes between dimensions of an image that are "integral" and those which are "separable." I have suggested that the rules for combining integral dimensions are those that lead to object perception, while the rules governing separability are those that lead to categorizing [Pribram, 1985].

The quantitative mathematical operations involved in categorizing will be detailed in another manuscript [Pribram and Carlton, in preparation]. Here, I want to address the neuroanatomical and neurophysiological evidence that makes the model plausible. I have already described the evidence for an inferotemporal cortico-collicular (and pretectal) pathway that could be responsible for the operation of segregation of image dimensions. In this instance, eye movements cannot have a role since electrical stimulation of the inferotemporal cortex does not result in eye movements. What must be occurring instead is a succession of computations of relationships among large portions of the visual field that are at any moment processed in parallel. In a sense, these momentary image patterns occurring in the striate cortex are put on temporary hold to operate as linear spatial filters which can be superimposed on one another. Much as IBM punch cards or the averaging techniques used in recording event-related electrical brain activity, successive superpositions allow commonalities among patterns to be enhanced, while irrelevancies (noise) are suppressed. Averaging is therefore one technique (perhaps the simplest) that can result in the production of adaptation levels. When more than one peak appears in the pattern, more than one generalization gradient, the several peaks become progressively more differentiated as more and more samples are processed.

Electrical stimulation of the inferotemporal cortex alters the receptive field properties recorded from neurons in the lateral geniculate nucleus and in the striate cortex: surround is enhanced with respect to center and effective receptive field size is diminished [Spinelli and Pribram, 1967; Lassonde et al., 1981]. These results can be interpreted to mean that the striate cortical microstructure has taken on a finer grain which allows sharper differentiation among the separable dimensions of the filter, the processing pattern. At the same time, the portion of the visual field being processed is relatively large: receptive fields recorded from the inferotemporal cortex are large and often extend across the midline [Gross, 1973].

Limitations of the Model

The weakness of the model as developed thus far lies in the fact that it does not account for the presence of visual receptive fields in the inferotemporal cortex; the fact that these fields are primarily visual, dependent on the integrity of the geniculostriate system and the forebrain commissural connections [Rocha-Miranda et al., 1975; Gross et al., 1977]; and the fact that in many cases neurons in the temporal cortex respond best to objects or other specific integral types of stimulation. These are the very data that support Mishkin's theory of the transcortical basis for hierarchy. The model under consideration must therefore take these data into account.

The receptive field properties of neurons are prime indicators of function. When that function is shown to be sensory-mode specific, it is reasonable to assume a fairly direct input from that particular sense. The transcortical connectivity to the inferotemporal cortex from the striate cortex involves at least two neurons—one to area 18 and another from area 18 to 19—before the final step from area 19 to 37 is completed. Even if one of these steps can be skipped, as perhaps is the case from the portions of the striate cortex that receive the most peripheral retinal projections [Ungerleider and Mishkin, 1982], the route remains an indirect one. In fact, one could trace an input to the inferotemporal cortex from the primary auditory cortex [see Pribram and MacLean, 1953; Dewson et al., 1969], the primary taste cortex [see Bagshaw and Pribram, 1953], and even the primary somatosensory cortex (see e.g., a pathway via area 7, Mountcastle et al. [1975]) in as few steps as those taken by the visual transcortical mechanism. Were the path from the peripheral retinal projection via the cortex on the medial surface of the monkey occipital lobe truly important, as Mishkin claims, this path would most likely feed into the cortical machinery involved in locating an object in space (the parietal cortex) and not the machinery involved in form and color discrimination.

Where, then, might a more direct input to the inferotemporal cortex originate? The short answer to this question is that I don't know. However, there are some leads that can be obtained from Gross et al.'s [1977] demonstrations of the dependency of the visual receptive field properties of the inferotemporal neurons on the integrity of the ipsilateral striate cortex and the forebrain commissures. They found that the latencies of response to visual stimuli were in the region of some 100 to 120 msec. (Striate cortex neurons respond at about 80 msec.) Resections of the occipital cortex and/or sections of the commissures were performed, and the monkeys were allowed a few weeks to recover. After unilateral occipital removal, inferotemporal units in both hemispheres responded only to stimuli in the hemifield contralateral to the intact striate cortex. After section of the corpus callosum and anterior commissures, inferotemporal units in both hemispheres responded only to stimuli in the hemifield contralateral to the recording site.

Some years back, I obtained some interesting results that may have a bearing on this issue. Using evoked potential techniques, experiments were carried out to determine the input to supplementary auditory cortical areas. In chronic experiments of the type used by Gross et al. [1969], I found that the input to the supplementary areas had disappeared. However, I obtained rather different results when I performed the experiments immediately after resection of the primary auditory cortex: potentials were evoked by auditory stimuli with only slight attenuation of amplitude. My conclusion was that in the chronic experiments, sufficient time had elapsed to allow degeneration of the medial geniculate input, and that the evoked potentials recorded from the supplementary auditory areas were dependent on the integrity of collaterals from the medial geniculate nucleus to these areas [Pribram et al., 1954].

It is possible that such collaterals also exist in the visual system and that some of them innervate the inferotemporal cortex. There is sufficient time for degeneration of the lateral geniculate to have occurred in Gross's and Mishkin's experiments [Chow and Dewson, 1966]. In the cat, all of what is now commonly called area 18 is innervated by the major projection of the lateral geniculate nucleus. This is not the case in the monkey, but the existence of collaterals has not been ruled out. Should they exist, they might well reach as far forward as the inferotemporal cortex.

An alternative route for a lateral geniculate input to the inferotemporal cortex would be via the pulvinar. The existence of massive geniculopulvinar connections is well established [Mehler, 1966], as is the existence of reciprocal connections between the inferior pulvinar and the inferotemporal cortex. Even this pathway is more direct than any known transcortical route.

But what, then, of the effects of section of the forebrain commissures? The role of the splenium of the corpus callosum in connecting the occipital cortices is well documented. Thus, the obtained effects of splenial section strengthens Mishkin's argument considerably. But this sectioning of the corpus callosum accounted for only half of the diminution of visual activation of inferotemporal neurons. What about the other half, which depends on the integrity of the anterior commissure? Are there fibers originating in the striate or prestriate cortex in the anterior commissure? I do not know of any. My guess, and at this time it is only a guess, is that the basal ganglia are involved, i.e., that a cortico-subcortical connection is important.

To summarize this section of my discussion: the hierarchical aspects of visual processing can be as readily attributed to systems of cortico-subcortical loops as to the operations of a transcortical mechanism. There is an abundance of evidence that cannot be easily subsumed under the transcortical theory. This evidence can be accommodated by reliance on a cortico-subcortical mechanism.

The Callosal Experiments

Within the framework of a cortico-subcortical hierarchical visual mechanism, what becomes of the results of the various elegant experiments detailed to us by Mishkin? He himself has pointed out some of the puzzling data that have emerged from his studies—but there is one fact that Mishkin rarely mentions. After all the extensive prestriate and inferotemporal resections and callosectomies, and chiasm and visual tract sections made in various combinations of laterality and order, the fact remains that many of these monkeys, after some prolonged period of difficulty, are able to perform the visual discriminations.

All of the transcortical pathways, and even much of the cortex that we have been discussing, are not *essential* to the performance of visual discriminations! In our published and unpublished experiments [Minturn, 1952; Ettlinger, 1959b; and especially Reitz-Blehert, 1968], we found this to be the case and Mishkin, in his review article [1966], notes in his second-to-last paragraph that parietal cortex (which Mishkin has relegated to spatial rather than to object vision) as well as prestriate must be removed in order for the deficit to appear.

Further, in our experiments we wondered if the recovery of function might be due to the prolonged period of testing, and that prolonged visual experience might in fact make the inferotemporal cortex inessential to the performance of the visual discrimination task. And we found just that. However, prolonged periods of testing, even with monkeys where resections in each hemisphere are performed in stages, ordinarily fail to impair the task when the resections become sufficiently extensive [Mishkin and Pribram, unpublished results]. We were therefore very surprised when our monkeys with huge bilateral prestriate and inferotemporal resections, unilateral optic tract and midline anterior commissure sections, *and* callostomy, performed readily and practically without deficit on visual pattern discriminations!

Our results immediately reminded us of James Sprague's [1966] fascinating experiments in which he was able to restore vision in a cortically produced hemianopic field by additional resection of the ipsilateral superior colliculus. As Hughlings Jackson had pointed out [1873], the several brain systems appear to be in balance and lesions often produce their effects by disturbing that balance. Sprague's remarkable experiments demonstrate that cortical-subcortical systems provide such a balance. Can this balance be restored as well by a procedure in which extensive visual training is provided between resections and transections which are performed in stages? It seems so.

The observations of Weiskrantz and Warrington [1975], and Warrington and Weiskrantz [1982] on blindsight in patients following unilateral occipital lobectomy also attest to the fact that a great deal of visual pattern processing occurs subcortically. The contribution of the cortex, per se, to each stage in the hierarchy of visual processes remains to be determined. Cytoarchitectural and receptive field considerations suggest that the cortex adds finer grain to whatever the subcortical mechanism is processing. The clinical observations suggest that, in addition to grain, reflective awareness of the resultants of the process depends on the integrity of the cortex.

My conclusion regarding the results of callosectomy in monkeys is therefore somewhat tangent to the interests of this conference. I am emphasizing the role of a hierarchy of precortical visual mechanisms (geniculate, collicular, pretectal) and suggesting that each of these mechanisms has a cortical component that improves grain and makes reflective awareness possible. It is, of course, the findings by Sperry, Bogen, Gazzaniga, Levy (see Levy, this volume) and their colleagues, of the role of the corpus callosum in reflective awareness that have proved so exciting. On this note I end my discussion.

REFERENCES

Anderson RM, Hunt SC, Vander Stoep A, Pribram KH (1976): Object permanency and delayed response at spatial context in monkeys with frontal lesions. Neuropsychologia 14:481–490.

Bagshaw MH, Pribram KH (1953): Cortical organization in gustation (Macaca mulatta). J Neurophysiol 16:499–508.

Barlow HB (1961): Possible principles underlying the transformation of sensory messages. In Rosenblith W. (ed): "Sensory Communication." Cambridge, MA: MIT Press, pp 217–234.

Barrett TW (1969): Studies of the function of the amygdaloid complex in Macaca mulatta. Neuropsychologia 7:1–12.

Blum JS, Chow KL, Pribram KH (1950): A behavioral analysis of the organization of the parieto-temporo-preoccipital cortex. J Comp Neurol 93:53–100.

Brody BA, Ungerleider L, Pribram KH (1977): The effects of instability of the visual display on pattern discrimination learning by monkeys: Dissociation produced after resections of frontal and inferotemporal cortex. Neuropsychologia 14(3):439–448.

Buerger AA, Gross CG, Rocha-Miranda CE (1974): Effects of ventral putamen lesions on discrimination learning by monkeys. J Comp Physiol Psychol 86:440–446.

Butter CM (1968): The effect of discrimination training on pattern equivalence in monkeys with inferotemporal and lateral striate lesions. Neuropsychologia 6:27–40.

Butter CM, Mishkin M, Rosvold HE (1965): Stimulus generalization in memory with inferotemporal and lateral occipital lesions. In Mustofsky DJ (ed): "Stimulus Generalization." Stanford: Stanford University Press, pp 119–133.

Carlton E (1985): On the formation of the retinal image. (in preparation.)

Chow KL (1951): Effects of partial extirpations of the posterior association cortex on visually mediated behavior. Comp Psychol Monogr 20:187–217.

Chow KL, Dewson JH III (1966): Numerical estimates of neuron and glia in lateral geniculate body during retrograde degeneration. J Comp Neurol 128:63–74.

Cohen NJ, Squire IR (1980): Preserved learning and retention of pattern-analyzing skill in amnesia: Dissociation of knowing how and knowing that. Science 210:207–210.

Cormier SM (1981): A match mismatch theory of limbic system function. Physiol Psychol 19:337–356.

Cutting J (1978): A cognitive approach to Korsakoff's syndrome. Cortex 14:495.

Dewson JH III, Pribram KH, Lynch J (1969): Effects of ablations of temporal cortex upon speech sound discrimination in the monkey. Exp Neurol 24:579–591.

Douglas RJ (1966): Transposition, novelty, and limbic lesions. J Comp Physiol Psychol 62:354–357.

Douglas RJ, Pribram KH (1966): Learning and limbic lesions. Neuropsychologia 4:197–220.

Ettlinger G (1959a): Visual discrimination with a single manipulandum following temporal ablations in the monkey. Q J Exp Psychol XI(3):164–174.

Ettlinger G (1959b): Visual discrimination following successive temporal ablations in monkeys. Brain 82:232–250.

Evarts EV (1952): Effect of ablation of prestriate cortex on auditory-visual association in monkey. J Neurophysiol 15:191–200.

Gaffan D (1974): Recognition impaired and association intact in the memory of monkeys after transection of the fornix. J Comp Physiol Psychol (in press).

Graff P, Mandler G, Haden PE (1982): Simulating amnesic symptoms in normal subjects. Science 218:1243–1244.

Gross CG (1973): Inferotemporal cortex and vision. In Stellars E, Sprague JM (eds): "Progress in Physiological Psychology, Vol 5." New York: Academic Press, pp 77–124.

Gross CG, Bender DB, Mishkin M (1977): Contributions of the corpus callosum and the anterior commissure to visual activation of inferior temporal neurons. Brain Res 131:227–239.

Gross CG, Bender DB, Rocha-Miranda CE (1969): Visual receptive fields of neurons in inferotemporal cortex of the monkey. Science 166:1303–1305.

Grueninger W, Pribram KH (1969): The effects of spatial and nonspatial distractors on performance latency of monkeys with frontal lesions. J Comp Physiol Psychol 68:203–209.

Hirsh RL (1969): The role of the hippocampus in information retrieval. Unpublished dissertation, Department of Psychology, Stanford: Stanford University.

Hirst W (1982): The amnesic syndrome: Descriptions and explanations. Psychol. Bull. 91:435–460.

Huppert FA, Piercy M (1976): Recognition memory in amnesic patients: Effect of temporal context and familiarity of material. Cortex 12:3–20.

Iwai E, Mishkin M (1968): Two visual foci in the temporal lobe of monkeys. In Yoshii N, Buchwald NA (eds): "Neuropsychological Basis of Learning and Behavior." Osaka, Osaka University Press.

Iwai E, Mishkin M (1969): Further evidence on the locus of the visual area in the temporal lobe of the monkey. Exp Neurol 25:585–594.

Jackson JH (1873): "Clinical and Physiological Researches on the Nervous System." London: J & A Churchill.

Jacobsen CF, Nissen HW (1937): Studies of cerebral function in primates. IV. The effects of frontal lobe lesions on the delayed alternation habit in monkeys. J Comp Psychol 23:101–112.

Kimble DP (1969): Possible inhibitory function of the hippocampus. Neuropsychologia 7:235–244.

Kimble DP, Pribram KH (1963): Hippocampectomy and behavior sequences. Science 139:824–825.

Kinsbourne M, Wood F (1975): Short-term memory processes and the amnesic syndrome. In Deutsch D, Deutsch JA (eds): "Short-Term Memory." New York: Academic Press.

Lassonde M (1977): Intracerebral influences on the microstructure of visual cortex. Unpublished PhD thesis, Department of Psychology, Stanford: Stanford University.

Lassonde M, Ptito M, Pribram KH (1981): Intracerebral influences on the microstructure of visual cortex. Exp Brain Res 43:131–144.

Lindsley DB (1984): Brain potentials, brain mechanisms, and complexity of visual information processing. In Froelich WD, Smith G, Draguns JG, Hentschel U (eds): "Psychological Processes in Cognition and Personality." Washington,: Hemisphere Publ. Corp., pp 231–245.

Malmo RB (1942): Interference factors in delayed response in monkeys after removal of frontal lobes. J Neurophysiol 5:295–308.

Marr D (1982): "Vision." San Francisco: Freeman.

Marr D, Poggio T, Ullman S (1978): Bandpass channels, zero-crossings, and early vision information processing. AI Memo 491, Artificial Intelligence Laboratory, MIT.

Mehler WR (1966): Some observations on secondary ascending afferent systems in the central nervous system. In Knighton RS, Dumke PR (eds): "Pain." New York: Little, Brown & Co., pp 11–32.

Milner B (1958): Psychological defects produced by temporal lobe excision. In Colomon HC, Cobb S, Penfield W (eds): "The Brain and Human Behavior." Proc of the Association for Research in Nervous and Mental Disease, Dec. 7–8, 1956, New York, pp 244–257.

Minturn WO (1952): The relation of partial amygdaloidectomy to food consumption and activity in the rat. Unpublished dissertation, Department of Psychology, Yale University School of Medicine.

Mishkin M (1966): Visual mechanisms beyond the striate cortex. In Russell RW (ed): "Frontiers in Physiological Psychology." New York: Academic Press, pp 93–119.

Mishkin M (1973): Cortical visual areas and their interaction. In Karczmar AG, Eccles JC (eds): "The Brain and Human Behavior." Berlin: Springer-Verlag, pp 187–208.

Mishkin M (1982): A memory system in the monkey. Philos Trans R Soc Lond [Biol] 298:85–95.

Mishkin M, Hall M (1955): Discriminations along a size continuum following ablation of the inferior temporal convexity in monkeys. J Comp Physiol Psychol 48:97–101.

Mishkin M, Malamut B, Bachevalier J (1984): Memories and habits: Two neural systems. In Lynch G, McGaugh JL, Weinberger NM (eds): "Neurobiology of Learning and Memory." New York: Guilford Press, pp 65–77.

Mishkin M, Petri HL (1984): Memories and habits: Some implications for the analysis of learning and retention. In Squire LR, Butters N (eds): "Neuropsychology of Memory." New York: Guilford Press, pp 287–296.

Mishkin M, Pribram KH (1954): Visual discrimination performance following partial ablations of the temporal lobe: I. Ventral vs. lateral. J Comp Physiol Psychol 47:14–20.

Mountcastle VB, Lynch JC, Georgopoulos A, Sakata H, Acuna C (1975): Posterior parietal association cortex of the monkey: Command functions for operations within extrapersonal space. J Neurophysiol 38:871–908.

Nissen WH (1951): Phylogenetic comparison. In Stevens SS (ed): "Handbook of Experimental Psychology." New York: Wiley, pp 347–386.

O'Keefe J, Nadel L (1978): "The Hippocampus as a Cognitive Map." London: Oxford University Press.

Olton DS, Becker JT, Handelmann GE (1979): Hippocampus, space, and memory. Brain Behav Sci 3:230–251.

Pribram KH (1954): Toward a science of neuropsychology (method and data). In Patton RA (ed): "Current Trends in Psychology and the Behavioral Sciences." Pittsburgh: University of Pennsylvania Press, pp 115–142.

Pribram KH (1958a): Comparative neurology and the evolution of behavior. In Roe A, Simpson GG (eds): "Handbook of Physiology, Neurophysiology II." New Haven: Yale University Press, pp 140–164.

Pribram KH (1958b): Neocortical function of behavior. In Harlow HF, Woolsey CN (eds): "Biological and Biochemical Bases of Behavior." Madison: University Wisconsin Press, pp 151–172.

Pribram KH (1960): The intrinsic systems of the forebrain. In Field J, Magoun HW, Hall VE (eds): "Handbook of Physiology, Neurophysiology II." Washington, DC: American Physiological Society, pp 1323–1344.

Pribram KH (1961): A further experimental analysis of the behavioral deficit that follows injury to the primate frontal cortex. Exp Neurol 3:342–466.

Pribram KH (1969): The amnestic syndromes: Disturbance in coding? In Talland GA, Waugh M (eds): "The Psychopathology of Memory." New York: Academic Press, pp 127–157.

Pribram KH (1977): New dimensions in the functions of the basal ganglia. In Shagass C, Gershon S, Friedhoff AJ (eds): "Psychopathology and Brain Dysfunction." New York: Raven Press, pp 77–95.

Pribram KH (1984): Brain systems and cognitive learning processes. In Roitblat HL, Bever TG, Terrace HS (eds): "Animal Cognition." Hillsdale, NJ: Erlbaum, pp 627–656.

Pribram KH (1985): Convolution and matrix systems as content addressible distributed brain processes in perception and memory. Paper presented at Ebbinghaus Memorial Symposium, Berlin Humboldt University, June 1985 (in press).

Pribram KH, Bagshaw M (1953): Further analysis of the temporal lobe syndrome utilizing fronto-temporal ablations. J Comp Neurol 99:347–375.

Pribram H, Barry J (1956): Further behavioral analysis of the parieto-temporo-preoccipital cortex. J Neurophysiol 19:99–106.

Pribram KH, Blehert SR, Spinelli DN (1966): The effects on visual discrimination of crosshatching and undercutting the inferotemporal cortex of monkeys. J Comp Physiol Psychol 62:358–364.

Pribram KH, Carlton E (1985a): Imaging. Paper presented at University of Lausanne, Switzerland, June 20–22 (in press).

Pribram KH, Carlton E (1985b): Object Perception. Paper presented at University of Bielefeld, West Germany, February 18–22 (in press).

Pribram KH, MacLean PD (1953): Neuronographic analysis of medial and basal cerebral cortex II. Monkey. J Neurophysiol 16:324–340.

Pribram KH, Mishkin M (1955): Simultaneous and successive visual discrimination by monkeys with inferotemporal lesions. J Comp Physiol Psychol 48:198–202.

Pribram KH, Mishkin M, Rosvold HE, Kaplan SJ (1952): Effects on delayed-response performance of lesions of dorsolateral and ventromedial frontal cortex of baboons. J Comp Physiol Psychol 45:565–575.

Pribram KH, Rosner BS, Rosenblith WA (1954): Electrical responses to acoustic clicks in monkey: Extent of neocortex activated. J Neurophysiol 17:336–344.

Pribram KH, Spinelli DN, Reitz SL (1969): Effects of radical disconnexion of occipital and temporal cortex on visual behaviour of monkeys. Brain 92:301–312.

Pribram KH, Wilson M, Connors J (1962): The effects of lesions of the medial forebrain in alternation behavior of rhesus monkeys. Exp Neurol 6:614–618.

Reitz SL, Pribram KH (1969): Some subcortical connections of the inferotemporal gyrus of monkey. Exp Neurol 25:632–645.

Reitz-Blehert S (1968): The relationship between primary visual cortex and the association areas. Unpublished doctoral dissertation, Department of Psychology, Stanford, California, Stanford University.

Rocha-Miranda CE, Bender DB, Gross CG, Mishkin M (1975): Visual activation of neurons in inferotemporal cortex depends on striate cortex and forebrain commissures. J Neurophysiol XXXVII, 1:475–491.

Spinelli DN, Pribram KH (1967): Changes in visual recovery function and unit activity produced by frontal and temporal cortex stimulation. EEG Clin Neurophysiol 22:143–149.

Sprague JM (1966): Interaction of cortex and superior colliculus in mediation of visually guided behavior in the cat. Science 153:1544–1547.

Stern ID (1981): A review of theories of human amnesia. Memory Cognition 9:247–262.

Stevens SS (1951): Mathematics, measurement and psychophysics. In Stevens SS (ed): "Handbook of Experimental Psychology." New York: Wiley, 31–32.

Talland GA, Waugh NC (1969): The pathology of memory. New York: Academic Press.

Tulving E, Donaldson E (eds) (1972): "Organization of Memory." New York: Academic Press.

Ungerleider L, Ganz L, Pribram KH (1977): Size constancy in Rhesus monkeys: Effects of pulvinar, prestriate, and infero-temporal lesions. Exp Brain Res 27:251–269.

Ungerleider L, Mishkin M (1982): Two cortical visual systems. In Ingle DJ, Mansfield RJW, Goodale MA (eds): "The Analysis of Visual Behavior." Cambridge, MIT Press, pp 459–586.

Warrington EK, Weiskrantz I (1982): Amnesia: A disconnection syndrome? Neuropsychologia 20:233–248.

Wegener JC (1968): The effect of cortical lesions on auditory and visual discrimination behavior in monkeys. Cortex IV:203–232.

Weiskrantz L, Cowey A (1970): Filling in the scotoma: A study of residual vision after striate cortex lesions in monkeys. In Stellar E, Sprague JM (eds): "Progress in Physiological Psychology, Vol 3." New York: Academic Press, pp 237–260.

Weiskrantz L, Warrington EK (1975): The problem of the amnesic syndrome in man and animals. In Isaacson RL, Pribram KH (eds): "The Hippocampus, Vol 2, Neurophysiology and Behavior." New York: Plenum Press, pp 411–426.

Weiskrantz L, Warrington EK, Sanders MD, Marshall J (1974): Visual capacity in the hemianopic field following a restricted occipital ablation. Brain 97(4):709–728.

Whitlock DG, Nauta WJ (1956): Subcortical projections from the temporal neocortex in Macaca mulatta. J Comp Neurol 106:183–212.

Wickelgren WA (1979): Chunking and consolidation: A theoretical synthesis of semantic networks, configuring in conditioning, S-R versus cognitive learning, normal forgetting, the amnesic syndrome, and the hippocampal arousal system. Psychol Rev 86:44.

Wilson M (1975): Effects of circumscribed cortical lesions upon somesthetic and visual discrimination in the monkey. J Comp Physiol Psychol 50:630–635.

Epilogue

This symposium has brought together a wealth of information bearing on its title **"Two Hemispheres—One Brain: Functions of the Corpus Callosum"**, with some papers bearing only indirectly on its title as they deal with mechanisms of higher level integration of the function of the two hemispheres in perception, learning, and motor control. The corpus callosum and anterior commissure are obviously of critical importance in the bilateral integration of midline perceptual and motor functions, though interaction and coordinated activation through interconnections in the brain stem play an important role as well, in maintaining the unity of self-awareness and states of reactivity of the brain as a whole.

Specialized functions of each hemisphere, even with regard to speech and language, appear to be only relative, and not exclusive, even though verbal behavior and awareness may seem to depend almost exclusively on the left hemisphere in left dominant split brain human subjects. However, such preparations may give a false impression of functional specialization in the intact brain when information from the two hemispheres becomes available to each. As Sperry has expressed it so well in his letter: "the gesture, personal honor, and all will be most gratefully remembered in both of my hemispheres working together as a bilateral entity, the function of which supersedes that of either hemisphere alone."

Herbert H. Jasper

Index